A STAND AGAINST TYRANNY

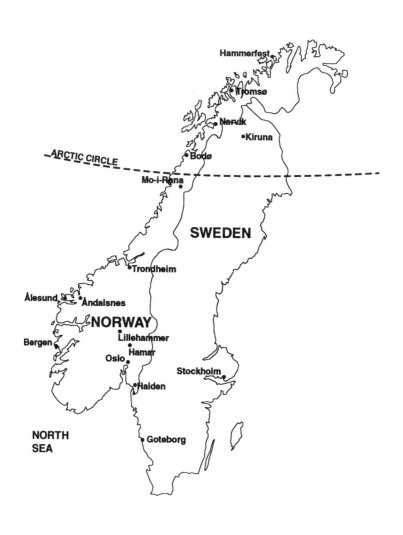

Hammerfest

Tromsø

Narvik

Kiruna

ARCTIC CIRCLE

Bodø

Mo-i-Rana

SWEDEN

Trondheim

Ålesund Åndalsnes

NORWAY

Bergen

Lillehammer

Hamar

Oslo

Stockholm

Halden

NORTH
SEA

Goteborg

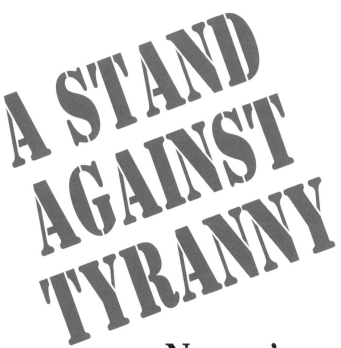

Norway's
Physicians
and the Nazis

Maynard M. Cohen

Wayne State University Press
Detroit

Library of Congress Cataloging-in-Publication Data

Cohen, Maynard M. (Maynard Manuel), date.
    A stand against tyranny : Norway's physicians and the Nazis / Maynard M.
Cohen.
        p.   cm.
    Includes bibliographical references and index.
    ISBN 0-8143-2603-X (alk. paper)
    1. World War, 1939–1945—Underground movements—Norway.
2. World War, 1939–1945—Personal narratives, Norwegian.   3. Physicians—
Norway—Biography.   4. Norway—History—German occupation, 1940–
1945.   I. Title.
D802.N7C64   1997
940.53'37—dc20   96-14957
ISBN 0-8143-2934-9

Designer: Mary Primeau

Cover art: A white rose, symbol of the resistance movement.

Contents

Norwegians in Nazi Concentration Camps

The March to Freedom

The Aftermath of War

Preface

The bitterness of five oppressive years of Nazi Occupation still hung heavily over Oslo when I first arrived in Norway in September of 1951. Rationing of sugar, coffee, meat, and butter along with the paucity of fresh fruits and vegetables were daily reminders of the suffering the nation had experienced. Foreign exchange was at a premium, causing imports to be severely limited. Oranges appeared on fruit stands only at Christmas time, and children had grown into their teens without seeing a banana or a pineapple. Traffic was leisurely, for most private vehicles of the 1930s were wartime casualties. The occasional new automobile was the property of a foreign diplomat or of the fortunate Norwegian who qualified for an import license on the basis of professional need. Local Nazis, collaborating opportunists, and any other individual who had consorted with the enemy remained excluded from normal society. For them employment was difficult and acceptance by coworkers impossible.

I had been well prepared for Oslo. Georg Monrad-Krohn, professor and head of the department of neurology, and wartime dean of the faculty of medicine of the University of Oslo, had been a recent guest at the University of Minnesota. He offered me the opportunity to teach neuropathology to his residents, and to lecture to Norwegian medical students. Sigvald Refsum, professor and head of the department of neurology in the newly formed medical school at the University of Bergen, then a visiting professor in our department, encouraged the move and provided encyclopedic information. Perhaps most convincing was my dear friend Robert Andersen. He was among the host of Norwegians who had involuntarily joined the Grini Society when imprisoned by the Nazi occupiers for "subversive" activities. Since 1948 he had been in Minneapolis, first in the music department of the University of Minnesota and then as a violinist in the Minneapolis Symphony Orchestra. He passed his enthusiasms on to me and provided introductions to friends in Oslo's musical community who would enormously enrich my stay.

But a few days were needed to organize my routine at *Rikshospital*, Norway's State Hospital and University Clinic. The neuropathology lecture series would begin some weeks off. Until then the first two hours of every morning were given over to rounds on the neurological service with Monrad-Krohn and his staff. I then made my way across the *Rikshospital* grounds to the University Institute of Pathology where I sat reading microscopic slides of nervous tissue with *Prosektor* Aagot Christie Løken.

It was from Aagot Løken that I had my first intimation of the underground activities of Norway's physicians. Reviewing slides, as we sat side by side at microscopes gave us considerable conversation time. Aside from diagnostic problems we spoke of many things, including the Occupation. Our inevitable dialogue was initiated by Aagot's offhanded remark that the attic above the very room in which we worked had housed an illegal radio receiver. Her own role, she told me, was inconsequential—offering her room for clandestine meetings—the participants masked to disguise identities even from comrades because anonymity was essential for survival. Even then, six years after the war had ended, little had emerged from participants in underground actions other than memoirs of dare devil agents such as Max Manus.

During my second week in Oslo Georg Henriksen, chief of the epilepsy service, extended the first of a string of dinner invitations. Once the meal had ended Kristian Kristiansen, chief of neurosurgery at the Oslo City Hospital (*Ullevaal Sykehus*), and I spoke extensively together. He lamented the state of neuropathology in Norway. The country's only fully trained specialist had departed for more inviting opportunities in the United States. Aagot Løken, although an excellent pathologist, had only a year of training to prepare for a specialized role in neuropathology. *Ullevaal Hospital*, the capital city's principal medical institution, with its three thousand beds, lacked a neuropathology laboratory completely. Kristiansen solicited my interest in establishing such a laboratory. A lifelong friendship and years of scientific cooperation began with that dinner conversation.

In the laboratory, and in Kristiansen's home I heard fleeting mention of medical personnel involvement in clandestine wartime activity—but very little was specific, and certainly nothing was personal. During the years of my continuing exchange with Norwegian colleagues, fragmented references to the Resistance recurred frequently, but the reticence and modesty of my friends always abbreviated the conversations. It seemed, indeed, that the contribution of Norway's doctors to the struggle against the occupying Nazis was significant and unique. Years passed, before I could put those initial intimations to any test.

In 1977 my teaching duties were sparse during the course of a five-month tenure as Fulbright Professor at the University of Oslo—a full quarter century after my curiosity had been piqued—allowing sufficient time for an earnest attempt to investigate the role of Norway's physicians in the Resistance. Interviews of medical colleagues and review of old newspapers made it apparent that physicians indeed had participated fearlessly, and contributed substantially. I continued to gather material over the next decade, aided magnificently by friends and colleagues. They would speak freely and with sincere admiration of the contribution of others—but only reluctantly of themselves.

The work that has finally emerged is a story based on personal interviews more than three decades after the actual events—gathered at a time when a number of the participants were no longer alive. What is remarkable is the clarity of recall and consistency of the various interviewees. In but a single instance was there a minor divergence.

As the interviews progressed it became obvious that, like other loyal Norwegians, many physicians carried out underground activities that could as well have been performed by others outside the profession. In other very important circumstances, however, medical qualifications were essential. These events and some that were facilitated by the physician's position in Norwegian society are described in the following chapters.

The interviews took place in Oslo and in Bergen, the home cities of protagonists who remained alive and were available. For the others both memoirs and biographies (particularly by colleagues and close friends of the biographees) were employed. All interviews were conducted in English. Portions of the interview appearing in the text enclosed in quotation marks are exactly as recorded on tape, or on rare occasion, in author's notes. Notes, tapes, and transcriptions are now permanently housed in the Archives of the University of Minnesota Library, Minneapolis, Minnesota. Quotations from source material have been translated by the author unless otherwise indicated. Also, I have maintained correspondence with many Norwegian sources for more than forty years, and have often drawn on these to complete the narrative.

As interviews progressed it became obvious that these acts of Resistance were, in many circumstances, intimately intertwined with the humanistic attitudes of Norwegian society. For that reason, along with the saga of her physicians, Norway's movement is traced from an inward-looking, often bigoted position to the respected one the nation now occupies in relation to humanitarian behavior. The influence of Fridtjof Nansen, as the most admired individual in the world of his time, was the single most important factor in this transition to enlightenment. Considerable attention, therefore, is devoted to the aspects of his life that not only placed his stamp on Norwegian character, but foreshadowed the catastrophic events that accompanied the Second World War.

Finally, in order to best understand the events that follow, a summary of pertinent Norwegian history is included.

I am enormously indebted to *Prosektor* Aagot Løken for awakening my interest and to my many treasured friends—particularly to Professors *Dr. Med.* Kristian Kristiansen, Leo Eitinger, Ole Jacob Malm, Jan Jansen, Leiv Kreyberg, Wilhelm Harkmark, Sigvald Refsum, Bertholdt Gründfeld, and Haakon Natvig; and to Tove Filseth Tau, and Dr. Hjalmar Wergeland—who provided detailed information based on personal experiences and gave so freely of their time. I am also grateful to Sigrid Helliesen Lund, Drs. Bjørn Foss, Viktor Gaustad, and Per Giertson for the openness of their interviews. Severt Stackland was most helpful in reconstructing eventful days in Buchenwald. I owe a particular debt to Marit Nansen Greve who was both generous and gracious in providing information on her father, Odd, and grandfather, the incomparable Fridtjof Nansen. Professor Johan Aarli discovered and directed me to original sources in the literature, and provided translation from *Landsmal* when my knowledge of *Riksmal* failed to suffice. Added to all the above I would like to acknowledge my gratitude to Jo Benkow, president of the *Storting*, for the interview he so graciously granted. Tom Madden, Donna Bergen, Alexander and Marion Karczmar, and Edward Dudley were helpful and critically effective readers. Richard Selzer and Charles Strozier generously shared their expertise in the preparation of the manuscript.

My gratitude to daughters Deborah and Nini, whose lively intellects and kind hearts were so important to me in completing this project.

I am grateful to the American Scandinavian Foundation for providing an award covering my 1951–1952 period in Norway, and for the Crown Princess Marte Fellowship supporting completion of *A Stand Against Tyranny*.

Finally, and most importantly, my wife, Doris Vidaver, who, in teaching me so much of her literary craft and knowledge in virtually every day of our years, has performed a major role in the shaping of this document.

This book is dedicated to all those appearing in the following pages—Norwegian, Czech, Austrian, and German—living and dead, who risked their lives to stand against Nazi tyranny—and particularly to the memory of Leo Eitinger and of Kristian Kristiansen.

A BRIEF HISTORY OF NORWAY

1. Introduction

Norwegians had prized their independence, the liberality of their celebrated Constitution, and the reputation they had enjoyed as defenders of peace, freedom, and human rights through the first four decades of the twentieth century. As guardians of the Nobel Peace Prize they had become the virtual conscience of the civilized world. Two of their countrymen, Christian Lange and Fridtjof Nansen, had themselves received the coveted distinction. A third Peace Prize was awarded to the League of Nations Office for Refugees, an office bearing the Nansen name and directed by Norway's Michael Hansson. Bjørnstjerne Bjørnson and Sigrid Undset had each received a Nobel Prize for literature, and like the immortal Henrik Ibsen, had supported human and individual rights through literary works.

The path toward truly fulfilling their liberal and humanitarian reputation was century-long and tortuous, however. The respect Norwegians enjoyed was not completely merited when Hitler plunged the Western world into war. Although the infamous Article 2 that had incorporated religious intolerance against Jesuits and Jews into Norway's Constitution in 1814 was rescinded in 1851,[1] solid remnants of bigotry still pervaded the country. Norwegians looked inward in the 1930s as—with the rest of the world—most turned their backs on the plight of the thousands fleeing Hitler's terror.

As the spring of 1940 neared its end Norway was a stunned and shattered nation. Air and naval encounters had swirled off the Norwegian coast since the early months of the Second World War, and the British destroyer *Cossack* had pursued its German prey deep into *Jøssingfjord* to liberate three hundred captured sailors.[2] Yet, the massive Nazi invasion in early April had caught the guileless Norsemen completely unprepared. Undefended, Oslo was quickly overrun and alien forces fanned out into the land. Britain hastily dispatched the few, poorly trained troops that could be spared as enemy might forced Norway's tiny army northward. French forces debarked in northern Norway, briefly turning retreat into

13

offense as the Arctic port of Narvik was stormed and retaken.[3] Norwegian elation was short-lived, however; the Nazis launched a fresh onslaught far to the south, threatening France itself. As Allied troops withdrew from Norway to meet the attack, beleaguered Norse forces were left to face the invaders alone. Before two months had passed, all organized military resistance against the Nazi aggressor had ended.

A pervasive sense of hopelessness gripped the distraught Norwegians as an unending string of German military successes was climaxed by the fall of France. Great Britain, however, remained unconquered and un-daunted, and the fugitive Norwegian authorities established themselves as a government-in-exile in London. That government resisted Hitler's pressure to conclude a peace, as King Haakon VII resolutely spurned the German demand that he abdicate. Determination then replaced dismay in Norway, nourished throughout five oppressive years of Nazi Occupation by the courageous underground Resistance movement, the civilian arm of which became known as the "Home Front."

The Home Front's fight for freedom and human dignity was unyield-ing. When the Occupation had ended and the postwar years had brought a sense of normalcy to the world once again, Norway had finally mea-sured up to her reputation as an enlightened leader among humanitarian nations.

Violence and sabotage were not the principal instruments of the Norwegian Home Front, for the Nazis responded savagely to such acts. Saboteurs were brutally tortured, and the assassination of a single German would set off a wave of executions in reprisal. As human costs mounted, the government-in-exile decreed that violent actions be the sole pre-rogative of British agents and of Norway's Britain-based troops. Norse commandos and saboteurs responded brilliantly, and at times crucially. The legendary destruction of the Norwegian heavy water plant during transport to Germany forestalled completion of the atomic weapon with which Hitler had hoped to achieve a final victory.[4]

Teachers, athletes, clergymen, lawyers, postal and transport workers, and a variety of professional and craft organizations participated in the non-violent Resistance. The role of Norway's physicians, however, was central to the effort—an effort for which they were uniquely qualified. As graduates of Norway's single medical school at the University of Oslo, doctors formed a closely knit group with a built-in communication network. They occupied the physician's trusted position in Norwegian society and, in the guise of the practice of medicine, could contact virtually any of their countrymen without arousing Nazi suspicion. Physicians maintained their automobiles, enjoying a freedom of travel denied to others, and could bypass curfews with impunity. Finally, under crucial circumstances doctors had access to the ultimate sanctuary, the hospital.

The saga of Norway's physicians during the Occupation—of their valor, dedication, and irreplaceable contribution to their nation's liberation—is not a tale to be told in isolation, for medicine is intricately interwoven into societal structure. The groundwork for the behavior of Norwegian doctors had been laid over eleven decades by countrymen who had devoted their lives to the battle against bigotry, and to the relief of human beings who had been uprooted from their homelands by tyranny and the terrors of war. What follows then is a story, not solely of Norway's doctors during their most trying period, but an account of a nation's growing compassion toward refugees and the persecuted, and the final fulfillment of the country's century-long progression from an official policy of intolerance to a true humanitarianism. Above all it is a memorial to those many Norwegians, native and refugee alike, and the handful of Austrians and Germans who placed their lives at risk in the service of mankind, and it is a testimonial to Fridtjof Nansen who, through a lifetime of service to his countrymen and the world, and the power of his personality, set Norway on her most admirable course.

2. The Separation from Sweden

For more than five centuries Norway had uneasily shared a monarch with her Scandinavian neighbors. Danish Queen Margaret had united Norway, Sweden, and Denmark under a common crown in 1398.[1] Virtually from that moment the three countries had scrapped like children born of the same mother. Swedes, in particular, battled the Danes until the sixteenth century, finally breaking out of the union in 1523—achieving an independence that failed to end the hostilities. For close to three hundred years the two countries warred across the separating waters. In time Norway became a bartering chip between her two sibling nations.

Sweden found new adversaries beyond the Scandinavian orbit—battling until early in the nineteenth century when she lost Finland to Russia. The Swedish Crown Prince, Karl Johan,[2] then invaded Denmark seeking other lands to compensate for the loss. In negotiating the Treaty of Kiel in 1814 the Swedes demanded dominion over Norway, forcing the Danes to yield sovereignty over its northern neighbor.[3]

Incensed, the Norwegians refused to comply—arguing that assigning a complete nation to another without consent of the governed was a flagrant violation of international law. On May 17, 1814, an assembly at Eidsvoll declared Norway independent and drafted a Constitution hailed for egalitarianism and liberality to this day, despite the flaw of bigotry. Sweden responded to the move toward Norwegian self-determination with an invading army. After initial skirmishes, the conflict was quickly resolved through peaceful negotiation. Norwegians retained a nominal independence, governing through their own Parliament, the *Storting*. They were, however, denied control of the administrative bureaucracy and foreign service, both of which remained firmly in Swedish hands.

The Swedish-Norwegian alliance was turbulent from the outset. Norway's massive shipping industry flew the national flag across all the earth's seas. Norse tonnage ranked fourth among the nations—far outstripping

16

that of Sweden. Mariners and land-living Norwegians alike chafed at Swedish control of the consular service, so vital to Norway's commerce, and rankled at a bureaucracy in "foreign" hands. As tensions grew toward the end of the nineteenth century, Alfred Nobel, founding giant of the Swedish explosive industry, left a legacy believed to be his effort toward bringing the scrapping sibling nations together. The award he considered of greatest import, the Nobel Peace Prize, was to be made by a committee of five selected by the Norwegian *Storting*.[4]

If indeed Nobel's intent had been to relieve tensions between the two countries his plan bore no fruit, at least at the outset. After ninety years of recurring disputes, the issue of some degree of control of Norwegian foreign policy brought the conflict to a head. Norway demanded sole responsibility for her consular representation at foreign ports of call. Sweden remained adamantly opposed. Norway's *Storting* followed with a declaration of independence, which was countered by a Swedish threat of war.

The consular dispute between the fractious Scandinavian neighbors simmered and erupted into a boil in 1905 when Norway's *Storting* passed a resolution requiring Sweden to yield its authority. King Oscar, sovereign of the two nations, refused to accept the resolution, and Norwegians turned naturally to their national hero, Fridtjof Nansen.[5] To his countrymen Nansen was the embodiment of a Norse God and the reincarnation of an ancient Viking. Tall, blond and fair-skinned, he was an exceptional skier who moved with the grace of a practiced athlete. His combination of a brilliantly analytical mind, a magnificent body, and an innate flair for leadership seemed to make no task impossible. Norwegians revelled in Nansen's Arctic exploits,[6] and the world added its unqualified admiration. Before his death in 1930, Fridtjof Nansen would gain universal gratitude for his humanitarian accomplishments as well. Nobel laureate Philip Noel-Baker was to write, "There is not a country on the continent of Europe where wives and mothers have not wept in gratitude for the work which Nansen did."[7]

It was but a small step for Nansen to expand his own sense of independence to that of the nation as a whole. That personal independence allowed him to serve as his countrymen's rallying point, but was to prevent him from becoming Norway's political leader once separation from Sweden had been accomplished. Fridtjof Nansen had maintained his own firm belief in God, but had withdrawn from the Lutheran Church—rejecting Norway's state-imposed religion. The national crisis brought his religious attitudes to the minds of the Norwegian people no less than did his fierce support of Norwegian independence. Nansen addressed the consular subject at an emotion-charged meeting of the Student Association on February 23, 1905. His speech supporting immediate action ignited the audience and led Sigurd Bødtker to spring to his feet and shout:

> You have written that we need men: you are right for you are a man; and you have the right to cry "Courage" for you have shown courage yourself. It is said that you cannot be Prime Minister because you have declared yourself outside the State Church. But I beg you to remember the words of Henry IV: "Paris is worth a mass". Take the helm, Fridtjof Nansen! At this moment you are Norway's flag.[8]

Appealing as it may have seemed, promise of the helm and the prime ministry could not dislodge Nansen from his beliefs and ideals as he turned Bødtker's appeal aside. The confidence Fridtjof Nansen inspired in his fellow man and his enormous talents were to serve the country in perhaps an even more significant manner. As Norway's spokesman, Nansen marshalled crucial support in European countries where admiration for his achievements and his person was unbounded. The article Nansen published in the *Times* (London) was lauded by an accompanying editorial, and appeared in leading newspapers in other European countries. His book *Norway and the Union with Sweden* clarified the Norwegian claim in English, German, and French, as well as in his native language.

Despite Norwegian insistence and the support Nansen had garnered abroad, King Oscar obstinately refused Norway's consular demands. On June 7, 1905, the *Storting* declared the union dissolved and Norway a sovereign nation. The Swedish monarch, the *Storting* reasoned, had made the union invalid by ceasing to function as Norway's king.

Norwegians overwhelmingly supported Nansen's view. The plebiscite that followed, dissolving the union with Sweden, was approved almost universally—only 184 negative votes were cast out of a total of nearly 400,000.

Sweden threatened war, and Norway mobilized the small forces she had available for the military confrontation. Once again Nansen's wisdom prevailed as he soothed the rising agitation in his country, and engineered widespread acceptance for a peaceful solution.

Perpetuation of the constitutional monarchy in Norway was by no means as universally desired as was independence itself. Norway's liberal press voiced strident objection to continuation of any vestige of hereditary rule.[9]

Fridtjof Nansen's skills were called upon. He met with Prince Carl of Denmark in July and again in August. Finally, Nansen returned to

Copenhagen on behalf of his government to tender the offer of the Norwegian throne. Prince Carl, well aware of republican ferment in Norway, requested a referendum, wishing to ascend the throne only as the people's choice. Norwegians went to the polls for a second time and by a majority of almost four to one they chose monarchy, with the young Danish prince as king. Prince Carl began his rule as Norway's constitutional sovereign on November 25, 1905, under the name of King Haakon VII. Thirty-five years later he played a decisive role in his new country's next battle for freedom—the struggle against Nazi tyranny.

Fridtjof Nansen's negotiating talents, linguistic ability, and unparalleled prestige made his presence on the diplomatic scene too valuable for Norway to allow him to concentrate on his personal love—science. He dearly wished to return to the Arctic, complete his conquest of the North Pole, then turn his attention to Antarctica and the South Pole. The needs of his country, then of the world, were to end his polar ambitions and allow him to return only sporadically to exploration, zoology, and oceanography.

Reluctantly, Fridtjof Nansen agreed to fill the crucial post of minister to Great Britain, and he served his country in London brilliantly for more than two years. He was compelled to reenter foreign relations during the First World War. From 1916 until the end of his life fourteen years later, he was involved almost continuously in international efforts to relieve the misfortunes of his fellow man.

Neutrality, together with a sound defense, spared Norway from the direct ravages of war. When the United States entered the conflict in 1916, however, Norwegians faced a danger of which Fridtjof Nansen had long warned—famine. A mountainous country, Norway has little tillable land—only 4 percent of its surface. Norwegians, therefore, depended upon imports for a major portion of their sustenance. Even in Nansen's time Norsemen produced only a third of the grain they consumed. When hostilities had cut off foodstuffs from Europe in 1914, Norway turned to America.

Once Herbert Hoover, as U.S. food administrator, set about husbanding American food in 1916, an embargo was placed on all exports. Norway was particularly vulnerable, since close to 100 percent of her vital import of foodstuffs came from the United States. On its part, the United States showed reluctance in continuing the supply since the threat to Norse shipping by marauding U-boats had forced Norwegians to continue export of a portion of their plentiful fish-catch to Germany.

An end to the delivery of American grain made the specter of famine a reality. Nansen was pressed into his country's service once again, leading a Norwegian commission to Washington. His title for the task, minister plenipotentiary on special mission, underscored the magnitude of the assignment. Herbert Hoover, the ultimate authority in the management of U.S. food exports was the only individual of the day whose accomplishments in relief of human suffering approached Nansen's. Millions of Belgians and French were already indebted to Hoover for rescue from starvation. The paths of the two humanitarians were to cross and recross over the next decade, to mankind's enormous benefit.

Hoover—generally a pacifist through Quaker upbringing—had come to share the prevailing American opinion, that the German aggressors must be defeated. He then volunteered his enormous capacities for the war effort. Hoover's extensive experience in Belgium relief made him an ideal choice to become the United States food administrator, empowered to regulate the purchase, price, distribution, and consumption of food, as well as its import and export. The final authority to grant Fridtjof Nansen's request for food lay entirely in Herbert Hoover's hands.

By early 1918 Norwegian stores were exhausted, and Norway's proposal had yet to be accepted by the food administration. Nine months in fruitless discussion had passed when Nansen decided matters should be entirely his own responsibility, telegraphing for just that authority. Lacking any reply he proceeded to negotiate on his own. Within days he had signed a treaty assuring Norway an adequate supply of flour, grain, corn, coffee, and sugar. Additionally, the U.S. War Export Board would allow a quarter million tons of iron and steel to be shipped annually. The prospects of famine had been alleviated; two days *after* the signing Nansen's official authority arrived.[10]

BETWEEN TWO WORLD WARS

3. Russian Prisoners of War

At twenty-five, Konrad Birkhaug had yet to achieve his goal of a degree in medicine when the United States entered the First World War. Another world war later, having become a physician, he was to face down the Nazis who were occupying Western Norway.

As a teen-ager Konrad had been driven from the family home in Bergen by his overbearing father's hatred of religion.[1] The youth had found faith at a revival meeting where, emotionally he had declared for a "life in the hands of God." He centered his future about his newly found beliefs and joined the Young Men's Christian Association, determined in every manner to conform to the morality of the Scriptures.

Forced on to his own when Constable Birkhaug uncovered his son's conversion to faith, Konrad found employment with *Prosektor* (an academic in Pathology; one who dissects) H. P. Lie in Bergen's Municipal Hospital. Exposed to the world of the hospital, and nourished by Dr. Lie's guiding influence the young Birkhaug became fascinated by the intricacies of medicine. Soon a medical career became the young man's passion. Without family support, however, hope of reaching that goal in Norway was but an illusion. Konrad Birkhaug looked to the riches of the New World for fulfillment of his ambition. His older brother Oscar, already a farm-hand in North Dakota, had lured the young man with tales of earnings huge enough to bring Konrad's dreams to reality.

Once in North Dakota, Konrad Birkhaug discovered he lacked the credentials to embark on his medical education. Farm labor, lucrative as it was by Norwegian standards, would never allow the new immigrant to accumulate sufficient savings to achieve his goal. Konrad's new-found religion was his salvation. The young believer had found the nearby Scottish-Presbyterian church more to his liking than his own Lutheran congregation. Through regular Sunday attendance Birkhaug soon became close to Grace and Charles Northrop—to the point of virtual adoption into the family. In great fondness for their young Norwegian friend, the Northrops arranged admittance to a college-preparatory course at their denomination's facility, Jamestown College, and a scholarship that would provide tuition throughout his entire education.

Konrad Birkhaug entered the college-preparatory course in 1912, and Jamestown College two years later. In the spring of 1917 he was notified of his acceptance to the first year class at the Johns Hopkins Medical School. Shortly afterward, on April 5, the United States entered the war against Germany. The young student felt driven to complete the naturalization process and, as a citizen of the United States, become commissioned in the Reserve Officers' Training Corps. "Flat feet and cardiac nervousness under stress"[2] doomed the application, and Birkhaug searched elsewhere for his fate.

Determined to aid somehow in the war effort, Konrad Birkhaug then enlisted in the YMCA program that was providing relief to Allied troops and prisoners of war. At the end of April 1918, Konrad Birkhaug received the assignment setting him on the road to Russia. The October Revolution gave control to the Bolsheviks, who quickly withdrew from their country's partnership with the Western Allies. Together with Louis Penningroth and Carl Yettru, he was to travel from Copenhagen to Murmansk in escort of twenty-two convalescing Russian officers who had been exchanged for wounded German officers held in England. After delivery of their charges, the young Americans were then to proceed to Moscow and aid the YMCA in servicing the ill and injured among returning Russian troops. On arrival in Petrograd, en route to Moscow, they were greeted by an astounded Donald Lowrie, Petrograd representative of the Y. Zealous Communist censors had intercepted all letters and telegrams so Lowrie had no inkling of their arrival. The hospitable Lowrie eagerly showed his unexpected guests the glories of Petrograd.

At a last stop Lowrie pulled his rickety Ford to a halt before the mounted statue of Peter the Great, where the guests stepped from the car to snap some photographs. A terrified mob interrupted the photo interlude, fleeing in disorder to escape the shots and bayonets of pursuing Communist soldiers. As he ran toward the car Konrad Birkhaug tripped and fell, then lay covered by others who, in turn, had fallen over him in a frenzied dash to safety. The shooting soon ended, and the troops set about carrying off the dead and the wounded. Birkhaug arose to find himself bleeding from the nose and mouth, but otherwise intact.

The Treaty of Brest-Litovsk had freed the Russians from the ravages of war, but had only compounded the problems of relief. Three million prisoners of war found freedom even more perilous than confinement after having been released from German internment camps and sent off to the Russian border. From that point the ex-prisoners were on their own, making their way home or to Moscow by every means open to them. Some three thousand passed through evacuation stations in Moscow alone. Konrad Birkhaug was given the task of organizing and supervising YMCA relief for the five hundred former prisoners who filled the beds of the Savoleski Red Cross Hospital.

Aside from the Y itself, Birkhaug found support from strange and diverse sources—from aristocratic anti-communist officers and devout peasants to Leon Trotsky himself. The young Norwegian found the means to stock canteens on every floor of the hospital. Tea, coffee, cocoa, and biscuits were continually available from morning until evening. A library and a game room with chess, checkers, and dominoes were established to ease the boredom. Russian aides wrote letters for the illiterate, and the Y posted the missives onward. Two barber shops helped preserve the prisoners' sense of dignity. Capping the achievements was the furnishing of a three-hundred-seat theater—aided, surprisingly but enthusiastically, by the hospital's Communist commissar. On discharge each patient was provided with a packet of sausages, dried smoked herring, hard biscuits, sweet cookies, tea, sugar, twenty cigarettes with matches, and the following message:

> This little gift is presented by the American Young Men's Christian Association, as a friendly expression of the Christian goodwill of America toward the Russian people. We thank you for the services you have rendered in the war. We sympathize with you in what you have suffered during your imprisonment. Now that these bitter days are past, we wish you Godspeed on your journey to a happy homecoming.[3]

Commissar Bjelenko Polikarp was permissive and almost grateful for Y relief efforts, even "robbing the rich to serve the poor" to outfit the hospital theater. He bridled, however, at nightly services and distribution of religious literature—countering with his own propaganda in the form of an atheistic magazine called *Bezbojnij* (The Godless). Konrad Birkhaug included an excerpt from one such magazine in his autobiography.

> You say: I am a conscious human being who doesn't believe in the priests' tall stories, and I don't admit the existence of God. It is well that you say so. But have you searched your heart? Have you not ikons hanging in your rooms? Don't you let the priest bless your Easter-loaves?
>
> Have you exerted influence on your wife to tear herself away from the priests' idiocies? Have you let your children grow up in freedom from

primitive fairy tales and without religious fear? Do you let your mother-in-law or other woman relatives, those living cadavers, poison your innocent child's mind with abominable priestly fantasies?

Comrade! Go on the warpath against the priests' worship of devils! It is most important that you express your godless conviction publicly, and above all with your own family! Henceforward, throw out the lifeline to others!

M.K.P.
The Communist Party's Atheist Society in Moscow[4]

Konrad Birkhaug's brief meeting with Leon Trotsky was to reinforce the Russian leader's positive feeling toward Americans serving with the YMCA, a feeling that was to prove life-saving before the young man left the country. At the time, Trotsky was the peoples' commissar of military affairs. He came to the Red Cross Hospital to see his nephew, a fatally wounded gunshot victim of a clash with the opposing Left-Social Revolutionaries. Birkhaug was enormously impressed by the vitality and power of Trotsky's personality. He was also relieved that Trotsky's American accent and fluent English, acquired during two years as a journalist in Brooklyn, made conversation in Russian superfluous. Commissar Trotsky expressed his gratitude and admiration for Birkhaug's colleagues, Jerome Davis and Crawford Wheeler, for having driven Red Cross ambulances under fire, as the vehicles filled with the wounded were guided to emergency stations during the October Revolution.

On July 6, 1918, yet another crisis erupted in the chaotic country that eventually forced all Americans out of Russia. Iakov Blumkin and Nicolai Andreyev, two zealots of the opposition Left-Social Revolutionaries, gained admittance to the German embassy through forged credentials. They were then shown in directly to the ambassador, Count von Mirbach. A fusillade of shots from their two revolvers dispatched the German emissary, then the assassins escaped, exploding grenades behind them as they fled. The two killers were captured, but the murder they had committed set off an unsuccessful attempt by the opposition to take over the Communist government, followed by bloody Bolshevik retribution.

On July 26, 1918, the remaining ambassadors of all Western powers fled from Petrograd to Arkhangelsk, 350 miles northeast on the White Sea. In concert with the diplomats' move, French and British troops moved in to occupy both Murmansk and Arkhangelsk. Western powers, at the same time, supported a Social-Revolutionary provisional government in opposition to the Bolsheviks. The position of all Westerners in Russia became untenable and on August 8, the U.S. State Department ordered all American citizens out of the Soviet state.

Inexplicably, the YMCA staff was dispatched southward to Nizhni Novgorod, barely ten miles from the Kasan Front where White Russian Forces faced Soviet troops. Leon Trotsky provided a letter of safe conduct that brought protection to the fleeing Americans and passage southward aboard the *Kersjenjets* on the Moskovskaja River.

On August 25 YMCA Secretary-General Ethan Colton received a troubling communication aboard the river steamer. The letter from Georgy Chicherin, Soviet commissar of internal affairs, ended on a note of at least partial reassurance.

> The entrance of United States' troops into the Arctic European Russia with hostile intent against the Soviet government has made untenable the position of American organizations and personnel in that jurisdiction, not excepting those of service character like the YMCA relief work under your supervision.
>
> The Soviet government has accorded diplomatic immunity to you and your American staff in recognition of the YMCA organization's valuable humanitarian work and great material help. A special train will be placed at your and your American group's disposition for exit from Soviet territory into Finland.[5]

The young men's concern upon being deposited in Finland—then occupied by the German enemy—was allayed by Chicherin's final point.

> The Finnish government has successfully interceded with the German Military Command, which permits passage of the special Wagon-Lit train with American citizens, from the Russian frontier to the Swedish border, in gratitude for the valuable American relief measures which have saved the Finnish populace from famine, and by sparing the Imperial German government from providing for them.[6]

The return to Moscow was uneventful, but all passengers were confined to the special cars that contained YMCA and U.S. consular personnel as well as other Americans with Soviet exit permits.

At noon on September 2, confinement was lifted, and the group was free to leave the train until the scheduled time of departure. Unmindful of his previous brush with death in Petrograd, Konrad Birkhaug agreed to accompany Frank Olmstead on a souvenir-hunting expedition in Moscow. As the two Americans stood watching a military funeral procession for "brave heroes who bloodthirsty British invasion troops have killed on the northern front at Murmansk and Arkhangelsk,"[7] they were overheard to be speaking English. Two policemen immediately confiscated their passports and hauled Birkhaug and his companion to Gorochovaja Prison.

Rather than immediate freedom, a copy of Chicherin's letter brought only the need to be "corroborated by authorities." Olmstead and Birkhaug were led into a darkened dungeon, already filled with Social-Revolutionaries. They rested only fitfully over the hours filled with comings and goings. Names were called out, the condemned were led away, and a volley of shots rang out. New prisoners were led in to replace the departed.

After sixteen hours the two Americans responded fearfully as their names were called. Their fears were for naught, as they were quickly set free and driven by the police to the Finland station. To their good fortune, the train that should have long since departed was delayed.

At precisely 2:00 P.M. on September 3, the refugee train started off for the Finnish border. Hours later, the American convoy trudged across the barbed wire-lined frontier, young and old, weak and strong alike, carrying their bags unassisted.

As Chicherin had promised, the twenty-four-hour journey across Finland was uneventful. The group, by then relaxed, reached safety in Stockholm. Three weeks of rest and recreation followed before Konrad Birkhaug and nine of his comrades were ordered to provide services to the twenty thousand Allied troops stationed in the Murmansk-Arkhangelsk area.

In Murmansk, the new arrivals found the YMCA club lacking in games and other equipment, so Birkhaug was dispatched on a purchasing expedition to Norway's nearest port of Kirkenes, just over a hundred miles across the Barents Sea. The passage was stormy and Birkhaug retired as quickly as possible after his arrival in the Norwegian port, at 11:00 P.M. on November 11, 1918. He was awakened by the tumult in the streets beneath the window of his hotel. The Germans had capitulated. On that very day, at 11:00 A.M., the armistice had begun.

Konrad Birkhaug's tenure in Murmansk was just long enough to experience the two months of complete darkness that annually envelops the Arctic Circle. On February 4, 1919, he was ordered, with three colleagues, to proceed to France to aid in the relief of Russian prisoners of war who had just been released in Germany.

After the starkness and violence of Moscow and Petrograd Birkhaug was astounded by the opulence that was Paris. The elegance of the shops, food overflowing from the French "horn of plenty," and the nighttime frolics of the French capital overwhelmed the young American. There was scant time for pleasure however, for the YMCA urgently needed relief workers. The prisoner of war camps were filled with thousands of Russian soldiers who had been exchanged with the armistice. Birkhaug was assigned the task of organizing relief for more than four thousand ex-prisoners in camps near Verdun awaiting transport back to their homeland.

The friendliness with which General Valentine greeted Konrad Birkhaug was replaced by flaming anger when the Frenchman read of the new arrival's assignment and said, "The devil take you and your benevolence for Russian idiots and communists."[8] Birkhaug himself had learned his disrespect for the Soviet system first-hand and replied, "I saw more than enough of the political idiocy of Marxism during my last year's stay in Russia. But on the other hand, I have great faith in the YMCA's Christian-humanitarian welfare work as a moral re-armament for intractable prisoners-of-war."[9] The general relented, wishing Birkhaug good luck in his effort to "beat common sense into the heads of these worthless bums who flatly refuse to help us clear away the city ruins."[10]

Konrad Birkhaug's faith was rewarded. The Russians joined in vigorously, helping in building canteens, reading rooms, playing fields, and a theater—then enthusiastically utilizing the facilities they'd helped to create. Morale climbed as the ex-prisoners streamed out on to the playing fields, as they staged comedies and drama, and as the theater rang with music.

The Russians remained unwilling to labor unpaid for the French—demanding the modest sum of a single franc a day. General Valentine, recognizing a great change in his charges, accepted the terms. Soon the Russians were hard at work clearing the ruins of Verdun.

Birkhaug was soon able to take time to visit the American cemetery at Romagne-sous-Montfaucon some forty miles to the north, where a fallen classmate lay buried. Conversing with the supervisor of American Graves Registration, he discovered that transfer of the U.S. dead from small cemeteries to Romagne-sous-Montfaucon was lagging due to the lack of French grave-diggers, and that an appointed deadline could not be met. Birkhaug was persuaded to entreat General Valentine to release about two hundred Russians for the task. Valentine, however, felt compelled to use every available ex-prisoner in clearing the ruins of battle.

Konrad Birkhaug decided to intervene on behalf of his adopted country. Through trusted Russians, Birkhaug passed the word that any ex-prisoner able to slip away from camp would be protected by the United States Army, and receive the sum of $10 a day. More than two hundred managed to accept the handsome offer. The task was completed on time.

On Memorial Day of 1919, along with a hundred thousand Allied troops, Konrad Birkhaug witnessed General John Pershing, commander in chief of Allied forces in Europe, as he dedicated the burial ground at Romagne-sous-Montfaucon.

His principal tasks completed, Konrad Birkhaug felt the time had come to return to the United States. He took leave of his ex-prisoners in Verdun in the spring of 1920, carrying with him a letter of appreciation and commendation from Captain W. C. Brigham of the American Grave Registration Service.

Konrad Birkhaug's departure from Verdun was commemorated by Russian and French alike. At farewell ceremonies in his honor Colonel Permikoff presented him with the Grand Cross of St. Anna on behalf of the Russian Army Legion's Committee in Liege. For his part, General Valentine offered dinner in the officer's mess in the citadel. Embracing Birkhaug at the dinner's end, the general placed the *Reconnaissance Fran-caise* gold medal on the young man's breast.

In September 1920, Konrad Birkhaug resumed his interrupted education at Johns Hopkins Medical School. Two decades were to pass before he would again face man's brutality in wartime—and then on his native soil. The task of repatriating Russian ex-prisoners of war, including those from whom Birkhaug took leave in Verdun, fell to Fridtjof Nansen.

4. Fridtjof Nansen in the League of Nations

Hundreds of thousands of prisoners of war remained confined to camps scattered throughout Europe after the First World War had ended. The largest number were in the Soviet Union where thousands of German and Austro-Hungarian captives had been held since the first years of war. Once revolution, then civil war, swept Russia, prisoners of war became forgotten men. Allied prisoners were still held in Germany and the Middle-European countries that had constituted the already dissolved Austro-Hungarian Empire.

The League of Nations was formed in 1920, nobly intending to make force obsolete as a means of solving disputes between nations. In one of its wisest moments the League requested Fridtjof Nansen to deal with the massive problem of repatriation of prisoners of war. Nansen hesitated, longing to return to the science he had missed so desperately. The council of the League clearly recognized no other human being to be so capable of carrying out the mission. Philip Noel-Baker, in the league's secretariat, was dispatched to Nansen's home in Lysaker to convince the revered Norwegian to lead the humanitarian endeavor—a task Noel-Baker promised would require but a month or two. Far from ending in two months, the mission Nansen undertook on April 11, 1920, led to continuous humanitarian efforts on behalf of the League of Nations for the entire decade remaining in his life.[1]

At the outset the problem appeared hopelessly complex. Former soldiers from twenty-six nations remained in prison camps, often under the most primitive of conditions. Dealing with the Soviet Union was particularly challenging. The civil war still convulsed Russia, and the ruling Bolsheviks were suspicious of the capitalist governments of the West. At first, Georgy Chicherin, Soviet commissar for foreign affairs, refused to deal with Fridtjof Nansen as representative of the League of

Nations—an organization Bolshevik authorities had refused to recognize. At that point Nansen ordered the relief train he commanded to prepare for departure in two hours. The perceptive Norwegian then softened his stance, offering to act, not as a functionary of the League of Nations, but only as representative of the individual governments involved. Chicherin was won over, agreeing to send at least two trainloads of prisoners weekly from Siberia and European Russia to the Soviet border. The same trains were to return filled with Russians who had been held in Germany and Central Europe.

Chicherin was true to his word and soon filled the relief camps at the border with returning prisoners. The newly freed men were deloused, bathed, fed, clothed, and sent homeward on the same trains that had brought Russian ex-prisoners from Europe.

Forging an agreement was the smallest part of Nansen's endeavors on behalf of the ex-prisoners. The League of Nations had authorized the repatriation efforts without the means with which to complete the project. Raising funds for transport, establishing transient camps, feeding and clothing the prisoners, and providing essential medical care fell entirely to Nansen. Neither Russia nor the defeated countries were in any position to guarantee the loans needed to carry out the exchange. Nansen's persuasions convinced the victorious Allies of the worthiness of the cause and of the economic benefits to be gained by reentering prisoners into a work force massively shrunken by wartime losses. Loans were provided and exchange proceeded. By the autumn of 1920, more than 150,000 ex-prisoners had been returned to their homes.

Weekly dispatch of two or more trainloads of prisoners by the Soviets failed to clear their camps before cold descended in 1920. Eighty thousand wretched captives were forced to winter once again in Siberia—many for the seventh time. The displaced prisoners were in desperate need. After more than three years of internal upheaval and with a war still in process, Russia had neither the means nor the desire to provide for their charges. The detained were declared Free Men and essentially left on their own.

Nansen Relief, a completely independent organization formed to carry the unfortunate captives through yet another Siberian winter, functioned under its namesake's direction. Adding to his personal efforts, Nansen led the International Red Cross and the YMCA in raising the necessary funds for food, clothing, and medicine—then cooperated in distribution with representatives of the Austrian, German, and Soviet governments.

Prisoners by the thousands, responding to the Free Men edict, fled the camps—struggling toward freedom in every manner possible. Fifteen thousand crossed Siberia, halting at the port of Vladivostock, unable to find passage to their homelands. American charitable organizations responded generously to Nansen's appeal, raising the million dollars needed to engage vessels to carry the ex-prisoners homeward.

During eighteen months of unceasing effort, Fridtjof Nansen, and his two closest aides, Philip Noel-Baker and the Norwegian Captain Finne, had assembled a host of assistants. Working in concert throughout that period they succeeded in rescuing more than 437,000 prisoners from a hopeless existence.

Before all Russian prisoners of war had yet been repatriated Fridtjof Nansen was appointed high commissioner for refugees of the League of Nations, a post which occupied him for the remainder of his life. The task of caring for stateless refugees was enormous—more than three times as many still floated about Europe and the Far East as the number of prisoners of war who had been rescued from internment—and the problem has remained unsolved until the present day. The unfortunates had been disenfranchised by changes in governments or through redrawing of national boundaries. Lacking papers they could neither work nor cross frontiers to find employment. Nearly a quarter million refugees had crowded into Constantinople alone—Russians, Greeks, and Armenians.

Fridtjof Nansen attacked the problem head-on, calling a conference of nations in Geneva in July 1922. He proposed issuing a certificate of legitimization, to serve in lieu of a passport. His proposal received wide support. The certificate approved by the conference—which carried the engraved photograph of Fridtjof Nansen and became famous as the "Nansen Passport"—allowed movement, employment, and security to hundreds of thousands of the stateless.

Nansen settled refugees in France, Bulgaria, Yugoslavia, and Palestine, but the problem was too massive for even the world's greatest humanitarian to solve in the time he was allotted. At the end of the decade, eight years after Nansen's historic appeal, a million refugees for whom the security of a permanent residence had yet to be attained, remained in Europe.

From its October 1917 birth in revolution throughout the early years of the 1920s, problems of even greater magnitude than those of prisoners-of-war occupied the Soviet Union. Armies of White Russians fought to retake supremacy of the polyglot nation, and Poland battled for independence from former Russian masters—both with the support of the capitalist West. The Soviets were mistrustful, to the state of paranoia, about an outside world aligned against them. They looked with suspicion at every contact with the Western powers even when survival of their own citizens was at stake.

By 1919 Nansen clearly recognized famine as a realistic threat in parts of the Soviet Union. In early spring he conferred with Herbert Hoover, and the two humanitarians agreed to submit a proposal to the Supreme

Council of the League of Nations to aid the Soviets with food and medical supplies. The United States was to advance the necessary credit. The Supreme Council accepted the proposal, with a codicil that guaranteed refusal—all hostilities in the Soviet Union must end. Soviet Foreign Minister Chicherin suggested that representatives of his government confer with the League over the matter. The Supreme Council held firm to the restriction, and the effort came to naught.

Fridtjof Nansen's fears became reality two years later when drought destroyed crops in the Russian breadbasket, the Volga Valley, and the Ukraine. Thirty-three million were faced with starvation. To add to the catastrophe, cholera and typhus menaced the region. On August 21, 1921, an international conference of Red Cross and other philanthropic organizations appealed to Nansen to undertake the relief of the famine- and disease-stricken area.

The artist Erik Werenskiold recognized Nansen's depression at the thought of again abandoning the scientific life for which he yearned. Werenskiold counseled his friend, "If I know you aright, you would never be at peace with yourself if you did not do that."[2] The judgement was correct. Fridtjof Nansen took on yet another monumental task.

Nansen had already achieved Chicherin's trust, and together they worked out the details of administering relief funds and obtaining an international loan. In the chambers of the League of Nations, however, the efforts proved futile. Political enmities came to the fore. Nansen pleaded before the assembly:

> In the name of humanity, in the name of everything noble and sacred to us, I appeal to you who have wives and children of your own, to consider what it means to see women and children perishing of starvation. In this place I appeal to the governments, to the peoples of Europe, to the whole world, for their help, hasten to act before it is too late to repent.[3]

The Serbian representative was unmoved, voicing the thoughts of many present—better Russians should die than their government be aided.[4] Nansen's eloquence and passion were ineffective. The assembly refused to act—adopting the common political subterfuge—referral to a conference. The Brussels Conference in turn set up a committee of investigation and unmeetable conditions, including redemption of all Czarist debts.

In the meantime, Nansen called on private organizations to relieve the desperate need. Bureaucratic bickering was fatal. Winter descended, waterways froze, and millions in the Ukraine perished of starvation and disease.

Fridtjof Nansen, appalled at governmental indifference, maintained his faith in people. He toured the Western world in January 1922, appealing to the goodness of man as he spoke passionately and exhibited photographs and slides he had taken himself of the horrors of starvation. His listeners responded magnificently. An American newsman commented, "The church towers bow down in the night as he drives by."[5]

Nansen's own country was first to act, dispatching fish and cod-liver oil worth 700,000 kroner. Denmark and Sweden followed. France provided 6 million francs, Great Britain 250,000 pounds and support for a quarter million children, Holland 4,000 tons of food, Italian Socialists 2.5 million lire, and the Pope 1 million lire and so on. From the United States, aided by the efforts of Herbert Hoover, came $60 million and support for 2.5 million children. Disregarding his own role, Nansen praised Hoover, "In the whole history of the world there is no humanitarian work that can be compared with the relief work organized by Hoover during and after the War, which had its climax here in Russia."[6]

Embarking on his Russian mission, and needing a trusted assistant, Fridtjof Nansen chose a young captain in the Norwegian military, fluent in Russian and experienced in the Soviet Union. Until assigned his humanitarian task, Vidkun Quisling had excelled in every undertaking. After finishing first in his class at the Norwegian Military Academy, he left the service to teach for a year, then enrolled in the Military High School, intending to become proficient in artillery and engineering. There he compiled the best record ever achieved in the hundred years of the school's existence. In 1911 he became a probationary officer on the Norwegian general staff. As officers on the general staff were required to develop particular expertise about some foreign country, Vidkun Quisling chose Russia. In his characteristically thorough manner, he became fluent in Russia's language, knowledgeable in its literature, and completely familiar with the country's economic and military potential.[7]

Vidkun Quisling chafed at the inactivity of the desk in the general staff office, requesting transfer to a post where use could be made of his knowledge and talents. An appointment as military attaché in Petrograd—still Russia's capital—followed in April 1918. Quisling's tenure in Russia was short-lived, for the dangers of the civil war led to closure of the legation in Petrograd, and transfer of Norwegian diplomatic efforts to the legation in Helsingfors, Finland. Vidkun Quisling became joint military attaché and legation secretary and was charged with the critical responsibility of Russian affairs.

Shortly after Quisling was ordered back to Norway in 1921 Andreas Urbye, Norwegian minister in Finland, responded to Fridtjof Nansen's

query with an enthusiastic recommendation for the former military
attaché.[8] Quisling was as effective in humanitarian relief as he had
been in every undertaking. He became secretary to the commission
in the Ukraine, with headquarters in Kharkov. Much of his work was
in the field, as he set up the huge Nansen Kitchens that nourished
the starved and swiftly lowered the mortality from both starvation and
disease.

Fridtjof Nansen was particularly moved by the desperate need of
children in the Ukraine. More than one million were bereft of one or
both parents, and the mortality rate of newborns approached 80 percent.
At Nansen's directive, children were afforded special attention at the
Kitchens.

Except for a brief return to Norway Vidkun Quisling continued his
humanitarian efforts in the Ukraine until September 1923. In that same
month he married a young Russian, Maria Vasilievna Pasek, and together they returned to Norway.[9] Quisling's extraordinary efforts earned
Nansen's gratitude and respect, and a plaque of recognition from the
Soviet government. For himself, Vidkun Quisling developed an admiration for the Soviet system, and for a time, at least, became an outspoken
supporter of communism in his own country.[10]

Of his travels in the Ukraine, Fridtjof Nansen was later to say, "The
things I saw are a constant nightmare to me," for he had not the means
to save all the starving. Far better, he was forced to decide, to save half
the people than all the people half the time. Nansen recognized that
mere relief of hunger must be only a temporary measure. Once the crisis
was alleviated a continuing supply of grain was essential. All seed corn
had been consumed to ease the pain of starvation, and farm machinery
that had deteriorated since the beginning of the war in 1914 needed
both replacement and augmentation. Nansen wrote of the problem in
1922, and Quisling saw to implementation. By the time the project was
completed in the fall of 1923, supplies of grain were rolling again from
the farms of Russia's breadbasket.

Fridtjof Nansen was awarded the Nobel Peace Prize in Oslo in December 1922 for monumental accomplishments in prisoner of war and refugee
relief that would have been denied to any other living man. As T. R.
Johnson, a colleague on the League of Nations Commission for Refugees,
described Nansen: "He always considered matters entirely apart from the
political and other aspects and thought exclusively of the welfare of the
persons with whom he had to do at the moment." It was this quality that
made him "the only man outside of Russia whom the Russians trusted."[11]
Fridtjof Nansen used part of the 122,000 kroner prize to establish two

large research stations in Russia to aid in the modernization of Soviet agriculture. The remainder, and an equal amount, matched by Danish publisher Christian Erichsen, was sequestered for humanitarian work in the future.

In the turbulent postwar world, Fridtjof Nansen was to have little respite. Before the task in the Ukraine was complete the Greco-Turkish war ended in the late summer of 1922 with a catastrophic defeat for Greek forces. Driven by the victorious Turks, 1.5 million Greeks and Armenians who had populated Eastern Thrace and Anatolia fled across the Bosporus and into Western Thrace in wild panic. Turkey held back about a hundred thousand male Greeks in "labor battalions."

Faced with a flood of refugees, many carrying typhus and smallpox and dying by the hundreds, the Greek government knew exactly where to turn for aid. A telegram was dispatched to Fridtjof Nansen at the League of Nations in Geneva. The League appropriated $18,000 to a relief effort, as Nansen was authorized to take charge of the operations.[12] The British led off contributions from various nations with £55 thousand. In the course of a single evening funds were raised, food procured, and ships engaged. Nansen mobilized the Red Cross, the Near East Appeal, and the All-British Appeal, then left for Macedonia to arrange temporary shelter and medical care for the refugees. The death rate plunged by 90 percent in a very short time.

At the beginning of October Fridtjof Nansen moved on to Constantinople to organize relief work in cooperation with several foreign humanitarian societies. While in Turkey he received a letter from Greek Premier Venezilos, pointing out that should the Turks continue to drive out Greeks in such barbarous fashion, Greece, although forced to act against her will, would have no recourse but to reciprocate by expelling Turks from Greek soil. The letter authorized Nansen to deal with the problem on Greece's behalf.

Fridtjof Nansen recognized the need for haste if any endangered Greeks in labor battalions were to be saved. Within a week he proposed an agreement between the two hostile countries and completed negotiations with the Turkish leader, Mustapha Kemal Pasha, and his representatives. No agreement could be forged that would eliminate hardship and suffering, but the conditions of Nansen's proposal gave Greek refugees the chance for survival. Turkey was to have the right to send all Greeks in Anatolia and Eastern Thrace to Greece. At the same time the Greek government could return all Turks from Greece to Turkey. The owners of property abandoned in either country were to be compensated in full immediately, and thus be able to purchase equivalent property in their new homes. In both countries displaced families were to move into the homes and work the land of their exchanged counterparts.

Nansen's plan was adopted at the peace conference in Lausanne. The accord came too late, however, to rescue the large part of the Greek labor battalions. In addition the Turks refused to compensate those Greeks who had already fled their land, "in accord with Turkish law."

His negotiations in Constantinople completed, Fridtjof Nansen drove through Eastern Thrace, where he passed a "whole nation on the highway"[13] a flood of refugees heedless of the grain they left ripening in the field. Nansen quickly secured funds from the Greek government, which he used to bring a pause in the race to safety long enough to allow refugees to harvest and carry some crops, livestock, tools, and other belongings along in the flight. The million in Asia Minor, however, made no such pause as they fled headlong across the Bosporus leaving virtually everything behind, carrying only the clothes on their backs.

A million and a quarter refugees wintered in makeshift shelters in Greece, supported entirely by funds raised outside the country. The American Red Cross alone provided for the maintenance of more than half the victims.

The government in Athens had no confidence the refugees could be settled permanently in Greece and voiced deep concerns for the future. Nansen, however, was certain not only of survival but that the refugees would prove an asset to the country over the years. To prove the point, his assistant, Colonel Proctor, settled ten thousand of the displaced in fifteen new villages in Western Thrace. Some tilled the land and others began new industry using skills they had brought, such as silk worm culture, and carpet weaving. Within a year the new villagers were self supporting.

With Nansen's hard evidence, the League of Nations set up a commission under the direction of Henry Morgenthau, former U. S. ambassador to Turkey, and later secretary of the treasury under Franklin Delano Roosevelt. The commission oversaw funds provided by the Greek government and by the League, and assisted in obtaining further funds through loan. A million and a quarter displaced Greeks were absorbed almost miraculously into an existing population of only 4.5 million. In the end, the new arrivals brought new skills and contributed significantly to the economy and security of their homeland.

On May 14, 1930, a day after Fridtjof Nansen's death, the Greek government was able to announce to the League of Nations, that the settlement of refugees in Macedonia was complete. The commission had accomplished its purpose, and all further administration would be in Greek hands.

5. Nansen in Armenia

The agreement Nansen had so delicately fashioned between Greece and Turkey excluded the long suffering Armenians. Unlike the Greeks, they had no land of their own, and no Turks to offer in exchange for their kinsmen. Somehow, Fridtjof Nansen hoped to protect the persecuted from near extinction in Turkey. He proposed that Armenian refugees in other countries be added to those already in Turkey and placed in an Asiatic Turkish homeland protected by geography. Nansen recorded the response:

> The Turks listened with their customary polished courtesy to this proposal and my explanations, which they pronounced extremely interesting; but it always ended the same way: the Armenians were best off where they were in Anatolia, and there was no danger of any trouble between the Turks and Armenians, who got on well enough with one another so long as the Armenians were not egged on by the Europeans.[1]

In what was to be his final relief effort Fridtjof Nansen took up the cause of those talented people who, as a target for extinction, had attracted international attention long before "genocide" became a watchword in the world press.

The Armenian nation had inhabited a land rich in history, commanded by the towering height of Mount Ararat, on whose slopes Noah was said to have perched his ark as waters receded from a submerged world. The Garden of Eden, as well, was claimed to have lain close by. The lushness had long since disappeared, for the Armenian people suffered the devastating inroads of hostile neighbors—Mongols, Arabs, Persians, and finally and most catastrophically, the Turks. From the fifteenth century onward Western Armenia suffered under Turkish domination. Armenia east of the Arax River was Persian domain.

West of the Arax, atrocities escalated throughout the years, culminating in the twentieth century in an official policy calling for the elimination of the Armenian race from Turkish soil. Armenian males from the age of eight were forced to pay a burdensome tax in lieu of military service until sixty. The most painful of the burdens, however, was the "boy tax." Thousands of male children between the ages of four and eight were taken from Christian families, circumcised, and raised as Moslems. They were then trained as Janissaries, Turkey's most feared and effective fighting force.[2]

When Abdul Hamid, son of an Armenian mother, became sultan in 1876, he raised Turkish cruelty to new heights against a people whose blood half-filled his veins. Indignation flared anew in the West, in 1895 as Gladstone spoke of Hamid as "the great criminal in the palace."[3] The aging British politician entreated Europe to act. If the combined powers of Great Britain, France, and Russia, who had definite obligations in the matter, were to yield to the sultan, they would cover themselves with shame in the eyes of the world. His incensed speech led to a resolution, but as before, no action.

A procession of Armenians, in the false hope of addressing grievances through a petition to the Grand Vizier, served as pretext for even greater outrage, with massacre of the unarmed marchers. Fridtjof Nansen recorded the proclamation following the incident.[4]

> All who are children of Muhammed must now do their duty and kill all Armenians, sack their houses and burn them to the ground. Not one Armenian is to be spared. Such is the command of the Sultan. Those who do not obey will be regarded as Armenians and killed also. Therefore every Musulman must show his loyalty to the government by first killing the Christians who have lived on terms of friendship with him.

By the beginning of February of 1896, from seventy thousand to ninety thousand Armenians were estimated to have been massacred by the Turks, and thousands more died of illness or starvation. Christians were given the option of conversion to Islam, and public circumcisions were held for those who accepted that choice. Thousands, however, refused. Headed by their priests, whole villages of Armenians went to their deaths. Other thousands managed escape over the frontier into Persia or Russian Armenia.

The three great European powers accomplished little on behalf of the persecuted. As diplomatic relations with Turkey became extremely strained, a new friend to Turkey slipped into the diplomatic vacuum. Kaiser Wilhelm II paid a visit to Abdul Hamid in Constantinople in 1898, and soon Turkey turned to Germany as the principal European contact, even to becoming her ally in the First World War.

The constitution that proclaimed equality for all races and creeds, and the aid they gave the "Young Turks" in deposing Hamid in 1898, brought Armenians only short-lived freedom from persecution. With the outbreak of World War I in 1914, the Young Turks unleashed savagery on the Armenians that outstripped that of Abdul Hamid, and became unresponsive even to the restraining efforts of their new ally, the Germans. On November 21, 1914, the Young Turks, scorners of all religion themselves, and who were not above using religious directives for political purposes, declared a holy war, a *Jihad*. It then became the duty of all Turks to murder any infidel who refused the Moslem faith.

The central committee of the Young Turks "decided to liberate the Fatherland from the tyranny of this accursed race," sending the following telegram to the Police Office in Aleppo on September 15, 1915.[5]

> It had already been reported that by the order of the Committee, the Government has determined completely to exterminate the Armenians living in Turkey. Those who refuse to obey this order can not be regarded as a friend of the Government. Regardless of women, children, or invalids, and however deplorable the methods of destruction may seem, an end is to be put to their existence without paying heed to feeling or conscience.
>
> Minister for the Interior
> Tala'at

Whole villages were dispatched on "deportation marches." Few marchers reached their destinations, however. Young males were massacred at once. Women and children, along with old men, were driven toward Syria and Mesopotamia. Leslie Davis, U. S. consul in the Anatolian town of Harput, reported that Armenian corpses lined the roadsides and their stench poisoned the atmosphere. In valley after mountainous valley he observed the remains of thousands littering the slope. Everywhere, he noted, were signs of enormous cruelty on the march and of the brutality of the murders.[6]

Notes of protest by their German allies failed to move the Young Turks. On December 18, 1915, Tala'at Bey, Turkish minister of the interior, prophetically remarked to the German ambassador, Count Metternich, that he was sure Germans would have done the same in similar circumstances.[7]

The massacres of 1915 and 1916 were calculated to have exterminated a million Armenians in Turkey. Fewer than four hundred thousand remained in that country in 1919. Two hundred thousand more survived in concentration camps in Syria and Mesopotamia, and another two hundred and fifty thousand had fled to Russian Armenia, East of the Arax River. Fridtjof Nansen wrote:

> These were atrocities, which far exceed any we know in history, both in their extent and in their appalling cruelty. It could hardly be otherwise when a nation whose public morality was that of the Middle Ages, became possessed of modern appliances and methods.[8]

He was not to live to see those atrocities exceeded by Turkey's former ally, and to involve citizens of his own homeland.

The Allies, banking on Armenian yearning for independence and security, offered a national homeland with their ultimate victory over the Turks and Germans in the First World War. Armenian volunteers fought heroically on the Allied side; more than two hundred thousand gave their lives for a cause they believed would bring freedom and safety to their people. The hope was never realized.

In April 1920, President Woodrow Wilson sought to govern Armenia temporarily through a United States mandate from the Allies. The U. S. Senate, however, refused to ratify the mandate. The Treaty of Sevres, signed by Turkey and the Allies in 1920 recognized Armenia, both east and west of the Arax, as a free and independent state. The Turks recanted that provision, however; and the Allies refused to take the necessary steps to enforce the treaty.

Armenians west of the Arax were left once more at the mercies of their Turkish persecutors. The British Foreign Secretary Lord Curzon, who had championed Armenian independence, characterized the abandonment as "one of the great scandals of the world."[9] East of the river, however, Armenians, recognizing they could not stand alone, joined the Soviet Union, with Yerevan as the capital of their state.

Armenians shared "deportation" with the Greeks in 1922, following negotiations between Fridtjof Nansen and the Turks. Unlike the Greeks, however, Armenians were returned to no homeland. Swept along with the refugee tide they remained as aliens in Greece, Bulgaria, and Syria. Nansen's unmatched abilities were called upon for aid to just those Armenian refugees.

When the League of Nations required Fridtjof Nansen's enormous talents on behalf of the oppressed yet again in 1925, he was loathe to undertake such a burdensome responsibility. He was, however, an easy prey when human beings were in dire need. He was persuaded to cooperate with the International Labor Bureau in an effort to aid Armenians barely surviving as refugees in several countries. The Council of the League of Nations had received a proposal that fifty thousand refugees be resettled in the Sardarabad Desert in the Soviet Republic of Armenia.[10]

Soviet Armenians had strained their resources to the utmost in accepting their fellows who had already escaped Turkish persecution. All arable land had already been put to use; only arid, desolate stretches were available as a new homeland to the refugees. The supplicants believed diligent Armenians could force the Sardarabad Desert to flourish through irrigation and cultivation, and had requested the League of Nations' aid in raising the 1 million pounds sterling estimated as necessary to complete the undertaking. Fridtjof Nansen's first task was to establish the feasibility of the project.

Together with the Council of the League, Nansen selected an international commission for the purpose. C. E. Dupuis, an Englishman and former adviser to the Egyptian Ministry of Labor, and the Italian Pio Lo Salvo were highly recommended as hydraulic engineers. The Frenchman G. Carle was experienced and knowledgeable in subtropical agriculture. Once again, Vidkun Quisling's organizational abilities and fluency in Russian were invaluable in his function as secretary to the commission.

Soviet Russia continued to regard the League of Nations with intense suspicion. After his extraordinary accomplishment in relief of the Ukrainian famine, however, Fridtjof Nansen had earned the trust of Georgy Chicherin, peoples' commissar for foreign affairs. The commissar agreed to Nansen's letter of request, with two stipulations. The commission, although led by Nansen, League of Nations high commissioner for refugees, must not serve as the League's official representatives in Soviet Armenia. The investigators were also to cooperate with the committee appointed by the Armenian government. Nansen most readily agreed, and his party was treated with the utmost cordiality throughout the investigation.

The first official task was conferring with the president of the Federation of the Transcaucasian Republics (Georgia, Armenia, and Azerbaijan) to consider where Armenian refugees could be settled should the Sardarabad Desert plan not prove feasible. The president pointed out a plain in Azerbaijan where, with proper irrigation, many thousands could be supported. Another one to two thousand could be accommodated in Abkhasia in Georgia, where several thousand Armenian refugees had already been settled.

In their Armenian travels, the visitors had come upon scattered, round, dome-roofed tents of Tatars from Azerbaijan, who had driven cattle into Armenian pastures for summer feeding. Prophetically, Nansen wrote:

I could not help thinking that in days to come with increasing prosperity
and larger numbers of cattle, there would be trouble; and the nomads that
have roamed these mountains from early times, would be none too ready
to relinquish their ancient rights.[11]

In the afternoon of June 26, 1925, Fridtjof Nansen and his commission met with Armenian authorities in Yerevan where they outlined the
results of their study, discussed options, and presented a realistic proposal.
Nansen had long experience cajoling contributions and securing loans
from governments and private institutions on behalf of the oppressed.
Despite the enormous debt owed the Armenian nation for sacrifice of
their youth in the Allied cause, the great powers unquestionably would
be unwilling to provide a loan of the size necessary to revitalize the
Sardarabad Desert. Reluctantly, Nansen advised the Armenians he could
not recommend such a plan. The commission found, however, that at
least thirty thousand acres of fertile land—mostly surrounding Yerevan—
could be cultivated and provide livelihood for upward of twenty-five
thousand Armenians. Drainage of swamps could also provide immediate
employment for over two thousand refugees. As a bonus, cultivating the
environs of Yerevan, would enhance both the prosperity and beauty of
the city.

Economic conditions in Europe were then unfavorable for raising
the lesser but still large sums needed through contributions from either
governments or private donors. Nansen, therefore considered a loan the
only possibility.

Before leaving Armenia, Nansen added to his enormous list of laurels,
being named professor at the new University in Yerevan.

The easiest part of Nansen's mission was accomplished in barely over
two weeks, and ended happily. The painful aspects were to follow at
the League of Nations. Nansen proposed the League provide Armenia
with a loan to carry through the recommendation he had made in
Yerevan—a loan to be guaranteed by the Armenian government, the
Soviet government, and the State Bank in Russia. British opposition,
however, made such a loan impossible. Fridtjof Nansen then proposed a
smaller loan, merely for transport of refugees, in the hope the Armenian
government would undertake the project on its own. This too was refused.

Indignant, and frustrated by the continuing abandonment of a needy
and long suffering people, Nansen tendered his resignation as high
commissioner for refugees. Delegates to the League rose up in protest.
Once again Fridtjof Nansen placed values above personal feeling, and
allowed himself to be persuaded to continue. He felt he had no other

course, firmly believing as he did, that a community of nations was the only means of civilized survival: If we do not succeed in reaching the goal along that road, then I see no way to salvation . . . then I am afraid that European civilization is no longer capable of development. It is really doomed to death.[12]

Fridtjof Nansen was unwilling to join his peers in Geneva in abandoning the Armenian cause. Accompanied by Vidkun Quisling, he continued his Armenian trip with a voyage through the Caucasus in search of vacant lands where Armenians could be settled. He found space for twelve thousand refugees, and just before his death, signed an agreement for their resettlement.[13]

During his early years in Bergen, Fridtjof Nansen, accompanied only by his dog, had skied nearly two hundred miles across the high Hardanger plateau between Voss and Oslo in the darkness of Norwegian winter—the first ever to achieve such a crossing. Then at the age of fifty-five, he repeated the feat. Nansen looked to one more passage—planning the journey for 1931, after having passed the age of seventy.[14] He was never to reach either goal, nor would he fulfill his intention to reach North Pole by Zeppelin and set up a camp for scientific observations.[15] The Nansen name, however, continued to bring hope to refugees even in the face of approaching war. His post at the League of Nations was renamed the International Nansen Office for Refugees, with the Norwegian Michael Hansson as high commissioner.[16] His personal banner was to be carried by his son, Odd, in a new effort to save refugees from the tyrant, who in his villainy dwarfed every predecessor.

THE SHADOW OF WAR

6. Quisling
Turns to the Nazis

On return to Norway in 1923, Vidkun Quisling confidently expected to reap the benefits of his accomplishments in the Ukraine. Fridtjof Nansen had expressed appreciation of his assistant's efforts, and Quisling carried home the following commendation from the Ukrainian Red Cross: "We consider that a large part of the success of the work of the mission may be attributed to your personal qualities, your tact, and your noble and sincere friendship for our country and our people."[1]

The qualities of tact and nobility seemed to have deserted Vidkun Quisling in Norway, and rewards for humanitarian efforts eluded him. To his chagrin, Quisling discovered that neither service with Nansen nor the period as military attaché in the Norwegian Legation would be credited toward seniority on the general staff. Whatever the reasoning behind the general staff's refusal, Quisling was compelled to stand by as younger and less accomplished officers became his superiors. His future in the military compromised, Vidkun Quisling left active service to be placed in the inactive reserve at half salary.

Toward the end of 1923, Fridtjof Nansen again sought Quisling's assistance in League of Nations humanitarian activities. As the League's high commissioner for refugees, Nansen was given responsibility for the repatriation of displaced Russians who had sought refuge in Bulgaria, a particularly difficult logistical problem since the two countries shared no common border. Once again, Vidkun Quisling performed effectively. After repatriation was concluded, he continued to operate in the Balkans, then concluded his efforts on behalf of the League of Nations in Soviet Armenia. After agreement was reached on the final proposal, Nansen and Quisling traveled together through the Transcaucus and up the Volga. In *Through the Caucasus to the Volga*, Fridtjof Nansen expressed his "hearty thanks to Captain Vidkun Quisling for his untiring kindness as a traveling companion, and for the valuable help he has given the author through his knowledge of Russian and his many sided attainments."[2]

The years from early 1926 to December 1929 found Quisling back in Moscow.[3] Initially he managed the office of Frederik Prytz, entrepreneur and former Norwegian chargé d'affaires in Petrograd. When diplomatic relations between the Soviet Union and Great Britain were severed in May 1927, Norway undertook to represent British interests. Vidkun Quisling was assigned that responsibility. He worked closely with the British, even to moving into their former embassy to have immediate access to their files. After diplomatic relations were resumed in October 1929, the British expressed their extreme satisfaction by awarding Quisling the coveted Commander of the British Empire, in what was to be a source of future embarrassment.[4]

At the end of 1929, once again in Norway, but unemployed and sustained only by a half-salary as captain in the Army reserve, Vidkun Quisling considered entering politics. He had, until that point, been much influenced by the power of Nansen's personality and his political thought. Both men had sympathized early with Russia's revolutionary government, but after Stalin became firmly entrenched, they viewed the Soviet Union as a threat to Western Europe. Each, in his own way, was fiercely patriotic, and both considered a strong defense a necessity in preserving Norwegian neutrality. Nansen, however, attributed value to every human life, irrespective of political persuasion, race, or religion. Quisling was soon to fall in line with racial theorists and to enthusiastically embrace a belief in the superiority of the Nordic race.

As he contemplated a political career, Quisling turned to Fridtjof Nansen for advice. Some Quisling biographers suggest that indeed Norway's national hero encouraged the younger man's move.[5] Nansen, however, was selective in his loyalties, and even more discriminating in welcoming colleagues into his inner circle of friends.[6]

In his memoirs, Fridtjof's son Odd, described his father's relationship to Quisling, and his own reactions.[7]

> I cannot say that I really knew Vidkun Quisling. But I saw him frequently between 1922 and 1925 when he was attached to Fridtjof Nansen's humanitarian relief action in Russia, Armenia and the Balkans, and greeted him when we met as he came to our home to confer with my father about the relief work.
>
> No condition of friendship existed between my father and Quisling. He never participated in any meal or in any form of social gathering in our home. The words and greeting that were exchanged were completely formal. He came and went like a foreigner—combative, taciturn and serious.

He rarely greeted anyone he met without being greeted first. When he was obliged to return a greeting he slipped his hat down the smallest possible distance in front of his face—then up again in its place, and avoided looking at those he greeted. He walked with quick, purposeful steps, with his head bowed, his gaze turned down, and with a repressed, grim expression on his face. I can never recall having seen so much as a suggestion of a smile on his stony face at any time. I never attempted to coax one forth either. I was, after all, a very anonymous young man and had nothing to speak of with Quisling at the time. My entire existence passed completely over his head. . . .

. . . secret political activity, while he was still engaged in humanitarian relief work was a violation of the conditions of his contract. He certainly never mentioned it to my father, but my father had some idea and it essentially contributed to undermining the trust my father had in him. To some extent that explained remarks my father made in private—more than once—when discussing Quisling and his cooperation. "I can never depend on that fellow. He never looks you in the eye."

Otherwise, Quisling received complete recognition for his outstand-ingly capable work from my father, and for the valuable help he had contributed, with his first-hand knowledge of the Russian situation.

Vidkun Quisling remained completely at the periphery of Norwegian politics until Fridtjof Nansen's death. Then, capitalizing on his previous association with the dead hero, Quisling published a series of articles entitled, "Thoughts on the occasion of Fridtjof Nansen's death." Quisling inferred himself to be the logical heir to Nansen's mantle, an inference that aroused a storm of protest from the Labor Party, those closest to Nansen's political views and from Odd Nansen. The articles thrust their author onto the national scene, however, and aroused some support for the opinions he claimed to have shared with Norway's hero.

The unsettled political situation in Norway led to both the fall of the Liberal government in 1931, and the mandate to one of Norway's smaller and more widely cooperative parties to form the new government. Peder Kolstad, leader of the Agrarian Party, astounded his peers and virtually all of Norway when he chose Vidkun Quisling as minister of defense. As the last word in the acrimonious debate in the *Storting* concerning the controversial appointment, Labor Party leader Johan Nygaardsvold wished the Agrarian Party the "joy of Quisling."[8]

Nygaardsvold's words were prophetic. Quisling's term began in con-troversy, which was to wax and wane but never to subside. The new party leader and his minister of defense clashed from the outset. Jens Hunseid, although strongly disposed to dismiss his stormy minister, felt compelled by politics to keep Vidkun Quisling in the cabinet. The two remained in bitter opposition throughout the tenure of the Agrarian government. Quisling, who had already earned the enmity of the Labor Party, then lost the support of his partymates. When he accused the Labor Party of treason by, among other things, being in the service of foreign interests, Labor demanded his resignation. The Agrarian Party, already in difficulty, hastened toward a fall in February 1933. Quisling, completely without support, lost the last position he would hold in a democratic government.

With the urging and assistance of his former employer in Moscow, Frederik Prytz, and a small group of opportunistic business men, Vidkun Quisling formed Norway's fascist party under the completely inappropriate name of *Nasjonal Samling* (National Unity). Initially, certain prominent Norwegians participated, in the mistaken belief the party indeed promoted unity among their countrymen. When the *Nasjonal Samling*'s true fascist nature emerged, and Quisling turned to anti-Semitic diatribe, virtually all fell away, leaving the aging Nobel laureate Knut Hamsun as the principal "reputable" adherent.

The *Nasjonal Samling* managed to collect only 2.2 percent of Norwegian votes in the first election it contested in 1933, failing to place a single candidate in the *Storting*. In succeeding years numbers fell, in many areas not even reaching one tenth of one percent of voters in the municipal elections of 1936. Party meetings and rallies, however, began to take on more of a strident tone and nazi character. Quisling, mimicking his nazi idol, called himself the *Fører* and gathered about as protection a corps of young rowdies he named the *Hird*, after the bodyguard of ancient Norwegian kings. *Nasjonal Samling* rallies frequently ended in violence, often to the point of riot, pitting jeering Norwegians against Quisling toughs.

Odd Nansen described the character of the sessions.[9]

Now and then throughout the thirties I attended "Nasjonal Samling's" meetings, mostly out of curiosity to see the "Fører" and his henchmen close up, to study their behavior, and listen to their violent speeches that now and then approached paroxysms of rage—in slavish imitation of Hitler.

They were not permitted then to wear uniforms, so the "Fører" and those closest to him, the "Hird," and the rank and file were dressed in sport clothes with knee-pants.

When the assembly had taken their places, a blast of trumpets announced that the Fører was approaching. He paraded in together with his higher leaders with his right arm raised in the Nazi salute, strode under a tent of sun-cross banners and Norwegian flags, up the middle aisle of the assembly hall to a long table up on the stage, where he sat, after renewed saluting and shouts of "Heil og sel." I must genuinely concede that this exhibition tickled one's funny bone. But it was unpleasant at the same time. They were actually deadly serious adults who played that game.

In 1939 Quisling delivered a series of lectures that he entitled "The Jewish Problem in Norway." I attended one of those lectures in the Engineers' House in Oslo and purposefully took a place near the podium.

Naturally it was "the Jew Hambro" [president of the *Storting*, C. J. Hambro, a practicing Christian although born of one Jewish parent] who received the worst going over. He was the most dangerous representative in our land for the worldwide Jewish-plutocratic conspiracy that undermined our society and played it into the hands of unscrupulous speculators. . . . He also took off on the Prime Minister, who, through a hair-splitting thought construction, that I have unfortunately forgot, called him the "artificial Jew, Nygaardsvold." He and his entire Labor Party were also prisoners of, and lackeys for the same Jewish-plutocratic world domination that was the world's greatest danger today—and not the least in Norway!

Finally he took off on the Jews generally, who were a plague and a danger to all countries in which they were found—and he was of the opinion that with the new glory about to dawn on the German and Norwegian races all Jews must be expelled immediately from the country.

Here I interrupted the lecturer and asked if I might ask him a question. I interpreted the angry rumbling I heard as giving me permission to speak.

"As you know, Quisling, today, tens of thousands of Jews, together with other refugees, have been pursued across the borders of Germany and other countries. They were robbed of everything they owned—their native country, their house and home—and found themselves in the utmost need without any means of existence. Every border is closed to them. From your many years in humanitarian and charitable service, you Quisling, better than most, know the refugees' horrible fate. You do not wish that we should turn them over to certain destruction without lifting a finger to help? To what do you think the Jewish refugees—and for that matter—all of Europe's Jews can resort?"

Quisling appeared troubled—so he said grimly: "They can go to Palestine, where they belong—or rather to Madagascar, for that matter, as long as we are rid of them!"

At the breaking off of the applause I answered, "You know just as well as I, Quisling that Palestine's borders are closed to the Jews—just as are all other borders. If they had been open, all of the banished and pursued Jews would travel there with pleasure and gratitude—yes to Madagascar also if the means of livelihood were arranged for them. But the problem today is, what will they do with themselves in the meantime—until such possibilities can be opened up for them?"

Quisling, who by now had approached anger because of this unpleasant interruption, replied curtly and dismissingly, "That doesn't concern me!"

After this refined reply to my question, which was followed by ear-splitting acclaim, I gave up. There was certainly nothing to reply to. He continued with his lecture, and was certainly untroubled by having one listener fewer in the packed hall.

After Quisling's electoral catastrophes in 1936, his following in *Nasjonal Samling* more and more comprised fringes of the radical right, and the uneducated youths that Prime Minister Nygaardsvold referred to as "a flock of juveniles."

Having lost any possibility of success through Norway's democratic process, Vidkun Quisling turned to Nazi Germany for his political salvation.

7. Johan Scharffenberg: First among the Anti-Nazis

To all appearances Johan Scharffenberg was a most unlikely Norse hero.[1] Tall, gaunt, and ungainly, with simian features and hair close-cropped to his balding head, he was a caricaturist's dream. Unathletic in a nation of hikers and skiers, he was an atheist among the devout, a republican in a sea of monarchists, a classicist in a country of mariners and farmers, and a prohibitionist in the land of the *skaal*. Yet his unyielding devotion to his country, his unassailable integrity, and the conviction that characterized his every utterance throughout four decades as physician, psychiatrist, criminologist, and journalist, stirred his audiences and won him the respect of all loyal Norwegians. They rose to his resounding call, and with that call, the Resistance took form.

Johan Scharffenberg was born in 1869 with hardly a trace of "true Norwegian blood." His German ancestors had immigrated from Mecklenburg and Pomerania, and by the time of his birth were established in Moss, just south of Norway's capital. Throughout his life, however, Scharffenberg represented what Andre Bjerke considered the best of the Norwegian folk character—"Driving against the stream." He was a loner among his fellow students, not as a consequence of ingrained anti-social tendencies, but because few shared his consuming devotion to philosophy, psychology, history, literature, politics, and the classics. Mockingly, his classmates dubbed him "Professor." He established stronger bonds to teachers than to students. His ties to a favorite instructor who shared his abiding interests, Johan Andreas Schneider, were especially strong and enduring.

The works of Henrik Ibsen influenced young Scharffenberg as profoundly as they had Fridtjof Nansen. The youthful "Professor" learned much of *Peer Gynt* by heart and was intrigued by *Brand*. It was *Ghosts*, however, that affected him most deeply. He read the play in secret at the age of twelve, when it was first published. He was shaken by that work, for he suspected a hereditary taint in his maternal forebears. The possibility of perpetuating a familial mental illness made any thought of marriage impossible for him. The clandestine reading of *Ghosts* initiated his lifelong interest in hereditary and congenital disease.

Scharffenberg turned to journalism early, publishing his first article in 1887 during his *gymnasium* years in the *Romsdal Messenger*, a liberal journal of which his former mentor, Johan Schneider, was editor. Scharffenberg's early contributions reflected distrust of the great powers and dedication to the rights of small nations like his own.

At the age of twenty, two years after his first appearance in print, Johan Scharffenberg's book of poetry, *The Outcast's Song*, under the pseudonym of Kai Lykke, was released by the radical publisher Olaf Husebye. Although the newspaper *Dagbladet* referred to the work as a "pretty little book that may be transformed into a Christmas or New Year gift for those who seek something inexpensive and good,"[2] a request for honest criticism from Johan Schneider brought a more sober response. Scharffenberg's one-time teacher commented on the formlessness that reminded him of the great Henrik Wergeland during his immaturity. Schneider held out different hopes for his young protégé, suggesting the neophyte confine himself to prose.[3] The advice was to be followed only in part. Although his future publications were to be principally journalistic or scientific, Scharffenberg's poems continued to appear in periodicals and newspapers.

Once more Johan Scharffenberg "drove against the stream" in selecting a career in psychiatry. The specialty suffered from severe neglect and commanded little respect in Norway at the turn of the century. "No other physician," Scharffenberg later wrote, "was so mistrusted, ridiculed and scorned as the psychiatrist, whose task was the most difficult and thankless of all; the mentally ill were often apathetic, dirty, incurable, and not uncommonly, violent."[4] Scharffenberg was motivated, however, by a deep yearning for greater insight into the psychological and philosophical problems that had absorbed him from early youth and by his preoccupation with hereditary mental disease in his own family.

Johan Scharffenberg entered the Royal Frederick University (now the University of Oslo) in 1888, the very year a young Fridtjof Nansen had fired Norwegian imagination with his Greenland exploit. He required nine years to complete the usual six-year course. Preoccupation with journalism and political activity interfered with his progression in an orderly fashion. For the same reason he achieved only mediocre grades, admitting that he had been "diligently average" in his studies.

Despite combining a student's life with journalism, Scharffenberg felt isolated. He described that isolation in a letter to his professor of zoology, Ossian Sars, in 1893, respectfully seeking the opportunity to attend the biweekly Sunday night sessions of the Sars-Circle.[5]

The Sars household was the intellectual center of liberal politics in Oslo. Even into her eighties Maren Sars, sister of the country's leading poet, remained witty and inspiring as she presided over a salon that attracted the most distinguished of Norse writers, artists, politicians, and educators. As a participant, Scharffenberg had the opportunity to meet with the Nobel laureate playwright Bjørnstjerne Bjørnson; Sigurd Ibsen, diplomat and son of the unparalleled Henrik; and Maren's son-in-law, Fridtjof Nansen. Even more important, he exchanged opinions with young politicians such as Halvdan Koht, who would become important to him in the troubled years ahead.

On completion of his medical studies, Scharffenberg entered practice as assistant to his eldest brother in Østfold. Even with the constraints of private practice he devoted considerable attention to scientific and social aspects of his profession. Stimulated by his encounters with the ravages of tuberculosis, then one of Norway's greatest medical problems, he devised an encompassing scheme of managing the disease, which included development and maintenance of sanitoria.

Formal education in psychiatry did not exist in Norway during Scharffenberg's younger years. Attendance at lectures at certain mental institutions, entirely on a voluntary basis, was the only training available, and he found that unsatisfactory and tedious. Scharffenberg attended the program at Gaustad Mental Hospital, Norway's state mental institution, for several semesters, but terminated as he found the presentations wanting. As was his custom he responded by proposing a number of reforms, including the establishment of a University Clinic for Psychiatry. It was not until Norway's first professor of psychiatry was appointed, however, that Scharffenberg's suggestions could be implemented.

Permanent posts in psychiatry were few and poorly compensated in Norway. Scharffenberg, who had already spawned both enemies and controversy, had difficulty in finding a position as psychiatrist. His dedication and his intellectual strength, however, brought him supporters as well, and he was able to survive intermittent periods of unemployment with a series of temporary positions. It was not until the autumn of 1919, when he was appointed physician to Bot Penitentiary, that he achieved some degree of security. Even so, the stipend was so small as to require supplementation through private practice. Only when he also became director of the psychiatry service at the Oslo Hospital did he become financially secure.

Johan Scharffenberg's medical and scientific writings were extensive and wide ranging—covering his many professional interests and their social implications. He recognized the importance of employing exacting statistical methods if any significant information were to be obtained on familial mental disorders. Consequently he recommended the mainte-nance of a central registry of mentally ill patients to serve both as a basis for scientific investigations and to provide the necessary data on which to base rational reforms.

The position as physician to Bot Penitentiary complemented Scharf-fenberg's interest in forensic psychiatry. He studied the relationship be-tween mental illness and crime in the inmates, just as he studied the relationship between psychiatric and creative manifestations in writers and other artists. He was fascinated by psychic disturbances in religious prophets as well as in political leaders, which he described in both scientific and lay publications. Wary of all fads and tenuous theories of treatment of mental disease, he was skeptical of Freud and psychoanalysis and particularly harsh in his criticism of Wilhelm Reich, who had taken refuge from Hitler in Norway until 1939.

As a medical historian, Scharffenberg was without peer in his society. Among the most important of his historical contributions was a seminal study of the life and accomplishments of Herman Major—Norway's first psychiatrist, the 1848 architect of laws governing the mentally ill, and the founder of Gaustad Hospital.

Henrik Ibsen recognized Johan Scharffenberg to be as eclectic in journalism as in medicine. In his formative years Scharffenberg had no possibility to contact Ibsen, who had long since forsaken his native land. The great playwright did return to Norway in 1891, however, and remained until his death in 1906. In pursuit of history, Scharffenberg wrote to Ibsen in Christiania (later Oslo) in 1895, seeking additional information on mental illness that the playwright had mentioned in a newly begun autobiography. Ibsen was quick to respond with an invitation to his home, for he had been intrigued by many of Johan Scharffenberg's columns in *Dagbladet*. "You are involved in very many things, Herr Scharffenberg,"[6] the playwright told his guest. Scharffenberg explained that he wished to develop a perspective about all life's circumstances—to which Ibsen responded that he too wished to do so, but had found it very difficult.

Scharffenberg wrote of social and political problems, of history, art, philosophy and literature, and of medicine and science in a journalistic career that began at age seventeen and ended with his last publication at age ninety-five. Although he contributed to journals and newspapers of varying political persuasions, his most frequent and influential articles appeared in the liberal press.

Despite the necessity to compose his columns during free time, each publication was as carefully prepared as if it were a scientific article— complete with references, quotations, and footnotes. Far from discouraging his readers by their scholarly and exacting nature, his writings were gripping and treasured by his countrymen for their thought-provoking content. Of the many subjects that Scharffenberg covered in his columns none were as recurrent as alcoholism, Norwegian independence, the powers of religious and political "prophets," and support for the persecuted and downtrodden.

Coupling scientific knowledge with journalistic expertise, Johan Scharffenberg was Norway's most powerful opponent to the use and abuse of alcohol. He rose in opposition only after long and careful thought, for he was most sensitive to any infringement on personal freedom. He concluded that alcoholic obfuscation of the senses was far greater an interference with individual freedom than would be prohibition. He abandoned his position of being, at most, only a moderate drinker—only on social occasions—when he tasted an alcoholic drink for the last time in 1902 at a student celebration of his departure from Denmark. Scharffenberg became particularly sensitive to alcohol's disastrous effects on his colleagues. He felt that a psychiatrist who was other than completely abstemious failed in his duty.

Alcoholism, as a disease, occupied much of Scharffenberg's writings in the early years of the twentieth century, for he was distressed at the 1907 law that considered drunkenness a punishable offense. The inebriated, he felt, should be treated by a physician, just as victims of any other poisoning. Whenever possible Scharffenberg photographed the imprisoned drunk, comparing "drunk tanks" to the madhouses of bygone days.

Johan Scharffenberg found himself at odds with Fridtjof Nansen, to some extent, in the matter of temperance, but it was in the realm of a hereditary monarchy for Norway that the two humanitarians differed most. They were united in their enthusiasm for Norway's assuming command of its own destiny through a government completely independent of Sweden. As early as 1890 Scharffenberg wrote, "Let us recognize our shame, Norway is, in reality, a province of Sweden."

The psychiatrist recoiled at the thought of the pomp and glitter surrounding a monarchy, and his atheist intellect shuddered at the consideration of a king serving symbolically as "The Grace of God." To the dedicated egalitarian, a hereditary monarchy negated the principle that innate privilege should exist for no one. Scharffenberg again "drove against the stream," finding only few of his own mind, like Halvdan Koht. Even Bjørnstjerne Bjørnson and Ernst Sars joined with Fridtjof Nansen in recognizing the reality of the situation. Scharffenberg was shattered as the Norwegian people overwhelmingly chose Prince Carl as their new king, Haakon VII.

The unyielding republican convinced a Labor member of the *Storting*, Alfred Eriksen, to introduce a resolution calling for abolition of Article 10 of the Constitution—setting certain procedures for the royal coronation. Scharffenberg himself wrote the scholarly historic background justifying the action, and Article 10 was rescinded by unanimous vote.

His interrelated columns on the power and evils of the political and religious "prophets," and his support of those victimized by the followers of those prophets, delivered Johan Scharffenberg's most powerful impact and influenced the lives of his countrymen. He considered prophets such as Mohammed, Swedenborg, and Joseph Smith, founder of the Mormon sect, to have been psychopaths. Even George Fox, who laid the groundwork for the Society of Friends, was included among those who now and then exhibited sociopathic behavior. The successful among the prophets, he believed, combined psychic disequilibrium with an extraordinary hypnotic capacity to direct disciples into following their leadership.

Adolf Hitler's aggressive behavior and mesmerizing power brought him to Scharffenberg's attention at the very outset of the tyrant's career. The psychiatrist's extensive article in the Oslo daily newspaper *Arbeiderbladet* in the summer of 1933, titled "Hitler—Saviour or Madman," branded *Der Führer* a paranoid psychopath who had taken unto himself a quasi-religious, prophetic role as a manifestation of his mental illness.[7] Dr. Scharffenberg, in his usual manner, relied only upon available data, and was precise in his documentation. He dated delusions of grandeur and persecution, and resort to hallucinatory intuitions, at least as far back as 1918, when Hitler had reported visions of the Virgin Mary during his hospitalization at Pasewalk.

Psychiatrists, together with historians, Scharffenberg believed, needed to acquire greater understanding, not only of the mass psychosis that led to Nazi cruelties but to other aberrations of human behavior in history, such as persecution of "witches" and dispatching the innocent on the fatal "Childrens' Crusade." In the years that followed publication of his insightful article Dr. Scharffenberg faithfully followed his belief, writing and speaking in public repeatedly on the despicable breaches of human rights in the Third Reich, dwelling particularly on persecution of the Jews.

The German minister in Oslo seethed over Scharffenberg's repeated attacks on Nazism and its leader. "The Apex of Caesar's Madness,"[8] in which the Norwegian doctor gave *Der Führer* the opportunity to see "what a psychiatrist who can trace his 'aryan origins' further back in Germany" than Hitler himself thinks about his mental condition and character, infuriated the minister and led him to take action. He protested to the Norwegian foreign ministry that the psychiatrist had defamed the chief of state of a "friendly foreign country."

Scharffenberg was little impressed by the Nazi charge, for he was no stranger to either controversy or legal action. His care in preparation and his meticulous documentation had cleared him on virtually every occasion; once again he escaped prosecution. A thorough investigation by the justice department failed to find cause for action, and on the advice of both the attorney general and the chief of police, the German minister withdrew the charges.

Indignation continued to simmer in the German legation over the next year. In 1935 the minister seized his opportunity to renew the complaint when the Labor Party took control of the government. He approached the new foreign minister, Halvdan Koht, demanding once again that Scharffenberg be prosecuted for his temerity in ridiculing Hitler. Koht, a longtime friend of the psychiatrist and a close, frequent collaborator in liberal causes, readily agreed. He cautioned the complainant, however, that Norwegian law was firm in allowing the accused an opportunity to prove the truth of his assertions. Since Scharffenberg had followed his usual meticulous pattern in description and documentation, the frustrated Nazi minister followed the wisest path and withdrew the accusations.

In a combination of chagrin and self-protection, the German diplomat reported to his own foreign office that Scharffenberg was acknowledged as a psychopath in Norwegian circles, and unfailingly reported as a great villain in the press. For himself, he added, he considered the Norwegian doctor to be a cunning Marxist. As peculiar and irrational as was the German's statement, its appearance in the records was to prove paradoxically helpful to the psychiatrist once the Nazis had invaded his country.

Having brushed aside German objections, Scharffenberg missed no opportunity to warn his countrymen of the perils of Nazi persecutions. He became enormously concerned by the danger that Hitler's stepwise aggression might plunge the world into war. By 1937 Scharffenberg considered a Second World War inevitable. He recognized Denmark's position to be hopeless, but continued to believe that, as in the First World War, both Norway and Sweden had the capacity to develop defenses strong enough to preserve neutrality. Along with Fridtjof Nansen he had aggressively supported the augmentation of his country's armed forces to meet an aggressor's threat, and repeatedly pressed the ruling party to strengthen Norway's defense. In early 1939 he proposed a plan for assigning a permanent watch at each of Norway's fortresses to forestall any German attempt to invade. Labor, however, as a government of anti-militarism, followed its appointed course—progressive dismemberment of the armed forces.

Scharffenberg grieved over the plight of the victims of Nazi tyranny. In 1937 he proposed that the government resettle five thousand refugee Jews on Norwegian soil. Not only would the persecuted be saved, he reasoned, but a greater presence in a country of but fifteen hundred Jews could only be enriching. He often spoke with regret of not having a drop of Jewish blood in his veins. Just as did his proposals for military preparedness, suggestions of aid to the persecuted found few official supporters. Shades of Eidsvoll in 1814 still swirled about Norway's capital.

8. Odd Nansen: In his Father's Footsteps

Fridtjof Nansen's unparalleled efforts brought legitimacy and security to millions of refugees. Hundreds of thousands of the homeless still circled through Europe and the Near East, however, at the time of his death in 1930.[1] Hardly three years later the rise of yet another tyrant produced a flood of the persecuted unmatched in human history. From the moment of Hitler's ascent to power, repressions began. Social Democrats, Communists, and Jews with foresight and the means to escape, streamed across Germany's borders, particularly into Czechoslovakia and Austria. Norway's authorities showed the same disinterest as did the governments of most other nations.

Concerned as they were attempting to emerge from the Great Depression, Norwegians exhibited little interest in the refugees' plight. No Norwegian Relief Society felt compelled to take up their cause. The National Labor Organization established the Worker's Justice Fund to help some beleaguered Social Democrats, and the tiny Norwegian Communist Party offered aid to a few of their endangered fellows through Friends of the Right of Asylum. Until Fredrik Paasche, professor of German at the University of Oslo, took up their cause, help for persecuted Jews came only from an enlightened few, and almost entirely on a personal basis.

When Paasche approached Fridtjof's son in the late fall of 1936 to lead an organization aimed at rescuing victims of Nazi persecution, it was almost more the Nansen name he wanted than Odd himself. Embarking on his profession, the young architect hesitated to become involved in so consuming an effort. Nobel laureate Christian Lange and Foreign Minister Halvdan Koht added their urgings, stressing the importance of the effort and the suffering to be relieved. Odd Nansen relented, and Nansen Relief stood once more as a symbol of hope for the persecuted.

Odd turned to a young friend of the Nansen Family, Tove Filseth, to fulfill the central function of secretary for Nansen Relief. Tove, who had been studying in England, regretted leaving a pleasant life, but the urgency of Odd Nansen's request convinced her of the overwhelming significance of the new endeavor.[2] She soon became indispensable to all Nansen Relief activities, directing the office, ministering to new arrivals in Norway, and working in the field. Sigrid Helliesen Lund, who had already distinguished herself in the battle for civil rights, joined in as a member of the board of directors and worker in the field. The board was rounded out with two professors, Georg Morgenstierne and Edgar Schieldrop, and an attorney, Fredrik Winsnes.

Paasche's intuitive recognition of the importance of the Nansen name was justified again and again, beginning with the establishment of the 10th of October, Fridtjof's birthday, as the annual Nansen Relief Day. The event was celebrated with entertainment, lectures, and above all, solicitation of funds. Money was hard to come by in Norway of the 1930s, and a good deal of Odd's efforts went to raising funds in any way possible. Since Social Democrats and Communists were receiving aid from their Norwegian colleagues, Nansen decided to provide assistance to those with nowhere else to turn, particularly the Jews. Anti-Semitism had not yet disappeared from Norway, however. Some who responded to Odd Nansen's pleas did so only with the proviso that their contributions not be used to help Jews. For those funds, however, he found still more than an ample supply of seekers.

In the beginning Nansen Relief managed to bring only a trickle of refugees into Norway, for the obstacles were formidable. The Norwegian government demanded guarantees that "none should fall as a burden upon the state," and required a thousand kroner—the equivalent of many months income for a Norwegian—deposited in the bank for each person brought into the country by the newly formed organization. Once in Norway the fugitives were denied the right to work by both unions and the government. Jobs remained reserved for native Norwegians. Despite the prohibition, employment was found for some, but wages had to be paid secretly, under the guise of living support from Nansen Relief.

Among the new arrivals was a gifted toymaker, under whose direction a small factory was established in Oslo. The resulting product far surpassed anything on the Norwegian market in quality and richness of concept—yet the government forbade open marketing of the toys. Nansen Relief was reduced to private and secretive sales.

Three decades later, Odd Nansen wrote, "Neither the Labor Unions nor the authorities can look back to that time without shame. Still today, thirty years afterward, indignation rises up in me."[3]

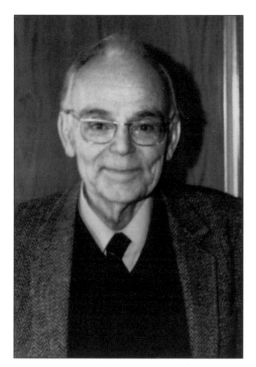

Leo Eitinger. Photograph
by the author, 1986.

Bjørn Foss negotiating
Quisling's surrender at
Bygdøy. Drawing from
Krigsinvaliden no. 1
(1964), p. 283. Used by
permission.

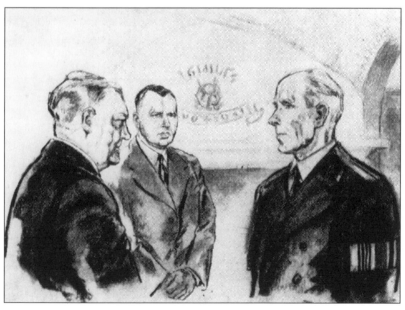

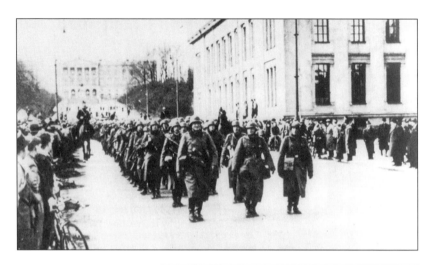

German troops marching into Oslo. Photograph from Krigens Dagbok (1984). Used by permission.

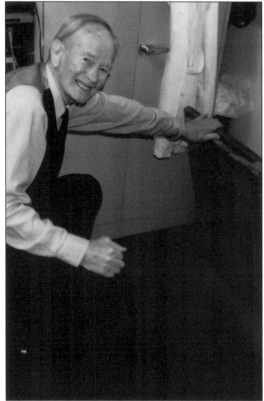

Per Giertson holding the trap door to underfloor hideout. Photograph by the author, 1987.

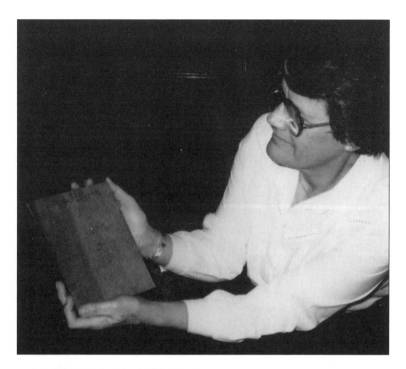

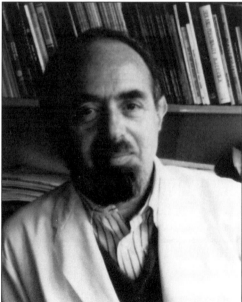

Marit Nansen Greve (daughter of Odd Nansen and grand-daughter of Fridtjof Nansen) holding the breadboard on which her father concealed his diary. Photograph by the author, 1987.

Berthold Gründfelt at his office. Photograph by the author, 1987.

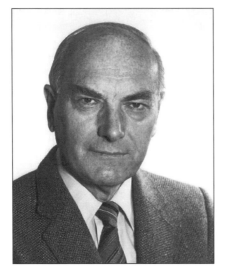 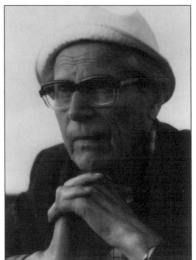

Wilhelm
Harkmark,
(above left).
Photograph
supplied by
Mrs. Ester
Harkmark,
used by
permission.

Jan Jansen,
(above right)
1982.
Photograph
supplied by
Professor Jan
Jansen, Jr.,
used by
permission.

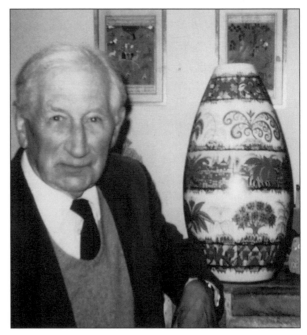

Leiv Kreyberg with vase–gift of Nikita Kruschev.
Photograph by the author, 1984.

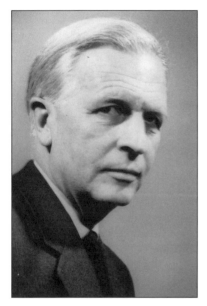

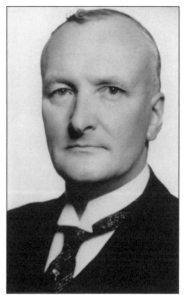

Kristian
Kristiansen (above
left). Photograph
by Rush Photo
Group 1978, used
by permission.

Erling Malm
(above right).
Photograph sup-
plied by Ole Jacob
Malm, used by
permission.

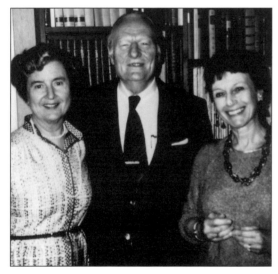

From left to right: Merete Malm, Ole Jacob Malm, and
Doris Vidaver in the Malm home in Oslo, May 1987.

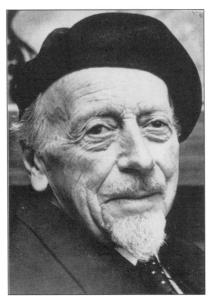

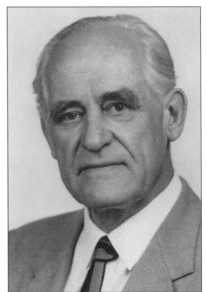

Georg H. Monrad-
Krohn (above left).
Photograph from
*Det Norske
Videnskapsakademi*
(1985). Used by
permission.

Odd Nansen (above
right). Photograph
supplied by Marit
Nansen Greve, used by
permission.

Fridtjof Nansen (right).
Photograph from
Farthest North (1897).

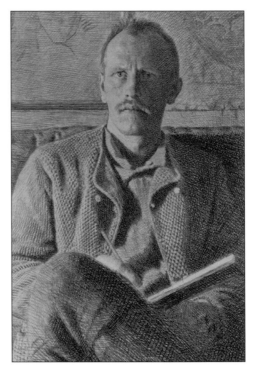

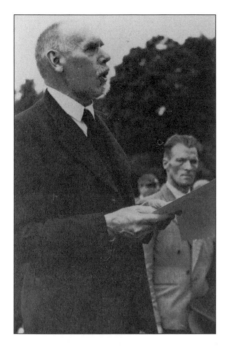

Johan Scharffenberg, from
Johan Scharffenberg (1977).
Used by permission.

Tove Filseth Tau and Haakon
Natvig with the author in 1986
in the Tau apartment in Oslo.
Photograph by Doris Vidaver,
used by permission.

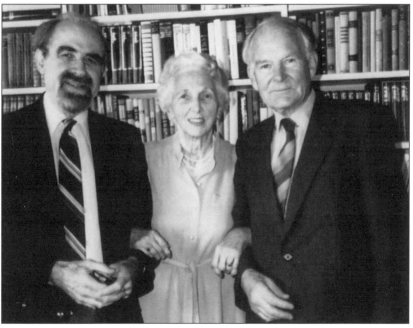

Caroline "Nic" Waal. Photograph supplied by Dr. Helge Waal, used by permission.

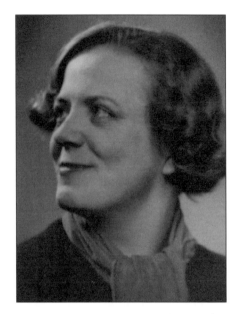

Villagers being driven from Telavåg by German troops. Photograph from *Norges Krigen* (1984). Used by permission.

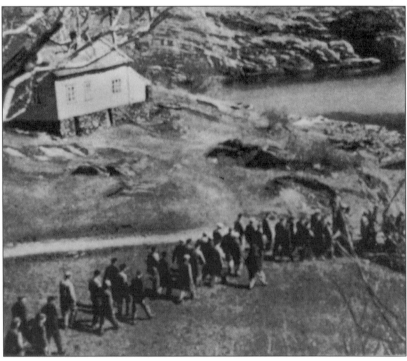

That indignation was minuscule, however, compared to that Nansen experienced once he decided to move his operations out into the field as well. Hitler's persecution had driven thousands of Social Democrats and Jews across the German border into Czechoslovakia and Austria, where large numbers of the two groups already existed and where many held distinguished positions. The Austrian *Anschluss* in March of 1938 doomed both fugitives and native Jews in Austria. With the infamous Munich Agreement that followed on September 30, Neville Chamberlain cast Czechoslovakia to the Nazi madman. In his misguided quest for "peace in our time," the British prime minister, in collaboration with French Premier Edouard Daladier, turned over the *Sudeten* regions of the Czech provinces of Bohemia and Moravia to the German dictator—with no Czechoslovakian participation, or even knowledge.

Once the British and French had abandoned the Czechs, the plight of political refugees and resident Jews became desperate in both Czechoslovakia and Austria. Odd Nansen then felt it imperative that Nansen Relief operate directly at the site of the problem. Tove Filseth and Odd's wife Kari were the first to leave Oslo for Prague, where they set up a small office in January 1939.

Queues of refugees formed daily outside the office to meet with the two women, and with Leif Ragnvald Konstad, chief of Norway's central passport office, whom they had prevailed upon to accompany them to the Czechoslovakian capital. Konstad was cooperative and efficient. When he had quickly issued a couple hundred entry permits, sufficient to exhaust Nansen Relief's available guarantee funds, he returned to Norway. Odd Nansen had remained in Oslo occupied, with Fredrik Paasche, raising funds through country-wide lectures and simply "begging" his more affluent friends and acquaintances. All the while he bombarded Norwegian authorities with pleas to allow entry to more refugees—but the government was unyielding. Financial guarantees were still required for each desperate fugitive.

After his strenuous efforts and those of Paasche had born some fruit in raising additional funds and they had obtained permission for transport of a new quota of refugees into Norway, Odd Nansen believed it was essential to travel to Prague himself. Not only could he share the heavy burden borne by his wife, Kari, and Tove Filseth in dealing with endangered refugees, but he could recount first hand observations and experiences as he continued an unremitting search for funds.

Passport Chief Konstad accompanied Odd Nansen, to once again expedite the issuance of entry permits, and to be certain that none should "fall as a burden on the state." Those in the direst need—the weak and the

sick—were excluded. Again Konstad was "effective . . . and not plagued
with sentimentality."[4] Within a few days the quota was filled and the
passport official returned to Norway.

The Nansens and Tove Filseth remained in Prague to prepare for
the transport of those issued Norwegian visas, to register refugees in
preparation for the next quota, and to organize what relief activities they
could. They abandoned their office in the city, holding daily interviews
in the lobby of the Hotel Esplanade, where they were lodging. Again
during office hours long queues would line the walks outside the hotel,
filled by the young and the elderly, all showing the face of misery, hunger,
and exhaustion—only few of whom would ultimately be saved.

The three Norwegians developed contacts in the city that would be
invaluable in the crises to come. Many Czech officials were concerned and
helpful, as were other relief organizations, particularly the International
Red Cross and the Society of Friends. A young Czech Army physician,
Leo Eitinger,[5] provided assistance to Nansen Relief in Prague. Before
the year was out, he too was a refugee and his own survival rested in Odd
Nansen's and Tove Filseth's hands.

Leo Eitinger, the youngest of four sisters and two brothers, had been
born into a religious Jewish family in 1912 in Lomnice, a small town to
the north of Brno in Moravia. To his friends he was known as "Shua,"
abbreviated from his middle name of Joshua.

While still a student at Masaryk University in the Moravian capital of
Brno, Shua Eitinger had been active in the League for Human Rights.
The old established organization had been politically neutral until Hitler
began his persecutions in the 1930s. The league was then restructured
as Jews throughout Western Europe joined to provide relief to their co-
religionists. The organization aided fugitives, often under intense Nazi
pursuit—to cross the border into Czech territory.

On completion of medical school in 1937, the young physician was
immediately conscripted into the Czechoslovakian army. The following
year, during the celebration of Bastille Day at the French Embassy
on July 14, Eitinger saw President Edvard Benes enter a closed room
with the French ambassador. The Czech leader appeared devastated on
emerging. Only later did Eitinger learn that the ambassador's purpose was
to announce his country's abandonment of Czechoslovakia. France had
embarked upon its fateful course of appeasement of the Nazis. She was
unwilling to confront Hitler and to join Czechs and Slovaks in opposing
the Nazis by force.

In March 1939, Nansen's contacts in the Slovakian capital of Bratislava
and in Vienna sent messages that persecution of Jews had escalated in

strength and cruelty, and they urgently appealed for help. In response, the three Norwegians set out for Bratislava, uncertain of what they might accomplish, but feeling the need to serve as witnesses, at the very least.

Slovakia had long been restive under control of the central Czech government.[6] The nationalistic Slovak People's Party, founded under the leadership of the Catholic prelate, Monsignor Andrej Hlinka, added to Czechoslovakian turmoil by agitating for Slovakian independence. In the chaos following the Munich Agreement the Czech authorities, yielding to added German pressure, allowed the Slovaks to form an autonomous government with only loose ties to the central administration. Virtually on the eve of realizing his ambition for Slovakia, Hlinka died. The new separatist leader, Monsignor Josef Tiso, was installed as premier. In Bratislava, the prelate surrounded himself with the HlinkaGuard, fascist toughs modeled after the German SS, and matching their Nazi counterparts in ferocious anti-Semitism.

The Nansens and Tove Filseth were met in Bratislava by their Slovakian contacts, and driven immediately to Rote Brucke, a park just across the Danube from the city. A small soda pavilion within the park was surrounded by barbed wire and patrolled by armed HlinkaGuard. The documents the Norwegians carried, obtained from Prague's highest authorities, brought them immediate admission to the pavilion. They were greeted by an appalling sight. Several hundred Jews lay packed tightly together on the concrete floor. They had been flushed out of their homes without warning, and imprisoned in the park with nothing but the clothes on their backs. In a fury, Odd Nansen left the two women to investigate further while he set out for a confrontation with Monsignor Tiso.

It may have been the Nansen name that brought Odd immediate entrance, for the prelate greeted him heartily, apparently confusing him with Fridtjof, "the Nansen whose humanitarian work he had heard of. . . ." In his later memoirs, Nansen described Tiso as a "fat thickset priest, in a floor length cassock, with a holy cross in gold dangling from a gold chain on his breast—and with a pair of staring dark eyes behind gold framed glasses."[7] The Slovakian premier inquired, "as innocent as God's lamb what he could be of service with."

Nansen's expressions of outrage were boundless: "How could it be possible that this unworthy and barbaric treatment of human beings could take place in a civilized country—and with his approval, he who was a priest in the holy Christian Church?" Nansen pointed to the gold cross which "had hopped up and down on his fat belly as he constantly made the sign of the cross and raised his eyes to heaven in order to show his great dismay."

Tiso played the role of an "indignant and despondent priest and friend of humanity," as he promised to investigate immediately, dissolve the camp, and set the matter right. "Had it not been for the piercing black gaze behind the glasses," Nansen recalled, "I could have thought that he was an honorable and straightforward man, and not a hypocritical father who sat there and lied right to my face."[8]

Tiso referred Nansen to the chief of police, dispatching the Norwegian to the encounter in the prelate's private Mercedes. The police chief declared that several camps had been established to protect certain Jews against the "agitated masses"—that he would investigate, and those who had forgotten themselves against the "Jewish friends and countrymen" would be punished.

Nansen heard no more from the Slovakians, and his telegraphed appeals for help to the League of Nations' high commissioner for refugees in London, to the International Red Cross, to the Norwegian authorities, and to other international organizations went unanswered.

Traveling on to post-*Anschluss* Vienna, the Norwegians found persecution of the Jews "legal" and thinly concealed. Despite this "legality," plundering and vicious acts still went on mostly in the dark of night. "Riffraff and uniformed bandits seldom showed themselves singly during the day," Nansen recalled, "but collections of troops marched continually through the streets singing their battle songs."[9]

As representatives of a small private organization from a small northern country, the three were powerless in the face of "legal" tyranny. Still, they met with the persecuted in the streets and in their homes, registered them in the small chance they could arrange safe transport to Norway, then carried within the horrible memories they would relate to their countrymen in hopes of obtaining money and visas to provide some small relief.

Odd Nansen resolved to stop in Bratislava on his return journey to Prague to accost Monsignor Tiso once again and remind him of his "golden promise." The city was darkened and under martial law when they arrived by train from Vienna late in the evening. The streets were emptied by the nighttime curfew, but the Norwegians could hear distant explosions and the sound of rifle fire. Nansen thought it best to send the two women onward to Prague on the same train, while remaining himself and attempting to fulfill his mission in the ominously darkened Bratislava. From his contact in the city Odd Nansen learned that the central Czech government had imprisoned Tiso, then released him, and the disorders had begun.

Precisely at 8 P.M. each evening the curfew was rigidly enforced. The HlinkaGuard would then raise the border-barrier at the bridge across the

Danube and join with the hordes of armed Germans and Austrians who poured into Bratislava to plunder and pillage the Jewish section of the city. That same night, from his balcony at the Hotel Carlton, Nansen could see fires flickering from the ruins of two synagogues some blocks away.

Odd Nansen called Tiso's office early the following morning, but the angry teutonic voice at the other end replied "*Sein Excellenz ist nicht zu treffen* (His Excellency is not to be met with)," and the telephone was laid down with a heavy hand before he could question further. A call to the chief of police brought the same response.

With lifting of the curfew at 8:00 A.M. Nansen's contact appeared, and the two walked toward the *Judengasse* in order to survey the night's plundering. Exhausted and dejected by the sight of smashed and looted shops, and dark patches of clotted blood on sidewalks and floors, Nansen returned in the afternoon to the Carlton, resolved to witness the nightly invasion by the Nazi mob. His friend had obtained a car with a permit to be out after curfew, and that evening they stationed themselves at the mouth of the square at the entrance to the bridge.

At exactly 8:00 P.M. the barrier opened and the shouting mob stormed across to meet with the HlinkaGuard. After a brief conference they set out "in full throat" to the *Judengasse* followed by trucks in which to haul away the booty. Nansen's entire being overflowed with outrage. "But what help is it to be outraged?" he wrote. "A complete people—yes all Europe's people allowed that to happen! Closed their eyes—and turned themselves away."[10]

On March 14 Slovakia made its final and disastrous move. Monsignor Tiso declared the province independent and separate from Czech Bohemia and Moravia.

Simultaneously, he became Hitler's vassal.

Odd Nansen arrived back in Prague on the evening of March 13, 1939, to find his wife alone at the Hotel Esplanade. Tove Filseth had returned to Oslo to assist the many new refugees Nansen Relief had sent to Norway from Czechoslovakia. Slovakia's secession the following day plunged Prague into an atmosphere of tension and uncertainty. Refugees crowded once more into the hotel lobby and filled the air with nagging rumors: "the 15th of March Hitler comes! the 15th of March Hitler comes!" It was just before that date but a year earlier that the Nazis had marched into Austria.

With Odd still in Bratislava, Kari had begun a new operation for Nansen Relief, aiding refugees in illegal flight across the Czech border to Poland—cooperating with both Czech and foreign relief groups, especially with the American and British Quaker organizations. In

addition, Nansen Relief had firmly set March 15—the fateful day of
the rumor—for a new transport of eighty refugees.

On the morning of March 14, Odd Nansen was called for a meeting
with Vladislav Klumpbar, Czech minister of social welfare and public
health, together with Director Podajski, representing the high commissioner for refugees, Drs. Kotek and Suhm of the Czechoslovakian Red
Cross, and a number of representatives of foreign relief organizations. All
agreed it was imperative to determine immediately how many refugees
would be at risk of death should the Germans invade. Klumpbar promised
every possible assistance to provide mass migration by train for the imperiled. The group dispatched a telegram to Lord Herbert Emerson, high
commissioner for refugees in London, appealing for money, personnel,
and a supreme effort to obtain visas from many countries for endangered
refugees. With that the meeting broke up, and the leaders of various
refugee groups agreed to assemble once more in the Nansen room at the
Hotel Esplanade at seven that evening.

Propelled by an sense of imminent catastrophe Podajski and Nansen
worked with the refugee leaders at fever pitch into the early morning
hours. They considered perhaps eight or nine thousand to be in the
greatest danger—half of the thirteen thousand who had fled Germany
to Czechoslovakia, and the rest Czech Communists, Social Democrats,
and Jews. They dispatched telegrams to various Western countries, urging them to accept the refugees, and repeated their plea for the high
commissioner in London to support their requests.

Just after 2:00 A.M. the last telegram was sent, and the Nansens decided
to reward themselves after the strenuous day with a drink at a café on
nearby Wenceslaus Place. They relaxed and ruminated over the day's
events until the break of dawn, then returned to the Hotel Esplanade for
a few hours sleep before gathering their contingent of eighty refugees for
transport to Norway.

The telephone shattered a sleep that had barely begun. Rudolf Kac,
leader of the Communist Refugee Group, was on the line, just a few hours
after leaving the meeting in the Nansen room.[11] He announced:

> Hitler came over the border four hours ago and will be in Prague by eight.
> The refugees are preparing to flee the city. I beseech you, Herr Nansen,
> to bring your influence to bear on the foreign legations and embassies—to
> get them to open their doors to the most endangered of us! Herr Nansen,
> I beg you, as urgently as I can, to handle it quickly. It is too late to await
> help from the outside. We have no time to lose. Before long the Germans
> will be here.

Nansen quickly dialed Klumpbar's private number, then Podajski's, but both were always busy. Odd Nansen turned the telephone over to his wife while he shaved and dressed. Finally Podajski's line cleared, and his voice could be heard. He too had been informed and would come by immediately to drive Nansen to the various diplomatic missions.

Then it was Klumpbar on the phone, quiet, almost jovial.

> I think I can reassure you, Herr Nansen, it is not yet fully so bad. There have been some disturbances at the border during the night, and the situation gave grounds for some anxiety—but.

At that point Nansen broke in, for as he stood razor in hand looking into the street he saw a sea of green soldiers with steel helmets—The Germans had come. It was the *15th of March*. Klumpbar's first response to Odd Nansen's report of catastrophe was *"Um Gottes Willen! Herr Nansen!"*.[12]

The lobby of the Hotel Esplanade reverberated with deafening shouts in German, and the constant movement of soldiers. In astonishment the Nansens recognized their fellow hotel guests of the previous weeks— "businessmen" now in their full Gestapo regalia. The streets were filled with troops, trucks, tanks, and motorcycles, and uniformed Germans directed traffic. Prague's large German population had rushed to the streets and windows, waving their German flags and swastika banners, while Czechs stared in disbelief—agonized at the fate of their country.

A cluster of anxious refugees had collected just outside the Esplanade, fearing they had become trapped in Prague. They had gathered early at the railroad station in preparation for their trip to Norway only to find the way blocked by Nazi soldiers and all trains suspended. Nansen could only promise to do whatever possible, and together with Podajski set out to Prague's diplomatic missions.

In complete shock, Odd learned firsthand what Fridtjof Nansen had meant in his Nobel Prize lecture when he described diplomats as "a sterile race that had brought mankind more pain than good throughout time."[13] The younger Nansen believed it a simple charitable duty to help those whose lives were threatened if one could do so without danger to one's own—yet no diplomat was willing to help. "It was incendiary, dangerous to life—material for political conflict—to offer aid to political refugees from a friendly country,"[14] one stated. A second telephoned his home government for instructions, but was cut off. A third pulled down the window shades, then refused. The fourth considered the consequences and found it safer to remain uninvolved, and the fifth stated he had

no right to expose his country to such a risk. Consul Hribek, at the
Norwegian consulate in Prague, had no such fears, however. He issued
visas—with or without authority from his government—for all who had
left passports in his possession.

Sickened by the diplomats' excuses and useless expressions of pity,
Nansen returned to the Hotel Esplanade to face a small crisis of his
own. The Gestapo had taken over the hotel, and the Nansens were to be
evicted. The hotel manager was apologetic yet powerless, so Kari Nansen
approached the Nazi billeting officer. Neither reason nor compassion
moved the German, nor even the final outburst of outrage and pent-up
indignation that had long been building within the two Norwegians.

Ten minutes later the Nansens found themselves on the street with
their luggage and no prospects for lodging in a city overrun with German
troops. The Esplanade's *portier* came to their rescue. He had a friend,
he whispered cautiously, also a *portier*, at the larger Hotel Alcron, who
for an English banknote would arrange a room. General Hoepner, the
Wehrmacht commander lived there himself, and was a decent man who
did not throw out hotel guests who had occupied quarters before the
German takeover. Odd Nansen parted with an English pound note as
the *portier* hailed a taxi and loaded their luggage aboard.

Entirely as promised the transfer went smoothly at the Alcron. The
friendly *portier* sent their baggage up through the rear, again cautioning
the Nansens to insist they had stayed long at the hotel if any German asked. They shared the elevator to their fifth floor room with the
Wehrmacht commanding general himself, who, Odd noticed, smiled and
seemed to show Kari Nansen more than the usual interest. In their room
Odd bridled at his wife's remark that the general could smile—he was a
human being.

Later as the Nansens sat in the Alcron's lobby drinking their tea and
planning strategy in the now dreadful situation, the German general
appeared and took a seat at a nearby table. Suddenly, Kari was struck with
the idea that her husband should approach the general for help. Odd was
appalled, thinking his wife absolutely mad. But her reason prevailed—for
with the Germans in complete command no other avenue existed. Odd
finally agreed, if Kari would arrange the meeting.

Odd rose to take a telephone call from Fredrik Paasche in Oslo,
who had been anxious about his friends' safety in Prague. Paasche had
conferred with Norway's foreign minister; Halvdan Koht, minister of
justice; Trygve Lie; and Prime Minister Johan Nygaardsvold himself, and
was given hope for many new entry permits. The crisis in Czechoslovakia
had brought more money flowing into the Nansen Relief office, and

within days Tove Filseth would be bringing a fresh supply of pounds and dollars to Prague. Happy and somewhat relieved by the news from home, Odd returned to the table to find his wife in conversation with the German general near the reception desk.

Winking, Kari introduced Odd to General Erich Hoepner, whom she'd already informed of their mission in Prague. Soberly the German officer accompanied Nansen to a table where they could speak together undisturbed. Odd Nansen began with a description of the refugees in Prague, how at that moment they lay in the snow beneath the open sky in the forest outside Prague, having forsaken their quarters in fear of the Gestapo. He spoke of the sick and the old, the women and children, who had fled from country to country and city to city to avoid their ever-following pursuers—adding that many were Jews. Nansen believed he detected a flicker of pain cross the general's face when he said the word Jew. Then Odd asked, "Perhaps the general had a wife and children himself and would understand." "I understand,"[15] said Hoepner, sorrowfully.

Nansen continued, "My country and many other countries are willing to help these human beings. With another word you will be rid of the Jews! What can be in the way of such cooperation?" General Hoepner declared his willingness to help, but nodding in the direction of a table filled with Gestapo, said he was afraid others would want to mix in.

Finally, Odd Nansen described the transport that should have left for Norway in the morning—how the mothers and children had been insanely happy—maintained by the thought of a haven in the north—and were then filled with boundless disappointment. Hoepner, still moved, promised to think the matter over and meet Nansen again at 1:00 P.M. the following day.

Odd Nansen appeared in the lobby at the appointed time to find a captain from the general's staff, who brought greetings and regret that his commander was unable to be present. The captain, however, would be at Nansen's service. The transport that should have left Prague would be allowed to depart—after the refugees were first seen by a representative of the police—a prettier name for the Gestapo. The captain reddened when informed that no refugee would fall for so obvious a ruse. The Gestapo could not be trusted with the fugitives' fate. The German officer then expressed the general's willingness to allow women and children with visas for Norway, or elsewhere, to leave freely.

Hoepner was good to his word. The transports departed, bearing the women and children, while Nansen Relief assisted the men in illegal flight across the Polish frontier. Nansen never saw the general again. Five years later, as Odd himself sat a prisoner in the Nazi concentration

camp in Sachsenhausen, he learned of his benefactor's fate. General Erich
Hoepner was hung on August 8, 1944, for his part in the generals' plot
to overthrow Hitler and end the war.

Tove Filseth arrived soon afterward with a stack of Norwegian visas
and bundles of English pound notes. Both were put to immediate use.
Several hundred refugees were shipped to Norway through "legal" channels, and even more fugitives were furnished with passports and money,
and illegally slipped across the border to Poland. In the beginning Polish
railroaders hid fugitives in locomotives and freight cars as well as beneath
the coaches.[16] The life-saving action was rarely performed on a charitable
basis, however. Transport to safety was almost always for a price that further depleted Nansen Relief's scanty resources. Mine shafts and tunnels
running beneath the border served as passageways to freedom for many
others.

Once in Poland the refugees assembled in Katowice and Krakow, from
where the Norwegian minister in Warsaw took over. Niels Christian
Ditleff obtained food and clothing for the fugitives, provided papers
where necessary, then transported them to the port of Gdynia, and started
them on their way to Norway.

Soon even "illegal" channels ran dry. Poles tightened their borders, and
military patrols turned the fleeing refugees back to ultimate destruction.
Day by day Odd Nansen waited for word from abroad. He could not
conceive that civilized nations would do nothing to put an end to the terror
and persecution that had spread from Germany to Czechoslovakia. Again
and again Nansen and Podajski telegraphed the high commissioner—
"Your presence in Praha urgently needed, please answer"[17]—with never
a reply. Finally Odd decided to seek out High Commissioner Lord
Emerson personally.

On March 26 Odd and Kari Nansen left Tove Filseth in Prague to
carry out their "legal" and "illegal" work. They traveled by train together to
Berlin then parted at Templehof Airport—she to continue on to Norway,
and he to fly to London.

Lord Herbert Emerson, the high commissioner for refugees, received
Odd Nansen graciously in his office on Northumberland Avenue. At first
the commissioner was indulgent—he had received the urgent telegrams,
but found it wisest not to answer because of "political consequences."
Besides, he questioned Nansen with characteristic British aplomb, were
not the telegrams a bit exaggerated?

Odd Nansen suppressed his indignation and, as quietly as possible for
him, described the events following the Nazi invasion, relief efforts by his
and other organizations, and what more might have been accomplished

had only the high commissioner come to their aid. Nansen ended his account, informing Lord Emerson how Polish soldiers turned hundreds of refugees back across the border to certain death if apprehended by the Gestapo. He urged the commissioner to travel to Warsaw or to send a representative who would convince the Polish authorities to allow free passage for refugees until their cases could be investigated.

The following day Lord Emerson dispatched an emissary to Warsaw. Within the week, Nansen's request was granted. Refugees crossing the Polish border had free passage until their status could be fully determined.

Before leaving England Nansen embarked on two more missions to secure assistance in rescuing fugitives from Nazi terror. First he sought out several members of the British Parliament to lay the problem before them. It was as if they and Nansen lived in different worlds—he detected no more reaction than a mere shrug. The response was far different in the Soviet embassy, although the final result was unvaried. Nansen found the Soviet embassy "royally furnished, . . . the least proletarian"[18] he had ever seen. A servant in gleaming red livery led him up a broad carpeted stairway to an audience with Ambassador Majskij.

Odd Nansen informed the ambassador of his experiences in Czecho-slovakia, and of Nansen Relief activities. He reported that Communists were in the greatest danger of all political refugees, then proposed that the Soviet Union open its border to its fellows in Germany, Austria, and Czechoslovakia. They existed in misery and hunger in those coun-tries. Other nations—Canada, the United States, and those in Western Europe—would have none of them.

Majskij maintained he must submit the proposal to Moscow before he could act. By that time, Nansen recognized, it would be too late. He tried reason with the ambassador, but Majskij preferred to speak about the great Norwegians—Knut Hamsun, Henrik Ibsen, and Fridtjof Nansen and his relief work during the Ukrainian famine. With each of Odd's attempts to lead the conversation back to the refugee problem, the Russian adroitly countered with Norwegian writers, the elder Nansen's expedition toward the North Pole, and his accomplishments as scientist. Odd Nansen knew he'd met defeat—his opponent was a true diplomat.

Once "independent," Slovakia found itself the target of Hungarian aspirations. Until the first World War had ended in 1918, Slovakia, like Hungary, had been part of the Austro-Hungarian Empire, although unwillingly so. Now that Slovaks had stripped themselves of the pro-tection of an effective Czechoslovakian Army, Hungary looked toward reclaiming some of its former territory. The Hungarians coveted Ruthe-nia at what was then Slovakia's easternmost point, as well as territory at the Hungarian-Slovakian frontier extending virtually to Bratislava itself.

On the day of Slovakian secession Lieutenant Leo Eitinger was a Czech Air Force physician, assigned to a military airfield in the seceded state. As a Czech from Brno in Moravia he suddenly found himself a foreigner in what had been his own country. With all Czech troops he was ordered out of Slovakia. As the young lieutenant completed packing at the end of April 1939, his assistant broke into the doctor's quarters in great agitation, shouting a warning—Hungarian bombers were approaching the airfield. Instinctively, Eitinger turned and plunged through the barracks' rear window. The assistant, however, raced toward the door, only to disintegrate in mid-stride, as a bomb exploded near the entrance. For the young Czech Jew, it was but the first of his escapes from death.[19]

Within days Hungary had accomplished its objective. Without the protection of the Czech Army, Slovakia had no means to stave off superior Hungarian power.

Together with all Czech troops stationed in Slovakia, Eitinger was returned to the German occupied territory, then discharged. Immediately, he sought the means of escape; Nansen Relief, however, had disappeared from Prague. Tove Filseth was last to depart, remaining behind until all her Norwegian visas were distributed. Visas alone were insufficient, for the Nazis still denied many fugitives safe passage from the country. Through clandestine connections, and the liberal use of bribes, she arranged illegal passage across the Polish border, then met her charges once more in Katowice. With Minister Ditleff's aid, she accompanied them first to the seaport of Gdynia, and finally to safety in Norway.[20]

Leo Eitinger joined the thousands of Jews attempting to escape from Czechoslovakia and from Nazi persecution. Long queues formed each day before foreign embassies, particularly those of Central America; for the most part the wait was in vain. Eitinger's family even attempted to purchase Chinese visas that would secure entrance to Shanghai, also to no avail. Leo Eitinger applied to the Norwegian consulate, then settled in to wait.

At the beginning of September 1939, Hitler set Europe aflame with his attack on Poland. Within the month the Poles were subdued and the Nazis began extensive roundups in Czechoslovakia as well as in Poland. Jews were simply stopped in the streets, loaded into lorries, and without any belongings driven away.[21] Some ultimately were dispatched to extermination camps in Poland, while others were emptied into the forests and simply left to perish. Dr. Eitinger hurriedly abandoned Prague for his home in Brno. Having been denied work in his profession it was dangerous to be unemployed and in the streets of the capital.

Odd Nansen had returned to Oslo from his mission in London to find Nansen Relief funds shrinking rapidly. The thousand kroner guarantee held fast, and more thousands had slipped away to support the unemployed refugees they had already brought to Norway. The demand for dollars and pounds for relief of those still outside the country continued to be heavy. The time had come, he reasoned, for the Norwegian government to do its share.

Nansen first approached Minister of Justice Trygve Lie, who was later to become the first secretary-general of the United Nations. Odd proposed that Lie place a request for a million kroner for refugee relief before the Norwegian *Storting*. Lie looked patronizingly at his visitor, saying, "You are not a politician, Nansen!"[22] He could not chance the government falling if the proposal were voted down. Nansen found it impossible to believe such a drastic result possible, but replied that should it occur, "it will in any case fall with honor."

Trygve Lie shook his head at such political naiveté, but agreed to talk further if Nansen could get him a majority on the matter. "But that, I believe, you can scarcely manage," he added.

Lie had not reckoned with Odd Nansen's skill and determination. Odd began with J. L. Mowinkel, former prime minister in the Liberal government, and a friend with a heart. Mowinkel underscored his intention to support the appropriation with a five-figure check to Nansen Relief. Nansen collared leader after party leader, and virtually all offered support. Only the Agrarian Party head withheld his commitment, but promised to abstain. A week later Trygve Lie stood at the podium in the Norwegian Parliament and spoke feelingly of the refugees' plight. Without a single dissenting vote a half million kroner was appropriated—to be divided between Nansen Relief and the Labor Justice Fund.

As October 10, 1939, the anniversary of Fridtjof Nansen's birth approached, Odd Nansen selected Johan Scharffenberg as principal speaker on the third annual Nansen Day. Certainly no other Norwegian was a more qualified or dedicated anti-Nazi. Scharffenberg, who freely accepted every opportunity to aid the victims of Nazi persecution, could be counted upon for an informed attack on the enemies of freedom. He was given complete latitude with the speech, as long as it was clearly concerned with refugee matters.

The tensions of preparation turned to anxiety for the Nansen Relief board of directors as the appointed day neared. They feared Scharffenberg would "go too far" in vilification of Hitler. Although Odd himself nourished no such misgivings, he yielded to the board's request to speak first with their distinguished orator.

As a youth, Odd Nansen and his circle of friends had considered Johan Scharffenberg a most peculiar personality, influenced as they were by his almost fanatical attacks on alcoholism and its evils. After the two humanitarians became united in a common cause, however, Nansen recognized both the perceptions and the courage behind the older doctor's stands. With a sense of awe, he entered Scharffenberg's quarters above *Botsfengslet*, the penitentiary where the physician-psychiatrist ministered to the inmates' physical and mental ills.

Odd Nansen was led by a young man into the study where he found Scharffenberg surrounded by books and magazines—piled from floor to ceiling and stacked on every available table and chair. An old-fashioned lorgnette with a black band dangled from Scharffenberg's nose, and Nansen marveled how like his many caricatures the psychiatrist appeared. Dr. Scharffenberg seemed slightly disoriented and failed to recognize his visitor. When Nansen introduced himself, however, and explained he had come on behalf of Nansen Relief, Scharffenberg brightened immediately and became the gracious host, assuring Odd it was kind of him to come. He was occupied, Johan Scharffenberg explained, preparing his Nansen Day speech.

Odd Nansen apologized, rather sheepishly, for having disturbed his host, then reluctantly explained his mission. Johan Scharffenberg appeared somewhat surprised, then laughed his characteristic "staccato laugh" and pointed to the clutter about him. "It is precisely why I sit here with all this material, in order to investigate and be certain that all I will say is in accord with the truth," he said. "It could happen that one may be uncertain, and with perhaps a slight mistaken memory, be proven not completely correct. Were I to do that I would fail, Architect Nansen. You need not be apprehensive about that!"[23] He then laughed his distinctive laugh again.

Nansen explained that he himself had no fear the speaker would go too far in his remarks about Hitler and Nazism. "I myself have been in Germany, Austria, and Czechoslovakia. I myself have seen and experienced persecution of the Jews at close quarters. I certainly know, as do you, that no word, no description is powerful enough to tell the truth about that which happened in the midst of us, without a finger being lifted to hinder it." Nansen added, "You have certainly heard more than enough from others and I can tell you nothing new."[24]

Scharffenberg was anxious to hear more from his visitor, but first he wished to assure the members of Nansen's board he would say nothing about Nazism, Hitler, or anyone else that was not absolutely true. Yes—

he would bring along enough evidence to document his statements on the spot. He shuffled off into the kitchen and returned with a tea service balanced on a small silver tray, then cleared away books and newspapers from two easy chairs, so they could sit while Nansen told his story.

Odd Nansen spoke of the persecution of the Jews he had seen in Bratislava and Vienna, of his meetings with Father Tiso and his police chief, of the drama that surrounded the invasion of Czechoslovakia, of General Hoepner's cooperation, of his meeting with the high commissioner for refugees in London, and finally about his shock in coming to a country "that still slept its sweetest Chamberlainsleep beneath a gigantic peace umbrella."[25]

When Nansen spoke of the woman pediatrician in Vienna whose entire day was spent patching together Jewish children who had been mauled by the Nazis he saw great tears roll down Scharffenberg's cheeks. Retelling was close to reexperiencing for Odd Nansen, and he paused frequently to control his faltering voice and collect himself so they should not sit and cry together.

The two Norwegians lost themselves completely in recounting the tragic events. Nansen noted:

> It was late before I finished, much later than I thought Scharffenberg in his ascetic life ordinarily allowed it to become. I was completely aghast when I looked at the clock, which had become past two, and apologized deeply and sincerely that I had kept him up so long. He brushed it aside, and assured me that it had been of the greatest value for him to listen to me.
>
> "I am very happy that you came to me," he said, and in his floppy slippers he followed me to the door, thanked me again that I came, and asked me to come again if he could be of any help in any manner or if I had any more to tell him.
>
> When I wheeled through the sleeping city and home to Polhøgda, in the fall night, and went through the thoughts the experiences that night had for me, I was convinced I had met a great and worthy human being—and had made a great and worthy friend.[26]

That evening had solidly welded the spirits of the two humanitarians together. In future difficulties Scharffenberg would replace the dead Fridtjof as counseling "father" to Odd Nansen whenever strength and advice were needed.

On October 10 as Odd Nansen stood at the podium in a University *Aula*, filled to the last seat, he became uneasy as the clock neared the announced time of 8:00 P.M. Scharffenberg had yet to show himself. Nansen let an "academic quarter of an hour" pass, then half of another before feeling obliged to set the evening's activities in motion.

While the performances continued, Nansen's hurried telephone call was unanswered. A special messenger returned, having found Scharffenberg's apartment dark and securely locked. Just as Odd Nansen began an apologetic announcement of the "unfortunate misunderstanding," Johan Scharffenberg rose from at the rear of the *Aula*, where he had been sitting together with a young man and a pile of books and papers. As the two struggled toward the podium bearing their burden the audience laughed and applauded.

Odd Nansen described Johan Scharffenberg and his effect:

> Scharffenberg had requested that before he began his speech, the audience should sing Bjørnson's "To the Wounded," to the music of Lammers. The text was enclosed in the program, and a small string orchestra, that had come in the meantime, played. Scharffenberg, psychologist that he was, wished to create just the atmosphere such a hymn would bring to the audience before the lecture began. Such was the feeling of awe in the hall before he had even begun.
>
> Scharffenberg was no great orator. His power and his entire subconscious being was not that of an orator. The words and sentences he formed as he spoke did not come easily and fluently from his lips, but the more obvious they were, and the more heartfelt, the more convincing they became. He both stuttered and stammered whenever he could not find the correct words immediately—or whenever he paused long enough to search for quotations he needed in his books and newspapers.
>
> Nevertheless his speech was one of the most impressive I have listened to at any time. None of those who heard it would be able to forget it. It was a song of praise for charity and truth and a fervent appeal to the Norwegian people to awaken from their "trance of neutrality." But at the same time it was a castigating condemnation of the irresponsible indifference of the times that allowed Nazi barbarism to have free rein.
>
> He could not resist sharp denunciations of Hitler. But on each occasion when he came forth with a denunciation or any reference to the tyranny of the Nazi attacks or to their crimes against humanity, he would duck down into his books, and newpapers, find evidence of the truth of his statements, then hold it forth before the audience with an outstretched arm and invite them to come and ascertain the truth for themselves.
>
> Far from destroying the unity and the crescendoing effect of his almost prophetic lecture, those interruptions worked in harmony with his somewhat naive "demonstration" quotations. The audience actually held its breath with suspense every time he paused to root about in his "evidence material."
>
> No one, not even those opposed to him—of which there were many about the room and who made notes for their *"Stimmungsberichte"* [The

Nazis hired individuals to prepare accounts of the atmosphere in Norway]
doubted that the apostle of the truth spoke the truth. The truth was Scharffenberg's religion, and speaking the truth was his foremost quality. He could
not tolerate hearing a lie or a "half truth." Not once could an inaccuracy
be stated, without his stepping in and correcting it, if it were possible.

Just as it was before he began his lecture there was a feeling of awe in
the hall when he finished. And silence was long before applause broke out.

Embarrassed and bewildered and unsure of what he should do with
himself, Scharffenberg stepped down from the podium. He was still more
embarrassed and even shamefaced when the gathering raised themselves
in unison to give him still more applause.[27]

Newspaper accounts of the meeting the following day were scant,
"chilly," and as Nansen had come to expect, some contained accusations of
hysteria and warmongering. Yet Scharffenberg's warnings and prophecies
passed out far beyond the walls of the *Aula*. The audience members
themselves spread the word of the inspirational speech on what was to be
the last and most memorable Nansen Day celebration.

With the Germans in complete control in Czechoslovakia, Nansen
Relief undertook a new and special task that continued even after Nazi and
Communist hordes had dismembered Poland—rescue of Jewish children.
Leo Eitinger and other contacts in the Jewish community had already
helped Tove Filseth locate families with the possibility of emigrating
to the West, particularly to the United States and Canada. While the
extended process of obtaining necessary documents continued, Nansen
Relief brought the families' children to a haven in Oslo, prepared to return
them to their parents the moment transport was imminent.

Leo Eitinger helped Sigrid Helliesen Lund gather groups of Jewish
children, sixty in all, whom she then led to safety in Norway. One of those
children, Berthold Gründfeld, maintains a still-vivid memory of the trip
across Germany.[28] He traveled from Bratislava with a half dozen other
children to meet up in Berlin with the larger group arriving from Brno
and Prague. It was his first real experience with a journey by train and
the excitement helped overcome the trauma of separation. The children
were met in the Berlin railway station by a rabbi, then slept in the Jewish
Cultural Center until the entire group was assembled. The rabbi and
Sigrid Helliesen Lund then led their charges to a second railroad station
from where they would depart on the next leg of their travel to Oslo.

It was a long walk, for public transportation was denied to Jews—there
could be no taxis, no trams, no buses for them. The children received
careful and detailed instructions. They were to walk always with their
heads turned to houses and walls. Never could they gaze into a German

face, for what might be considered a "provocation" would bring beatings or other harassment. As the fleeing children made their way to the station, passers-by spat upon the ground, and even on the children. One tearfully asked why the Germans spat on him. "Perhaps, it was only the wind," Sigrid Helliesen Lund replied in order to soften the blow.

The group of tiny fugitives traveled by train to Sassnitz, from where they crossed by ferry to Trelleborg in Sweden, and for the first time in years, freedom from peril. After another train ride they were in Oslo. Nansen Relief was anxious to provide each child with a home life, and sought foster families throughout Norway. Their goal was a home for every child by Chanukah of 1939, or where the foster parents were Christian, by Christmas.

Well into the summer of 1939 Eitinger finally received his visa for Norway, only to be faced with an even more formidable obstacle—obtaining an exit permit from the occupying forces. The invasion of Poland on September 1 compounded his problem, for all Czech physicians were declared essential for service in the German Army. The edict was sheer nonsense, since Jews were excluded from military duty with the Nazis.

Emigration from Czechoslovakia, although tightly organized by Adolf Eichmann, was still possible for those who held visas to neutral countries. After seemingly endless completion of papers, an exit permit was issued. Then, accompanied by his small nephew, Dr. Eitinger set off by train across Germany, heading for Norway and safety—for the time being.

The two refugees arrived in Oslo on November 17, 1939, to be greeted by Tove Filseth and provided assistance, including eighty kroner a month from Nansen Relief. Initially Eitinger lived with other Jewish-Czech fugitives and friends with whom he had worked in the League for Human Rights—and occupied himself aiding the refugee children who were still awaiting placement in Norwegian homes.

The young doctor approached Jørgen Berner, secretary-general of the Norwegian Medical Association about the possibility of work in a local hospital. It was necessary, he was told, to first learn the language of the country. Eitinger immersed himself in study for two months, then returned to the association headquarters. He was then provided a position as unpaid volunteer at an Oslo hospital, beginning his duties on February 1, 1940. For two months the refugee-physician occupied himself diligently, reviewing case histories and improving his Norwegian. In another two months Leo Eitinger was ready to resume his medical career. He received a work permit, and on April 5, 1940, was appointed to a position above the Arctic Circle, in Bodø, at what was then Norway's northernmost mental hospital.

9. Goliath in the North: The Russian Attack on Finland

Leiv Kreyberg, professor of pathology at the University of Oslo Medical School, thrived on confrontation.[1] As an activist and man of principal, he had little hesitation in speaking his mind, writing demanding letters, or expressing indignation in the press. He would travel virtually anywhere in support of causes he held dear—justice, human rights, and above all, the independence and neutrality of his nation. In 1936, sensing Hitler's insatiable desire for power and inexorable drive toward conquest, he sought both Norwegian and American support for a plan of international cooperation in pursuit of peace. The proposal received little support at home or from the American Civil Liberties Union, but the president of Smith College wrote, "I think that Dr. Kreyberg's idea is quite sound and might be effective. . . . It is alarming that a Scandinavian should feel this way, and I suspect that he is right in believing that we are soon to face a life and death struggle for liberty."[2]

In anticipation of a German invasion of Poland, Kreyberg resolved to see some of that country before its destruction. He managed to obtain an invitation as guest of the Krakow Fishing Club through Ladislas Neuman, then Polish minister to Norway. Once in Poland, in the summer of 1939, he traveled widely, fishing and using the subterfuge to speak with colleagues and Poles from all walks of life—students, farmers, artists— and particularly with refugees who streamed across the Polish frontier with Germany and Czechoslovakia.

Dr. Kreyberg's worst fears were confirmed, as he sensed the imminence of the conflagration Hitler was about to ignite throughout Europe. He described his journey and added personal observations in the newspaper *Dagbladet* on his return.

On September 5, 1939, four days after Germany had plunged Western Europe into war by invading Poland, Kreyberg suggested that his own country look to preparedness. At the same time he submitted an evacuation plan for the Institute of Pathology to Rector Didrik Seip of the University of Oslo. Since the Institute of Pathology serviced *Rikshospitalet* (Norway's state hospital) and its clinics, Kreyberg sent a letter to the director of that hospital on October 3, with suggestions for the institute's operation in the event of mobilization. Both missives remained unanswered.

When the Soviets sliced off Eastern Poland for themselves on September 17, 1939, the encircled country's fate was sealed. The Nazi siege of Warsaw ended on September 28, and by October 5 the last sporadic guerilla action had ceased. Within weeks of sharing a dismembered Poland with Germany, Stalin turned his attention to Scandinavia.

Signature of the Russo-German non-aggression pact in late August 1939 did nothing to alleviate Soviet distrust of Hitler. Fearing a German offensive against his own country, Stalin moved to eliminate Finland as a possible staging area for an attack against the Soviet Union. Clearly, capture of the Arctic port of Petsamo (ceded to Finland by the USSR in the Treaty of Dorpat in 1920) was of primary importance to the Soviets. Overrunning Petsamo would serve to protect the water route to the ice-free port and naval base at Murmansk—and once Finland was invaded, foreign aid could be prevented from reaching the beleaguered country via the Arctic route.

The Russian invasion of Finland on November 29, 1939, brought death and destruction close to the Finnish-Norwegian border, an area that had known only peace for centuries. The banks of the Pasvik River, separating the two countries, had been sparsely peopled by a mixture of Finns, Norwegians, Lapps, and Russians. To them the river represented no closed border. Rather it was a bridge for communication, which the inhabitants frequently crossed to meet with relatives and friends on the opposite bank. There had been, however, a change in 1918, when Finland was liberated from Russia. Incoming Finnish farmers constructed more modern and efficient buildings, and civil servants arrived to organize a new Finnish administration. The initial tensions between new settlers and the established though widely separated community persisted in 1939. Looking back to earlier times, the sympathies of many older inhabitants continued to lay with the Russians.[3]

Johan Scharffenberg and Leiv Kreyberg alike were shocked by the unprovoked Soviet attack on Finland and were mobilized to action, each in his own characteristic manner. Scharffenberg defended his fellow

Scandinavians and castigated the Soviets in newspaper articles and flaming speeches. If ever right were on a single side in wartime, he proclaimed, it was with the Finns, for Finland protected every value the Soviets had renounced—freedom, truth, justice, and human rights. Scharffenberg urged his own government to allow the Norwegian unemployed to work as civilians in Finland, thus freeing young Finns to enter military service.[4]

Leiv Kreyberg, as a member of the military reserve, volunteered to travel to Kirkenes in East Finnmark immediately after the Soviet aggression. Using that remote vantage point—above the Arctic Circle and close to the Finnish border—as a base he planned to observe medical problems in the field. No land route traversed the rugged mountains between Oslo and Kirkenes, so on December 9 Kreyberg boarded the night train to Stockholm, then traveled north to the Kiruna Mines, and then west back across Norway to Narvik on the railway constructed to carry Swedish iron ore for transshipment from that North Sea port.

As Leiv Kreyberg strode about the deck of the coastal steamer bearing him from Narvik to Kirkenes, he encountered "a middle-aged man at the rail, clad in a raincape and wearing a six-pence cap."[5] It was Otto Beutler, the new German vice consul to Kirkenes. The "diplomat's" role in the tiny town was unmasked when he installed an elaborate radio apparatus and strung his antennae between two birch trees outside his hotel room. Beutler attributed his desire for a powerful radio to a love of German music. During a later political discussion, the unbemused Kreyberg, only half in jest, offered to wager a case of whiskey against Beutler's single bottle that "Germany will attack our country before St. Hans Day"[6] (June 23rd). For his frankness, Leiv Kreyberg received a mild reprimand from his commanding officer, Colonel Faye, for "offending a diplomat of a friendly power."[7]

Initially the intruding Russian forces swept the outnumbered Finns before them. By the time Dr. Kreyberg's tortuous route brought him to Kirkenes on December 17, the tide had begun to turn as the intruders were forced back. It was an eerie battleground that he observed across the Pasvik River. The sun had made its annual withdrawal to the south nearly four weeks earlier and would not reappear for more than a month. The temperature hovered around -25°F, and the wintry countryside was faintly lit by the luminescent reflection of the moon on glistening snow. Professor Kreyberg described the scene on that Christmas day.

> I was out early to ski, in that morning light that was neither night nor day. The landscape resembled a pale, ink-drawing, but life-and-death were also there. Cannons thundered beyond Fjorvatnet and Hoyhenjarvi.

I skied half-way out onto the river ice to follow the details of the attack—
Russian tanks against Finnish artillery. In the interim Russian planes
dove in, dropped their bombs, raised themselves, then swung east over
the wooded ridge. Finnish patrols attacked on the flank, but later were
driven partly back. To the north I saw the smoke of campfires and burning
farms. . . . Again on the ice in the morning, and I followed a hand-to-hand
Finnish attack on the Russian camp. Throughout the afternoon exhausted,
wounded Finns arrived. They had lain half the day in the severe cold,
hidden in the rushes at the water's edge. They were disarmed and tended.[8]

On the 11th of January Kreyberg experienced double indignation—
the first at the downing of a Norwegian reconnaissance plane by a Soviet
aircraft that had pursued it across the border. The second followed the
arrival in Kirkenes of the freighter *Lake Halwill* en route from England to
Murmansk. Leiv Kreyberg was astonished to learn that while ostensibly
supporting the Finns, the British were shipping tin, nickel, rubber, and
copra to the Russians in Murmansk.

Throughout the early fighting the League of Nations had urged member states to assist the Finns. Large quantities of supplies, weapons, and
ammunition were dispatched from Sweden, France, and Great Britain,
and lesser amounts from Norway, Italy, Denmark, Belgium, Hungary, and
the United States. Many of the weapons were obsolescent or arrived too
late. The Finns employed all their ingenuity and determination to turn
back the Soviets. They lay in foxholes chiseled from the frozen earth and
hurled flaming, gasoline-filled bottles against advancing Russian tanks—
and the "Molotov Cocktail" was born. The poorly equipped military
of a nation of but four million could not withstand the Soviet might
indefinitely. The fighting front had become static at the end of January.
In February the tide turned once again—to favor the Soviets. By March
Finland had capitulated.

During the lull in the fighting at the end of January 1940, Leiv
Kreyberg returned to Oslo. Incensed with British double-dealing in
shipping war materials to Russia while ostensibly supporting the Soviet's
enemy, he poured his bitterness into a letter to Sir Cecil Dormer, the
British minister in Oslo. The English diplomat first claimed the delivery
was the contractual completion of an exchange of goods—the British
having already received the Soviet shipment. A second letter from Dormer
retracted the admission, however, claiming all deliveries, on both sides,
had been completed before the outbreak of war in Finland. He also
requested further information on the ship Kreyberg had mentioned.
Although that material was sent on to the British diplomat, Leiv Kreyberg
received no reply.[9]

Indignation flared at the Soviet aggression in the Arctic, and concern for their neighboring Finns gripped all of Sweden and Norway. The two countries united in sending a delegation to the United States under the direction of Folke Bernadotte. As a Norwegian representative, along with Trygve Hoffe, Odd Nansen was to work in the "Finnish Relief" program under the direction of Herbert Hoover, past president of the United States and the great humanitarian with whom Odd's father had cooperated one war past.

The committee's frustrations were deep and the disappointment keen at having accomplished so little before the Finns were compelled to capitulate on March 12, 1940. Odd Nansen made his way homeward and arrived just a week before Norway became another victim of the tyrant's might.

A NO LONGER
NEUTRAL NORWAY

10. The Perfidious Invasion

I

While Leiv Kreyberg was still in Finnmark, German militarists were at work planning the invasion of his country. Norway's enormous strategic importance made her a prime target for both Britain and the Nazis. Free passage through the Norwegian coastal waters of the North Sea was vital to the German war effort. Swedish iron ore from the Kiruna and Gallivare mines first traversed Norway by rail to reach Narvik, from where it was transferred to the German freighters that skirted the coast in neutral Norwegian waters before slipping into German ports on the Baltic sea. Much of the Nazi war machine was built of Swedish steel. Hitler could tolerate no British effort to interfere with those shipments. Churchill, on the other hand, was developing his plan to mine Norway's coastal waters at the very moment the Nazis were finalizing their own attack. Despite all clear indications of danger from both combatants, the Norwegian government remained blind to the country's vulnerability. Norsemen still depended on their traditional policy of neutrality to carry them unscathed through a conflict they regarded as none of their own.

Norway's significance to the Germans went far beyond safeguarding supplies of iron ore, as irreplaceable as the metal was to the Nazi war industry. Were Germany to strike most effectively at Allied shipping with their deadly submarines, forward bases were essential. The fjord-protected port in Trondheim provided ideal shelter for that purpose, and Narvik could become an admirable base for supply and other support vessels. On his part, Grand Admiral Erich Raeder considered the war as virtually lost for Germany were the Allies to occupy Norway.

When Vidkun Quisling, by then turned fascist, appeared in Berlin December 1939,[1] Raeder considered the Norwegian Nazi's visit a stroke of extraordinary good fortune. Quisling's initial encounter with the Nazi theorist Albert Rosenberg in June was followed by the December meeting that included Admiral Raeder. The Norwegian traitor intimated that

Britain had forged a secret agreement with Norway, allowing the British to set up a base near Kristiansand. To counteract the possibility of his country offering aid to Germany's enemy, Quisling suggested that a new Norwegian government be formed with himself at the head. As "legitimate leader" of his countrymen, Quisling himself would then invite the Nazis into Norway as "protection from the British."

The Norwegian turncoat convinced his Nazi hosts that many Norwegians in crucial positions were favorable to his proposal. Should that fail, however, Quisling promised that an invasion of Norway would be welcomed, particularly by the masses of local Nazis and Nazi sympathizers he claimed to exist in the country.

Desperate to protect their steel supply and to exploit Norway's military value, the Nazis already had plans for an attack on their drawing boards. Hitler, when he personally met with Quisling on December 18, was anxious to believe his visiting Norse sycophant. *Der Führer* gave orders to set Operation *Weserubung* (Weser Exercise), the code name for the invasion of Norway, in motion.

On a February afternoon in 1940, Leiv Kreyberg stopped at a coffee shop near the Solli Post Office to buy some chocolate. He was greeted there by Vidkun Quisling, seated conspicuously alone at a table.[2]

Leiv had met Vidkun years earlier—in 1916—through his brother, Jørgen Quisling. Kreyberg's friendship with Jørgen continued through their student years, and on occasion Vidkun was included in their social functions.

Ten years had passed since their last meeting when Leiv Kreyberg telephoned Vidkun Quisling in Moscow. Professor Kreyberg, together with his wife, had just attended the Scandinavian Pathological Congress in Helsingfors and had followed the scientific sessions with a sojourn in Leningrad and in Moscow. Leiv was intent on visiting Lenin's tomb, but was on the brink of disappointment—restoration was in progress and the memorial was closed. Kreyberg telephoned Vidkun Quisling, who temporarily represented British interests in Moscow. Quisling excused himself from aiding the Kreybergs, claiming his abundance of mail needed immediate attention making him unable to provide any assistance.

With characteristic determination Leiv Kreyberg sought the chief of security at the dead leader's tomb. Exhibiting a stamp-bedecked Norwegian passport, Leiv explained he had traveled three thousand kilometers to see Lenin, and hoped not to be disappointed. The guard-commander was sympathetic. The President of the Free Port of Danzig would make an official visit in some hours. The Kreybergs attached themselves to the visiting party, and Leiv's wish was fulfilled.

The following evening the Kreybergs were guests, together with Norwegian Consul Krane, at an elegant dinner in the home of Vidkun Quisling and his Russian wife. After the meal the guests were stunned as Quisling led them through the appalling Ukrainian famine of the early twenties with a personal account and photographs.

Vidkun Quisling invited Professor Kreyberg to a cup of coffee. Quisling then began a long, rambling monologue—about Germany, England, Russia, and Norway; the future; the momentous times; and so on. Leiv, too, was concerned with similar problems but he was "not grabbed by his [Quisling's] great vista. I was too earthbound." After half an hour, Kreyberg excused himself and returned home.

Describing the meeting to his wife Leiv added, "You know we owe Quisling a better dinner. In the last years it has not been possible to invite him because of his idiotic politics and now he is completely on the outside, and he sat there so forlorn in a shabby winter-coat." "If we have waited ten years," Mrs. Kreyberg firmly replied, "we can wait another ten years."

Professor Leiv Kreyberg, in the meantime, became a member of the Oslo Rifle Club. Each Sunday in the course of the winter he practiced—aiming at cutouts of human figures, always uncertain whether the targets represented Germans or Soviets. When purchasing Zeiss binoculars from a German concessionaire in Oslo he was required to sign a declaration that his purchase would never be sold to any of Germany's enemies. He did so, adding a proviso "with the exception of Germany attacking us."[3]

On April 6, 1940, Johan Scharffenberg wrote of Hitler again in a long feature article, referring to a Roman saying, "Those whom God will destroy, He first makes mad."[4]

Preparations for Operation *Weserubung* gained momentum in the early months of 1940. While invasion plans were germinating Great Britain continued her mastery of the seas beyond Norway's neutral zone. Using that mastery British naval forces steamed into Norwegian waters in a rescue mission that accelerated Nazi preparations for attack.

Acting on information that captured British seamen were in Norwegian waters, the destroyer *Cossack* set out to liberate the captives. The tanker *Altmark*, a service vessel for the pocket battleship *Graf Spee*, steamed homeward along the coast of Norway carrying a cargo of three hundred British prisoners captured by the German raider. On interception by the *Cossack* the *Altmark* fled into *Jøssingfjord*. Disregarding the warning by Norwegian torpedo boats that pursuit would violate Norway's neutrality, the destroyer pushed into the fjord and sent a boarding party aboard the *Altmark*, killing several German seamen in the process of liberating British prisoners.[5]

Hitler's fury was boundless. Preparations for the forcible entry into Norway commanded his first priority.

By the end of March all arrangements were in place. As a final preparatory step Vidkun Quisling was summoned to Copenhagen. On April 3, in the Hotel d'Angleterre the Norwegian turncoat met with Colonel Piekenbrock of the German Intelligence Service.[6] The Nazi officer found his informant anxious to provide all he knew of Norway's defense. Satisfied with his service to the Nazi cause, Quisling returned to Oslo to await the onslaught, confident he would soon control Norway's government himself.

The vanguard of slower ships in the multipronged Nazi attack force set out from their home ports on April 2, 1940. On April 8 the German troopship *Rio De Janeiro* was torpedoed off the coast of Bergen by the Polish submarine *Orzel*,[7] operating in concert with Allied naval forces. In Oslo that same night, Johan Scharffenberg pondered news of the sinking. With mounting concern he had read reports in an April 4th Swedish newspaper of German ships gathering in their home port, but he remained puzzled as to the exact significance of the event.[8]

The moon was new on the 7th of April as the Nazi aggressors moved into place. In the dark of the following night the invaders entered Norwegian waters and prepared for an air attack as well. Early on the fateful morning of April 9, 1940, German planes and paratroops landed unopposed at Oslo's Fornebu airport, then swept rapidly into the virtually unprotected city. Seaborne forces quickly subjugated the coastal ports of Arendal, Egersund, and Bergen, and penetrated even to the northern harbors of Trondheim and Narvik.

At sea, the invading Nazis met costly opposition from both Norwegians and the Allies. In the first days of the invasion obsolete cannon and ancient torpedoes from Oscarborg Fortress in Oslofjord ripped into the hull of the *Blucher*, newest of Germany's heavy cruisers, setting it ablaze to become the funeral pyre of a thousand Nazi troops—among them administrators hand-picked to manage the military government once Norway had fallen. British naval forces had followed the Nazi movement at sea closely, without the slightest awareness of the real purpose. British warships welcomed the chance to engage the enemy and devoted all their strength to the fray. By the time the fighting had ended three Nazi cruisers were destroyed, three others heavily damaged, and ten destroyers, fully half those in the German fleet, sunk or useless.

The traitorous Vidkun Quisling saw the invasion as his opportunity to seize the power he had sought long and unsuccessfully. With the support of Hans Wilhelm Scheid, head of the northern section of the German foreign ministry who was then in Norway—and to the complete amazement of Germans and Norwegians alike—Quisling, with a handful of Norse Nazis, broke into Oslo's state radio station. He took to the air waves, reporting to his countrymen that their government had fled. It was the duty and the right of the *Nasjonal Samling* to take over that government, he proclaimed, as he named himself Norway's head of state and minister of foreign affairs.[9]

The following day, April 10, unfounded rumors of impending British air attacks sent civilians flooding out of Oslo in disorderly panic. Dr. Ole Jacob Malm,[10] driving against the stream to reach his hospital, was shocked to see the signs of panic—strong men dragging women, children, and old people from their places on truckbeds whenever the traffic slowed or stopped. Once reaching his destination he spent several days treating those wounded during skirmishes in the wooded hills to the north of the city—Norwegian and German alike.

Small, poorly trained, and inadequately equipped with only obsolete weapons, the Norwegian army was no match for the superbly disciplined, heavily armed German swarms overrunning its country, yet it resisted. As the fighting moved northward to Gudbrandsdal, Ole Jacob Malm felt he could serve more effectively where action was continuing. Another junior colleague, Arne Homb, joined Dr. Malm. Together they met with Axel Christensen, chief of the medical service, to inform him of their intent to travel north. Dr. Christensen responded in a fury, warning the young surgeons they would have no place at Aker Hospital *if* they should return. As the two walked quietly toward the door they heard a sharp "Wait!" Malm and Homb turned to see Christensen's back as he stood facing the window. "If I were your age, my men," the older man said, "I would do just the same."[11] Malm would think of that moment often—after Axel Christensen had cast his own lot with the Nazis.

Ole Jacob Malm obtained passes from the local Red Cross for himself and Arne Homb, painted a Red Cross on his car, and drove off toward the battle line. In the course of the long day they crossed several German checkpoints. To Malm's astonishment the Nazi guards passed the vehicle with little more than cursory inspection. It might have been his "school-German" or the white coats on the back seat, Ole Jacob thought, but more likely, he felt, it was his handsome German car—an Adler Cabriolet—that impressed the Nazi troops as an officer's car.

In Lillehammer the two doctors joined two other colleagues, Eivind Platou and Halvard Scheie. Together they requisitioned the Lillehammer Tourist Hotel, borrowed instruments from Einar Murstad of Lillehammer's Community Hospital, and by the next day had set up their field hospital. The one hundred and sixty beds were filled to capacity with wounded Norwegians, Germans, and some Britons who had been hurriedly sent to Norway's aid. One wounded German sergeant-major insisted on keeping a machine-pistol at his side in bed. Sheie, however, with a foreboding face and a crackling *Waffen Heraus!* (Weapons out of here!), disarmed the soldier on the spot. Malm described his first encounter with Nazi racial-fanaticism by "an SS soldier with a high thigh amputation. He would only permit blood transfusion from another Nazi of the same breed."[12]

Within four weeks all action in the vicinity of Lillehammer had ended, the remaining patients were transferred, and the two young surgeons made their way back to Oslo. They returned to their duties at Aker Hospital without a solitary comment from Axel Christensen.

II

On the day of the German invasion King Haakon VII had gathered the remnants of his government, with the few troops he could muster, and fled northward from Oslo, under continual aerial bombardment. Virtually beneath the very noses of the Nazi vanguard, bankers Nicolai Rygg and Christian Dons hastily requisitioned a fleet of twenty-six trucks—then sent 1,534 crates and barrels containing $55 million of Norwegian gold reserves lumbering northward toward a temporary haven in Lillehammer. Thirty recruits from Jordstadmoen shepherded the treasure through Gudbrandsdal on a train attacked repeatedly by Nazi aircraft before reaching Åndalsnes. At the port, transfer of the precious cargo to a British cruiser began, only to be cut off at mid-point by the warship's hurried departure to avoid approaching German aircraft. The remainder of the gold was driven northward then loaded on small fishing smacks that set out immediately to sea.

The Norwegian government paused briefly in Hamar, seventy-five miles north of Oslo, then fled a few miles to the northeast to regroup at Elverum. On April 10, Dr. Curt Brauer, German minister to Norway, met with King Haakon VII and Foreign Minister Halvdan Koht, pressing Hitler's demands. Haakon VII must recognize Vidkun Quisling as Norway's premier, the Nazi diplomat insisted, in accord with specific instructions from Hitler. If not the German military would take over the administration.

The Norwegian monarch stood firm. He would not use his constitutional authority to turn his government over to a man his countrymen abhorred. Norway's leader must have the confidence of the people, and Norsemen had no such trust in Quisling. Besides, he added, that matter required action by the cabinet. Shortly afterward King Haakon made it clear to his cabinet that were such an action to occur, he would have but one response—he would abdicate.

The government remained loyal, and with the king fled toward Norway's western coast, constantly harassed by Nazi planes. At Molde on April 29, they boarded the British cruiser *Glasgow* that carried them above the Arctic Circle to the port of Tromsø. After seven hazardous weeks en route, constantly evading Nazi aerial attacks, the gold-laden flotilla of fishing smacks reached the same port and discharged its cargo. The Norwegian gold reserves were shipped to safety, first in London, then in New York.

On the battlefield the Norwegian position was desperate from the moment of attack. Not only were the Norsemen poorly equipped and badly outnumbered, but troops that could be ill-spared were sorely needed at the Pasvik River on the northeastern border. Russian forces had moved in to replace the Finns at the river once Finland had capitulated. Tenuous as it was the German-Soviet Pact remained in force, and Norwegians feared their new neighbors in the north might have designs on Norway as well.

The British were first to send aid to the beleaguered Norwegians. The newly arrived troops were inadequately trained "territorials," undisciplined and poorly supplied. Much of their materiel had been lost to German attack. Those Britons fled the battlefields in panic, and already exhausted Norwegians were recalled to the front.

The outlook improved as troops of the French Foreign Legion arrived in northern Norway on May 13. Just over two weeks later bombardment from British warships neutralized German artillery at Narvik. French and Norwegian troops stormed in and retook the city—the first decisive victory in the six-week-old war—and Norsemen rejoiced. The die had already been cast, however. France itself had come under German attack. Allied troops were withdrawn to meet the threat in the south. Again, Norway stood alone. The only alternatives were surrender or continuation of combat from bases in Great Britain. King Haakon and the Norwegian government chose to resist from abroad.

On June 7, King Haakon, Crown Prince Olav, and the remnants of Norway's legal government boarded the British cruiser *Devonshire*, bound for England where the Royal Norwegian government-in-exile remained a steadfast ally for the balance of the war.

Over Radio Oslo, Vidkun Quisling called upon the thousand Norwegian merchant vessels scattered worldwide to return to Norway, or enter a neutral port, preferably Italian or Spanish. The British Broadcasting Company carried a countermanding order from the Norwegian Seaman's Association. The mariners paid the traitor no more heed than did their countrymen at home. Virtually all Norwegian ships headed for Allied ports. The Norwegian Trade and Shipping Mission (*Nortraship*) was formed on April 18, placing the entire merchant flotilla under a single administration. Despite U-Boat harassment, those thousand ships became critical to maintaining Allied supplies throughout the war. During the course of the conflict almost half *Nortraship*'s fleet fell victim to German torpedoes and aerial bombs, and more than thirty-seven hundred seamen were lost. Proudly, using income from *Nortraship* Norway paid all her military expenses throughout the entire war, the only American ally to do so.

III

In the afternoon of April 8, 1940, a day before Norway became an occupied country, Leiv Kreyberg[13] found it difficult to concentrate on a lecture delivered to the Genetics Society by Dr. L. Hogben of Great Britain. Kreyberg found his thoughts wandering despite the excellence of the presentation. When the speaker had concluded, Kreyberg was persuaded—half against his will—to join the group having a light repast with the guest. Kreyberg picked up a newspaper as they neared Blom's Restaurant in a small courtyard off Karl Johansgate, just a block from the University. Noticing Kreyberg's agitation, a colleague suggested he "Take it easy, and don't be nervous."[14] Kreyberg wondered if the questioner really understood what was happening—then made his excuses and left the gathering.

At 5:00 A.M. the following morning Kreyberg was awakened by a telephone call from a cousin. The caller reported that her brother in Bergen had informed her moments before that the streets were filled with Germans. Shortly afterward Kreyberg saw swastika-marked planes in the skies above his home. At the police station he discovered war had broken out. "With whom?," he questioned. "I don't know," the police replied.[15]

Leiv Kreyberg, as a reserve officer in the 6th Division then stationed in Kirkenes, was convinced of his duty. He collected his Colt revolver, an old Savage hunting rifle, and the backpack he had kept filled in readiness. After he deposited his wife and four children in the Landåsen Hotel, Leiv headed north. At the Oppland District Hospital in Lillehammer,

Dr. Murstad, the chief physician, responded to Kreyberg's concerns for Norwegians wounded in encounters with Nazi troops. Murstad collected instruments and essential medications, especially morphine. Open trucks were covered with canvas, and straw was spread over the flatbed floor to convert a number of vehicles to ambulances. Five units, headed by physician volunteers and directed by Dr. Helge Granrud, were dispatched into the field.

On April 12, Captain Kreyberg met the commander of Norway's forces in the field. General Otto Ruge recalled that Leiv had served as observer in the border region of Finnmark just months earlier during the Russo-Finnish War. Ruge, whose staff was without a medical officer, invited Kreyberg to help organize the medical service. Kreyberg accepted and immediately drew up a table of organization and a plan for action.

Kreyberg then telephoned the Landåsen Hotel, directing his wife to bring the children to Lillehammer. Following a day's respite he sent his family northward, planning to rejoin them sometime later in Bud.

After a conference with Ruge, Kreyberg reconnoitered the district, seeking out the means and personnel for handling refugees and the wounded if needed. He found that the local physicians had already taken the initiative.

In the afternoon of April 15, Leiv Kreyberg met up with the district physician, Dr. Gunnar Seland, who informed him of a ferocious encounter between Norwegian soldiers and a group of German paratroopers in the vicinity of Dovre. Many had been killed or wounded. The two set off toward Dovre to provide medical assistance to their wounded countrymen.

All was strangely silent when the two physicians reached the vicinity of the fighting. They left their auto carrying a small flag marked with a Red Cross and walked slowly forward—at the same time calling out *Medical Corps.* Suddenly the Norwegians found themselves surrounded by armed Germans who had erupted from the roadside ditch. The doctors explained they had heard of the skirmish, and of the wounded who needed help.

Dr. Seland, who was still in civilian clothes, was led away blindfolded to the German headquarters, while the uniformed Kreyberg was held at their car by a young lieutenant and an enlisted man.

"Warum schiessen sie doch, die dumme Bauern?"[16] [Why are they still shooting, the dumb farmers?], the young German officer demanded. Kreyberg responded that the German farmers would also shoot if armed foreign soldiers plummeted from the skies. But we are friends, the lieutenant protested, who had come only to protect Norwegians from the

British. Captain Kreyberg suggested that if the English arrived in the same manner, they would have earned the same welcome.

The talk then turned personal—first to fishing then to common friends in the German's home city of Hamburg. Kreyberg learned that his captors were engineers on a mission to disrupt rail connections with Trondheim.

Dr. Seland returned presently with four wounded Norwegians. Two, with injuries in the lower limbs, were placed on the flatbed of a truck, and the others accompanied the doctors in Seland's car.

The young German officer, Lieutenant Herbert Schmidt, wrote of his encounter with Kreyberg in 1942, *"Hier fiel mir zum ersten Male die gute Haltung der Norweger auf, die ich spater noch schätzen lernte. Ein grossartiger Menschenschlag, ritterlich kampfend, mit anständigem Denken und Fühlen."* [Here, for the first time, I felt good attitudes on the part of Norwegians, that I later learned to value. A grand race of men, fighting chivalrously, with decent thoughts and feelings.]

On April 16, Professor Johan Holst, the newly appointed chief of the Royal Norwegian Army Medical Corps, arrived to take over his duties. Kreyberg delivered his report then prepared to travel to the 6th Division in Kirkenes.

In Pollfoss Kreyberg arranged for the daughter of the *Lensmann* to care for his car for the duration of the Occupation in return for a pair of skis. He set out by foot, then traveled by bus and boat as he headed first for Ålesund, then Molde.

After a conference with Fredrik Harbitz, chief physician of the Molde Hospital, Kreyberg proposed a ship be outfitted as a floating hospital. The vessel would transport soldiers wounded in the campaign in the north who had managed to reach Åndalsnes to hospitals near the coast, where they could be treated more effectively. Professor Holst approved the proposal and Kreyberg set his scheme in motion.

Leiv Kreyberg located Bernt Fauske's 340-ton cruise vessel, the *Brand IV*. The ship's seating capacity could be enlarged to two hundred, and the salon was ideal to fill with beds for sickrooms. On April 25, a large Red Cross was painted on either side of the stark white hull of the *Brand IV*, as well as on the deck, roof of the bridge, and even the smokestack. A Red Cross banner flew from the mast. Aside from Dr. Kreyberg, personnel included Dr. Gisela Lyng, five nurses, three young members of the Women's Defense League, eight Boy Scouts, and the Swedish artist, Helge Wahlblom.

The wounded 103 Norwegian and British soldiers, 9 German troops and 3 civilian refugees—who were loaded aboard the *Brand IV* on April 26 reached Ålesund without incident. While the ship was fast to the pier, however, an aerial bombing attack showered the vessel with fragments of stone. The hospital ship pulled away and circled the harbor for two hours until the Nazi planes had disappeared.

On her next call to Ålesund, on April 29, Navy Captain Puntervold requested that the *Brand IV* carry 120 cartons of canned meat to Åndalsnes. Kreyberg refused, stating, "That is contrary to the Geneva Convention."[17] Puntervold countered, "Do you believe the Germans respect it?," to which Kreyberg replied, "That I don't know, but I sail under the mark of the Red Cross." Puntervold pressed his point until Kreyberg gave him a final option—should the captain immediately paint the ship gray and provide a machine gun for defense, he would transport the tinned meat. The wounded could be carried on a warship—but he would not yield and set sail with contraband as cargo on a distinctly marked hospital ship. The vessel departed with the cartons still on the pier.

Nearing noon under the bright sun of a cloudless day three German planes passed low over the *Brand IV*. Before the enemy aircraft became little more than specks in the distance they turned toward the ship once again. Captain Kreyberg set the vessel on a steady course and ordered all personnel and patients to don life jackets and proceed below decks. Three bombs fell a scant thirty yards away. On the attackers' next pass Kreyberg heard a thunderous crash and the sound of shattering glass. He remembered kneeling with blood pouring down his face. He closed one eye at a time—found he could see from both—then felt his head and discovered no hole. He rose to see Dr. Arnoldus Blix, who had been added to the medical personnel, swaying and calling out, "Bring a tourniquet, my arm is gone."[18] The wounded physician dropped into Kreyberg's arms—dead. A nurse appeared, announcing five dead on board—including a Boy Scout.

The unmistakably marked hospital ship was damaged, but operable. Bernt Fauske made for Bjørnøya (Bear Island), where Kreyberg ordered everyone to disembark and take cover. The circling planes swooped low again and again, spraying the island with machine-gun fire. As the planes circled to return and strafe again the Norwegians spread out to new cover and retreated into the island. When the Nazi pilots finished with the already wounded, they bombed the oil storage tanks on the opposite side of the island and disappeared.

Two of the scouts returned to the ship for brandy. Kreyberg downed his allotment shortly after a nurse had swathed his head in a turban. The tension of the ordeal melted away. Everyone fell into a deep sleep. Soon another vessel arrived from Ålesund to speed the wounded to the hospital.

Bernt Fauske took the shattered *Brand IV* to harbor for repairs. Kreyberg was doubly happy he had not contraband aboard to serve as pretext for the bombing.

At the hospital in Molde, Kreyberg sought out Major Kusserow, one of the nine wounded Germans in the first *Brand IV* transport. "I am ashamed as a German," Kusserow responded on hearing of the outrage.[19]

Cast upon his own initiative once again, Kreyberg resolved to move northward to find his parent 6th Division. Along the way he managed to contact his wife, and arranged to meet his family in Bud on May 1. Reaching the District Hospital in Bodø, Leiv suggested moving the operating rooms to the basement in the event of a bombing raid. The chief physician, Dr. N. Friis, was irritated by the proposal. Bodø was an open city, he declared and as such was safe from attack. Before the month was out Bodø had been destroyed by enemy bombs.

Dr. Kreyberg found there was no need for his skills in Bodø. After discussing possibilities with journalist Per Bratland, he decided to make for Sweden and publicize the tragic events in his home country. In Stockholm on May 10, he began his press conference, "Today we Norwegians bow under a heavy burden."[20] He warned the Swedes to take care lest one day they too bow under the same yoke. The warning had little effect on the Swedes, but his words rang loud over Norway, France, and England. Through German broadcasts, Kreyberg's countrymen heard him condemned to death for his description of the lawless bombing of *Brand IV*. Return to Oslo under Nazi Occupation had become impossible. On the day of the German broadcast Dr. Axel Øwre, Leiv's faithful friend, carried Kreyberg's valuables, including his irreplaceable art collection, from his home to safe hiding in Ullevaal Hospital.

Despite his generally friendly reception from Swedes and from his countrymen who had sought refuge in Stockholm, Kreyberg felt an oppressive sense of isolation. Once the propaganda mission was complete he returned to his embattled country to rejoin the still resisting Norwegian forces. Hans Jacob Arnold, Leiv's eldest son, had been depressed as a stranger in a foreign land, so the fifteen-year-old youth accompanied his father to Norway.

After crossing the Pasvik River into their native country, father and son hired a taxi to carry them further into Kirkenes. The driver responded bitterly to questioning—launching a tirade against Kreyberg's former commander, Colonel Faye. In Kirkenes Dr. Alf Palmstrøm supported the cabbie's opinions. Faye had allowed German Vice Consul Otto Beutler to roam about unchallenged, even after the Nazi invasion. The German agent lived with the military staff at the *Turisthotel* and freely dispatched telegrams to his superiors—despite General Lindback-Larsen's orders for the German "diplomat" to be interned.

From his experiences in the Winter War of 1939 Dr. Kreyberg had been convinced that Beutler was an enemy agent. The population of Kirkenes now shared his conviction. On April 12, Norwegian troops in the Pasvik region sent a letter of protest to the high command in East-Finnmark concluding, "Let him (Beutler) have the protection consistent with the 'protection' Germany has offered us."[21] Finally, on April 20, Beutler was escorted across the border to Finland.

The two Kreybergs proceeded on to Tromsø where the elder rejoined the 6th Division, then met with King Haakon. The Norwegian monarch was much moved to receive the supportive greetings Kreyberg had carried from the United States Minister to Norway, F. J. H. Harriman, who was then in Sweden.

Once the crucial decision to move king and government to England had been made, General Ruge invited Captain Kreyberg to join the royal party aboard the British cruiser, *Devonshire*. The invitation, the general stressed, was not an order. Kreyberg was free to follow his own course, but he should leave Norway where he would be in unceasing peril until the Nazis were ejected from the land.

Buoyed by Ruge's gesture of confidence, Leiv Kreyberg chose not to follow his monarch. Only the navy and air force would engage the enemy from Great Britain, and he was an army captain.

IV

German aircraft touching down at Fornebu airport on April 9 were obscured from Odd Nansen's view at his residence some half-mile away only by a line of trees. At the time Odd, and his family still lived in his father's famous home, *Polhøgda* (Polar Height). In the days immediately following the Nazi invasion British aircraft struck the airport repeatedly, so Odd Nansen felt it safer to move his family into Oslo, at least temporarily. By April 20, when the bombing appeared to have ended, the Nansens moved out to *Polhøgda* again.

On the fourth night following their return the Nansens were awakened by the thunderous roar of a bomber just over the rooftop followed by an explosion that shook the entire building. Parents and children dressed quickly and hurried into the cellar for safety. When an hour had passed in quiet, Odd climbed the stairway to the tower where he could see the moon-bright landscape. The skies over the airport were illuminated by flickering flames that brought to mind a St. Hans Day bonfire, outstripping in its enormity the thousands that burn throughout the dusky night to celebrate the longest day of the year. Three decades later Odd Nansen described his emotions in his memoir.

> I will never forget my first personal encounter with the war. It was strange that it should take place at home, on the tower at Polhøgda. It was just beneath me that my father sat and worked in his tower study. He gazed over the same landscape from his window, with Baerum Ridge in the west and the fjord in the south, narrowed by the land of Nesodden and Hurum on either side, down against Drobak Sound that allows you to feel the sea behind. A marvelous, beautiful landscape that had given him so much inspiration and strength through the years. He brought forth those qualities to his fellow human beings in an almost mystical radiation of his personality—unbroken as long as he lived—of simple humanity, of benevolence beyond bounds and of courage and strength to rebuild a world torn asunder.
>
> How much hope and faith had its source in the room down below? How many tens of thousands of human beings were rescued, salvaged, and made secure from there? And how many thousands' thoughts had turned toward Polhøgda in gratitude for what he had done?
>
> And today, ten short years after his death, every hope has failed, all faith shattered, rolled over by Hitler's war machine, as an added irony of fate, the room stands empty and forsaken in his home, in the center of a war-zone, and awaits bombs that will obliterate it all. I wonder if that will come to pass?
>
> One must judge you almost fortunate, father, not to have experienced this.[22]

The following day, Odd Nansen and his family moved back to the other side of Oslo. Soon afterward he was given confidential information that the Nazis were about to requisition *Polhøgda* for use as a field hospital. After continual frustration Nansen ended up in the office of a high-ranking German officer named Gortz. Odd explained *Polhøgda*'s status as protected national property, with a museum, a library, irreplaceable archives, and the burial plot of Fridtjof Nansen. Gortz promised his assistance. No Germans appeared at *Polhøgda*, and after a period of time a large placard was nailed to the door of the main entrance:

> *Eigentum und Wohnung des beruhmten Polarforschers Fridtjof Nansen. Eintritt und Beschlagnahme verboten!* [Property and residence of the famous Polar explorer Fridtjof Nansen. Entry and seizure forbidden!]

11. The Resistance Begins

The recurring indignant complaints from the German Legation accusing Johan Scharffenberg of unrelenting attacks on Hitler and Nazism in the press led the Norwegian physician to expect immediate arrest once the Germans had occupied Oslo. Characteristically the aging psychiatrist did not panic but continued with his medical duties and faithfully vented his opinions in Oslo's newspaper. He pointed critically at the Nygaardsvold government, blaming it for "Norway's greatest shame and misfortune."[1] His article on May 17, Norway's traditional Constitution Day, concluded: "Without democracy and respect for human rights we cannot celebrate the 17th of May in truth and in spirit."[2]

The German administration attempted to ignore Scharffenberg, but his defiant defense of free expression and a free press inflamed the Nazis and cost him the freedom to publish. His challenging articles in the daily newspaper *Arbeiderbladet* on May 25 and 28 employed anecdotes from Plutarch and quotations from the Bible to stress the need to protect one's principles and one's country, even in the face of physical violence and threats to life. He wrote:

> More dangerous and effective than physical violence is the intellectual assault through censorship, one-sided propaganda, or direct lies. . . . Suppressing opposing criticism does not bear witness to strength, but to cowardice. . . .
>
> That there is an intellectual guardianship by people who are hardly my superior, I feel as a slow suffocation. If that be the condition in Norway for long, then, as often before, the words *"Vivere non est necesse"* lie before me. . . .
>
> When freedom of the press is so greatly restricted . . . remaining silent about subjects that have been termed "taboo" deserves greater consideration than my personal safety.[3]

Johan Sharffenberg's original manuscript concluded with Henrik Wergeland's poem *Sandhedens Arme* (Army of the Truth), perhaps the

most powerful of the works written in the poet's unceasing battle to
gain Jews admittance to Norway. That poem, Scharffenberg's specific
references to the Jews, and a great deal more of the article he had originally
submitted was deleted by the editors of *Arbeiderbladet* as being too risky.
Their most important responsibility was to keep the paper operating
during the occupation.

The challenging tone, and particularly references to "people who are
hardly my superior," infuriated the Nazis and they forbade Scharffenberg from publishing further. The newspaper remained open, but only
temporarily. In August 1940 *Arbeiderbladet*'s doors were closed for the
duration of the Occupation.

Unaccountably, Scharffenberg remained free of prison. He shifted his
attack to the speaker's podium, where he stood again and again stirring
his countrymen through emotion-laden words to defend freedom and
human rights.

Almost from the moment Odd Nansen took his leave from Johan
Scharffenberg following their emotional meeting in the psychiatrist's
apartment at Bot Penitentiary, the young architect had come to consider the older man a source of comfort and advice—for his qualities of
compassion and understanding were similar to those of his father. With
the Germans in control of his destiny Odd Nansen had repeated need for
Johan Scharffenberg's knowledge and sage counsel.

Prior to the invasion Odd Nansen had served as architect for construction then in process at Oslo's Fornebu Airport. When British bombing of
the airport appeared to have ceased late in April, Odd Nansen, together
with other architects, engineers, and construction foremen on the project
was summoned to a meeting. The assembled group was informed by Nazi
officers that Germans would take over direction of the construction, and
the *Luftwaffe* would replace the community of Oslo as builder. The airport
was to be completed as well as enlarged to meet Nazi military needs.[4]

As spokesman for the assembled group, Odd Nansen requested and
received a break for private discussion. After a brief conference Odd
Nansen announced the group's unanimous decision. Norwegians would
discontinue their efforts on the project, in accord with the Hague Convention. Since their country was at war with Germany they could not freely
and willingly continue to carry out work important to their enemy's war
effort. The Nazi officers took Nansen's report back to their superiors.

Odd Nansen sought out Johan Scharffenberg for advice and support
and to clarify the words and intent of the Hague Convention resolution.
Scharffenberg knew exactly where the Hague Convention report lay on

his bookshelf, and quickly found the pertinent Resolution 57. It was quite clear that the convention forbade use of civilians of an occupied nation, without their consent, to perform work important to the war effort of the enemy.

At a subsequent meeting Odd Nansen found the Nazis to be completely unconcerned with international law, as they demanded that work be carried out—by force, if necessary. Under that circumstance the Norwegians demanded the Germans state in writing that work was to be carried out under duress. No German word other than *Zwang* (force) would suffice, Nansen contended and insisted that each man receive a copy of the order containing that specific word.

Der schwierige Herr Nansen (the difficult Mr. Nansen), as he had come to be known, was summoned before *Luftwaffe* General von Kitzinger. The general thundered his displeasure at the difficulties Nansen had caused, and at the loss of time when every minute counted for the Germans. If he were Nansen, the General offered, he would end the discussions and resume work the following morning. Were the German officer in Odd Nansen's own position, the Norwegian countered, he could not comply without committing treason against his fatherland—it should not be necessary to explain the significance to a German officer.

Odd Nansen had struck a vital target; the general yielded—in principle, if not in actuality—agreeing to issue the order for Norwegians to resume work—if necessary, under *Zwang*. Having achieved at least that objective, Nansen asked further what would happen should there be refusal to follow the order. "I would not advise you to experiment with that, Herr Nansen," the general warned. "People have been shot for less. You must remember that we are at war, and do not tolerate impediments being placed in our way. We are compelled to do away with these in the one way possible."[5]

In despair, Odd Nansen hurried once again to Johan Scharffenberg, to report on the situation, and to be advised as to his best course of action. Nansen's counselor thought the Germans unlikely to carry out their threat—for the grave breach of international law would cost them dearly. There was, however, no guarantee Odd would escape with his life—the Germans were well known to have committed heinous crimes in both World Wars. "It would be absurd," Johan Scharffenberg concluded, for Odd to allow himself to be shot.[6] Following Scharffenberg's recommendations, Norwegian workmen took up their tasks, after receiving orders containing the word *Zwang*. Their efforts benefitted the occupying Nazis little, however. British bombers and Norwegian sabotage prevented the task's completion.

The invading Germans had overrun Oslo with the same terrifying efficiency as they had Prague, and had moved quickly to establish their dominance. Once the capital had fallen the Nazis expected a compliant Norwegian government to respond to their every demand. Indeed, Vidkun Quisling had already reassured Hitler that masses of Norsemen would flock to the Nazi flag.

Quisling's bungling attempt to take command, followed by King Haakon's resolute rejection of the traitor as his prime minister, shattered Hitler's expectations. Curt Brauer, having automatically become the *Reich* plenipotentiary on the Nazi invasion, seized the opportunity to depose Quisling, whom he saw as an ineffectual leader and a threat to Brauer's own authority.

With the remnants of Norway's legal government still resisting in the north, some central authority was required in Oslo to negotiate with the conquerors, as well as to prevent economic disaster and bureaucratic chaos. The single remaining authoritative body, the Supreme Court, briefly undertook the responsibility. Able diplomat as he was, Curt Brauer recognized the court's inadequacies and felt the need for a functional administration. Under Brauer's urgings the court appointed an Administrative Council, intended solely for executive function—with no semblance of legislative or political responsibility. The Supreme Court, continuing to work toward a reasonable working arrangement, selected a council from among Norway's most prominent citizens, including Rector Didrik Seip of the University of Oslo and State Health Commissioner Dr. Andreas Diesen. From his refuge in the north, the king, still officially at the government's head, refused to yield to Nazi convenience—rejecting the council as illegal.

Hitler's response was cold fury. Quisling, whom he had supported, had been deposed and the Administrative Council had failed to satisfy the king and become a legally functioning body. The unfortunate Brauer was dismissed on April 21—less than two weeks after reaching supremacy in Norway through German conquest. On May 6 he was called to active service in the *Wehrmacht* and on the 15th of the same month dispatched to the Western front.

Der Führer then turned to one of his own ilk. At Hermann Göring's suggestion the infamous *Gauleiter* of Essen, Joseph Terboven, was appointed *Reichskommissar* on April 24, to rule over the defeated nation. On arrival in Oslo the tyrant made his alternatives clear. Norwegians would form a government acceptable to him or he would impose a German military administration—with all its consequences. He pressured the reluctant Administrative Council to join with the *Storting*'s presidential committee in urging their king to abdicate. Without the monarch, Terboven planned to form a new "legal" government composed principally of Norwegian Nazis and sensitive to his every demand.

Vidkun Quisling immediately engaged the new *Reichskommissar* in a struggle for power. Joseph Terboven attempted to form a *Riksraad* (State Council) that would be subservient to him. When that move proved unsuccessful, orders from Hitler allowed Vidkun Quisling to emerge victorious. Although the *Reichskommissar* obstinately avoided naming Quisling head of state, the *Nasjonal Samling* was designated Norway's official party—and Quisling controlled that party and all cabinet appointments. Terboven then informed the conquered nation that self-determination could only be achieved through the *Nasjonal Samling*. The announcement, however, was little more than a charade, for the Nazi remained the supreme authority in the land.

The new order swelled party membership with malcontents and opportunists. Soon the *Fører*, as Quisling named himself, began replacing local officials throughout Norway with his party members. Despite the growth of *Nasjonal Samling* membership, the traitor was still unable to muster sufficient replacements of even the most modest capacity, and loyal Norwegians held sway, particularly in small towns and villages.

The Norse tyrant was quick to mimic his Nazi ideal. Jews and political opponents became targets of persecution. By order of Ragnar Skancke, newly appointed minister of church and education, all books written by Quisling's political opponents or by Jews were removed from library shelves. On December 12, 1940, the entire Supreme Court resigned in protest of *Nasjonal Samling* policies.

Once the initial shock of invasion and Occupation had passed, and their own authorities had fled to England, Norwegians sought new leaders. At that critical moment, according to Odd Nansen, Johan Scharffenberg assumed the major role. It was thus the respected psychiatrist to whom Nansen turned again as he considered assembling a group to take action and formulate policy for Occupied Norway.

Together, the two patriots selected nine committed Norwegians to join them in a meeting at *Polhøgda*[7] Jacques Worm-Müller, professor of history; Paal Berg, chief justice of the Supreme Court; Harald Gram, mayor of Oslo; Andreas Diesen, state commissioner of health; Eivind Bergrav, bishop of Oslo; Gunnar Jahn, director of Norway's bank, and former minister of finance; Didrik Seip, rector of the University of Oslo; Hans Gjerlow, *Morgenbladet*, editor; and Herman Reimers, attorney.

Odd Nansen considered the meeting a great success. All invitees attended and spoke. Nansen was elected chairman. Bishop Bergrav was the most voluble of the speakers, expressing his displeasure at Foreign Minister Halvdan Koht and the general ignorance of the government-in-exile in London about matters in their home country. Everyone agreed that one task of those present was to keep their government informed.

The group's principal concern, however, was the future of the acting government at home. Gunnar Jahn accurately anticipated that the Nazis would remove Norway's Administrative Council then demand the *Storting* be summoned to depose the king and government-in-exile. With many of its members having fled the country, Parliament could not be legally called to session, Scharffenberg noted. Even the Supreme Court could not remove the king; Haakon must abdicate of his own free will. Johan Scharffenberg's interpretation was supported by Chief Justice Paal Berg. Professor Worm-Müller reported that the process had already been initiated. The executive committee of the *Storting* was just then under pressure from the Germans. The Nazis wished to replace the Norwegian Administrative Council with a State Council, which in turn would recommend the king abdicate. Odd Nansen described the events that followed:

> That announcement . . . brought about a commotion in the assembly. I had my hands filled keeping order in the management of the debate, which grew louder and louder, and angrier and angrier. . . .
>
> Everyone uniformly condemned the Executive Committee's request to the king, but in return agreed that the king never should accede to the Executive Committee's request. . . .
>
> I thanked everyone for their attendance, and cautioned against the keeping of any record. . . . I would call the next meeting after consultation with Scharffenberg. "The Group" divided itself into small units that carefully disappeared into the summer night. . . .
>
> The king's answer came on the 3rd of July, but it was July 8th before it was first sent out over the BBC. Perhaps it was on that occasion that the announcer at the BBC questioned the king as he sat and awaited his turn at the microphone. She asked: "Pardon me, but of what country did you say you were king?" . . .
>
> Quietly, objectively, and in the best majestic manner, he rejected the Executive Committee's request, which he understood, of course, was the result of German threats.
>
> The king reminded us that he had come to the country in response to the Norwegian people's wish and desire. In the years he had served the country as king he had come to love both the country and the people. He neither could, nor wished to accommodate the Executive Committee's request when he was convinced it was not the will of the Norwegian people.

That was like a cleansing. It was good to be a Norwegian again, and to be able to look one another in the eye and say with pride that we had a king.

That event, the greatest and most joyful of the entire year, was celebrated with a codfish dinner at Worm-Muller's.

During the dinner, Scharffenberg rose and spoke. Emotionally he confessed that, as a convinced republican he had opposed the institution of a monarchy in 1905, and had opposed King Haakon in speech and writing since that time. Each of the many opportunities to meet with the king were rejected. "I am," Scharffenberg admitted, "to be blamed for narrow-mindedness." He paused, then continued with a voice broken-tearfully, at times. "If King Haakon—I mean *when* King Haakon returns to Norway after the war, I will go up to him at my first opportunity. First I will tell him what I have said here, then I will say to him: 'If Your Majesty might have use for me and the service I can render, I am at your Majesty's service as long as I live.'" King Haakon the 7th, *Skaal*.[8]

King Haakon's valorous refusal to comply with Nazi wishes were reproduced by the underground press in Oslo, then quickly distributed throughout the country. His duty, the monarch had reported, was to maintain the sovereignty of his nation until Norway was once again free, and a government could be formed through constitutional processes. The stirring speech rekindled the resolve of a faltering people. The *Storting* refused to turn over the powers of state to Nazi puppets.

A climactic speech delivered by Johan Scharffenberg to the University of Oslo Students' Association on September 21, 1940, marked the turning point in the Norwegian stand against Nazi tyranny. Abandoning his anti-monarchist stance of three and a half decades, he pointed with pride to the freedom of the Norwegian *Storting* in choosing the Danish Prince Carl as King Haakon in 1905. He continued, contrasting the openness and free will of that choice with Nazi attempts to press a puppet, Quisling government on an unwilling people.

The University *Aula* reverberated with the students' shouting acclaim, bringing Johan Scharffenberg back to the podium with a final warning. He admonished his enthusiastic audience to be clear about the obligations that went with their approval: "Let them [the Nazis] know that Norway's youth will defend freedom and independence, no matter the cost to us all."

In many Norwegian eyes, the Resistance movement was born in that moment. Arne Skouen wrote in *Dagbladet* thirty years later: "a stroke of genius, professionally executed at exactly the right second. A front was formed by the stroke of a hand and these five words, '*Husk! En slik tislutning forplikter*.'" (Remember, with such an approval you obligate yourself.)[9]

The furious Nazis arrested Johan Scharffenberg, finally unable to tolerate his taunts, and exhortations to resist. The Students' Association was dissolved and its chairman arrested as well. Ample warning of impending arrest gave Scharffenberg the opportunity to disappear underground, had he so chosen. Two Germans sought him at his home on September 25 and 26. Johan Scharffenberg awaited the third visit in his home. When the Nazi agents appeared he demanded to see their authority. They had none, for they needed none, he was told brusquely.

Once Scharffenberg was placed in a cell in the infamous prison at *Møllergata 19*, Kristian Kristensen, the police physician, arranged to have his colleague transferred to the prison dispensary.[10] The stay, however, was only temporary. The Gestapo would have none of this favored treatment and returned Scharffenberg to an ordinary prison cell with a bed so short for his lanky frame that he had difficulty sleeping. His countrymen expressed their support and admiration through cakes and masses of flowers delivered to the psychiatrist's cell—until the exasperated Gestapo forbade further delivery.

Despite his constant and longstanding flaunting of German authority, Scharffenberg was treated courteously during imprisonment and not subjected to the Nazis' usual barbaric interrogation techniques. He owed this favored treatment only in part to his own courage and deportment. He refused to surrender his dignity to German intimidation. On one occasion, during distribution of water rations to the prisoners, a Nazi guard roared the German equivalent of "Move it, man."[11] Scharffenberg was seen to walk slowly toward the guard, adjust his lorgnette, ask distinctly and piercingly, "What do you mean?" then move two steps closer and ask again, "Do you mean something, perhaps?" Chastened and intimidated the guard moved backward in silence. For the duration of his imprisonment, Scharffenberg was no longer the object of his captors' "roars."

Johan Scharffenberg's favored treatment, in greater part, seemed due to the intercession of Pastor V. H. Gunther of the German Lutheran Church in Oslo, who was given the mission of sounding out Norwegian thoughts of a future government for their country. Gunther, in pursuit of his goal, had spent many hours with Scharffenberg, and in sympathy with the psychiatrist, convinced the Gestapo that the septuagenarian physician was senile.

The six-year-old report from the German minister in Oslo, Scharffenberg's public attacks on the occupying Nazis, and his absolute fearlessness during interrogation led his captors to accept the validity of Gunther's contention. Scharffenberg had responded to questions about his statements of Hitler being mentally ill by insisting they were not *beskylding* (accusations) but *unnskylding* (excuses), for the German leader was hallucinating and thus not responsible for his actions. The psychiatrist continued, saying he would rather discuss Hitler's mental status with qualified professional colleagues.

The Gestapo found it wisest not to pursue scientific aspects of the matter, and they had no desire to convert a Norwegian folk-hero into a martyr.

The atheist Johan Scharffenberg was not without his sacred beliefs, for the truth was his religion, a religion that was to be sorely tried during his interrogation. Among Norwegian patriots, however, he let no deviation from fact lie unchallenged. Eivind Bergrav had unearthed an ancient resolution that gave the Bishop of Oslo the privilege of "bishopric visits" to the prison at *Møllergata 19*. Bishop Bergrav chose to exercise that right while Scharffenberg remained an inmate at No. 19. The imprisoned journalist-psychiatrist was the subject of his sermon.

At a time when Norway was in great need and in great distress, the bishop declaimed, a Norwegian who had written two newspaper articles took the lead—referring to Scharffenberg's stirring contributions in *Arbeiderbladet*, "*Vivere non est necesse* (to live is not necessary)" and "*Navigare necesse est* (it is necessary to navigate)." The titles, Bergrav said, were taken from an inscription above the city gates of Hamburg.

Scharffenberg, who had sat straight-faced during the entire sermon, threw his arms about the bishop at the conclusion, and tears coursed down the cheeks of the two comrades in Resistance. In the midst of the embrace Scharffenberg's tears ceased as he quietly informed Bishop Bergrav, "It was not the city gates of Hamburg, but in Lübeck where the inscription was written."[12]

In November 1942, Johan Scharffenberg was summoned to Gestapo Headquarters on *Viktoria Terasse* and questioned about a Norwegian engineer who had given refuge to members of the Home Front, three of whom Scharffenberg believed had been in mortal danger. "Completely calmly I denied any knowledge of these occurrences, not with respect to me, but to the engineer. *It was my duty to lie*,"[13] he reported later (emphasis mine).

When Johan Scharffenberg was released after six weeks at *Møllergata 19*, he was forbidden to speak in public. In the following year he was removed from his position at the Oslo Asylum.

Despite the attention he received from the Gestapo following his imprisonment, Scharffenberg was unwilling to give up his own personal battle against the Nazis. He continued to voice his opinions, shifting to the clandestine press. He had begun illegal newspaper activities while still imprisoned at *Møllergata 19* as he aided in the publication of *Nitten-titten*

(Looking in at 19). Oslo's populace anticipated Johan Scharffenberg's strident articles with the same interest as they had before the Occupation.

For a time the group formed by Nansen and Scharffenberg remained active under the psychiatrist's leadership. He was completely unsuited for the seclusion and the secrecy necessary to the organization that had become the very foundation for survival of the Home Front, however. He was frequently shadowed as he went about the city. With great regret the Resistance movement proceeded on its course excluding the great personality that had set it into motion. The original group was then superseded by other clandestine bodies.

12. Nazi Pressures Mount

The resignation of all justices of the Supreme Court in protest of Nazi coercion in December 1940, removed the last semblance of legality from the occupying forces. Joseph Terboven, however, remained unopposed as the sole power, and Quisling danced to his tune. The Norwegian turncoat pandered to every Nazi wish, and whatever small authority he was given was applied cruelly and vengefully. The Norse sycophant was rewarded with the empty title of minister-president in February of 1942, but never did he emerge from Terboven's shadow.[1] Despite the complete impotence of his administration, the Norwegian Nazi's name became a noun acknowledging his infamy throughout the world. Both Monsignor Josef Tiso in Slovakia and Ante Pavelic, the Nazi-designated puppet head of the Croatian Free State, far outdid the ambitious Norwegian in power over their dominions and the extraordinary depravity of their acts. The sound of their names lacked melody, however, and failed to capture the imagination of their enemies. Only "Quisling" remains defined in today's dictionaries—a traitor who serves as puppet of the enemy occupying his country.

In the autumn of 1940, Nazi authorities made several inept and completely unsuccessful attempts to obtain the cooperation of Norwegian trade, sporting, and professional societies. When *Reichskommissar* Terboven, in frustration, moved to stifle all opposition through restrictive measures, the Norwegian organizations responded in a united front with the medical association at the fore.

Local Nazi leaders began their move against Norway's physicians beginning with Dr. Rolf Gjessing, director of Dikemark Hospital.[2] There were then only twenty-three members of the *Nasjonal Samling* at Dikemark Hospital, the psychiatric branch of the Oslo Community Hospitals, but their leader, newly appointed male nurse Camillus Wassdahl boasted, "there will be more." Former Chief Male Nurse Murvold had worked beyond his retirement age because of the institution's need. On March 25, 1941, however, Thorleif Østrem, director of Norway's Health

Service, had ordered him retired and replaced by the irascible Wassdahl. Gjessing resisted, for as hospital director, his was the authority to fill such positions—through royal mandate. Department heads of the Oslo Community Hospitals also insisted that such an important and responsible position be declared vacant and filled only through open competition.

Østrem was unyielding, ordering Gjessing to name Wassdahl chief male nurse on April 22. The order included transfer of a second quisling, Ingvald Fedje, from the psychiatric service at Ullevaal Hospital, to replace the capable Assistant Chief Male Nurse Eggan at Dikemark. The second appointment was as unfitting as the first. As chief of the psychiatric service at Ullevaal Hospital and Fedje's superior, Dr. Haakon Saethre had reported him to be unbalanced and unreasonable. Although he could be comforting at times, Saethre reported, patients frequently complained of his loss of self control and explosive behavior under more trying circumstances.

Wassdahl, with the complete support of Østrem, attempted to widen *Nasjonal Samling's* influence at Dikemark Hospital and advance his own cause.

On April 25, Lars Hordnes, a painter in the hospital, in full Hird uniform and accompanied by half a dozen of his ilk, brushed aside admonitions that the doctor was interviewing a patient, and burst into Gjessing's office, placing him "under arrest." The quislings treated Gjessing crudely and impudently as they drove him to Hird Headquarters. After transfer to the prison at *Møllergata 19* he was suspended from his position at Dikemark. Gjessing spent an anxious week in confinement until he was released on May 3.

Norwegians rose in angry protest against the illegal imprisonment of Gjessing—the country's most distinguished and influential citizens and all quarters of the medical profession, a few of whom were themselves members of the *Nasjonal Samling*, joined in.

Rector of the University of Oslo Didrik Seip and Bishop Eivind Bergrav were among those signing letters of support for the beleaguered doctor. The Norwegian Psychiatric Society and the Norwegian Medical Association added their own protests. Finally and most effectively, all department heads of the Oslo Community Hospitals expressed four demands in the course of their lengthy and comprehensive protest to the Police Department:

1. The vacant position as Chief Nurse at Dikemark will be announced in the usual manner, and the appointment will be made in accord with the regulations in force and on the exclusive basis of professional qualifications.

2. Mr. Wassdahl and Mr. Fedje will retire from their new positions.

3. The suspension of Director Gjessing will be lifted.

4. Assurance will be given that tyrannization of the hospital on the part of either the Hird or their leadership will not occur in the future.[3]

Furthermore, the doctors warned, should these demands not be met, all physicians in Oslo's Community Hospital would strike. The protest concluded with a declaration of solidarity, with confidence that physicians throughout Norway's hospitals were united in the same cause.

The *Nasjonal Samling* commission formed to examine the matter found in Gjessing's favor. Indeed, the members stated, "Gjessing's relationship with the *Nasjonal Samling* can only be characterized as above reproach."[4] Camillus Wassdahl and Ingvald Fedje were demoted to their former status, and Lars Hordnes was removed from employment at Dikemark Hospital.

In November 1940, Norway's Nazis had made their clumsy attempt to gain control of the Norwegian Medical Association. Few physicians had any stomach for the quislings, and but two doctors of prominence had enrolled in the *Nasjonal Samling*, Klaus Hansen, professor of pharmacology at the University of Oslo, and Dr. Axel Christensen, Ole Jacob Malm's chief at Aker Hospital.[5]

Hansen met with two association officials, Dr. Christian Krohn, vice president and Berner, secretary-general, on November 2. The Norwegian Nazi laid out the Occupation force's intention. First he asked that all Norwegian physicians swear loyalty to the new government. A number of professional guilds were then to be formed, among them Norway's Guild for Health and Hygiene. Hansen proposed the medical association become a member of that group. Clearly the guild was to have a political role and be led by quislings.

Although Hansen and Christensen had come to the forefront by declaring themselves members of the *Nasjonal Samling*, it was unclear at the time exactly how many turncoats were among Norway's physicians. Ole Jacob Malm, then a board member of the Young Physicians Association, decided to "smoke out" certain of his colleagues by placing the following notice in the daily *Aftenposten*: "The undersigned members of the *Nasjonal Samling* physician group, Oslo and Akershus District, hereby urge their colleagues to join the *Nasjonal Samling* and work in keeping with the new time." The eighteen names that followed included those of Axel Christensen and Klaus Hansen. The editors, noting their disgust, placed a heavily black-bordered advertisement just above the announcement:

ROTTER

La ikke rottene ødelegge De-
res elendom og spise op Deres
matforråd.
Vi foretar utrydding med
anerkjente sikre preparater.
GÅRDEIERFORENINGENS
DESINFEKSJON A/S
Tollbugt. 25.   Tlf. 10662

[**RATS**, Do not let rats destroy your property and eat your food supplies.
We exterminate with recognized safe preparations.]

The article served its purpose. Those named who were not quislings or
were fence-sitting demanded the retraction that was printed the following
day. The others were clearly identified as having gone over to the enemy.[6]

Secretary-General Berner was soon arrested, and the Norwegian Medical Association could no longer function freely and independently. As
members ceased paying dues and boycotted meetings the real association
became dormant for the remainder of the Occupation.[7] The skeleton
Nazi organization that succeeded the legitimate society was virtually
functionless. Fewer than one hundred physicians were estimated to have
participated.[8] Individual physicians turned to clandestine operations to
continue their struggle for freedom and independence from Nazi rule.

On Norway's National Holiday, May 17 1941, with the medical
association in the vanguard, leaders of forty-three professional and trade
societies signed a letter protesting Joseph Terboven's attempts to Nazify
their organizations. Five weeks later, the signatories were collected by
the police then addressed by a menacing *Reichskommissar*. Nine of the
leaders were arrested, and Terboven declared the majority of the societies
dissolved. The Opposition then moved underground.

Norwegians were inexperienced in clandestine operations, and the
Resistance movement developed slowly and unsteadily. Soon after Terboven's speech in June 1941, plans for leadership of the new underground,

the Home Front, were made at a meeting at the home of Professor Werner Werenskjold. Five subsections were formed under the direction of the R-Group, as it came to be known (R from råd, the Norwegian word for council).[9] Two were led by physicians. The liaison group, directed by Dr. Bjørn Helland-Hansen, functioned in cooperation with national bodies such as Labor and the Farmers Organization. Johannes Heimbeck was placed in charge of the finance group.

Heimbeck was perfection itself for his job. To his medical colleagues he was flippant and disrespectful. Dr. Ketil Motzfeldt, chief of medicine at Aker Hospital, referred to Heimbeck as "Norway's handsomest and dumbest internist," and in reverse compliment, "the best mountaineer among internists and the best internist among mountaineers."[10] Dr. Heimbeck's dynamic mien, his overwhelming self-confidence, and off-handed responses helped to disguise his underground work. No one would believe he could be involved in any serious activity.

Johannes Heimbeck's task was enormous. Not only did the Home Front procure funds for illegal activities, but it provided support for each family losing a breadwinner through imprisonment, escape to Sweden, or disappearance underground to elude the Gestapo. When persecution or pressure by the Occupation Forces resulted in loss of income for loyal Norwegians, Heimbeck's finance group stepped in to provide the funds necessary for economic survival.

The R-Group turned to such prominent Norwegians as Chief Justice Paal Berg, former Finance Minister Gunnar Jahn, Bishop Eivind Bergrav, and Dr. Johan Scharffenberg for advice and support. The first three remained as leaders of the Home Front throughout the Occupation. Scharffenberg, as previously noted, was soon excluded. Despite their admiration, the Home Front leadership could not risk including him in their underground deliberations—and the exclusion embittered the zealous doctor.

Bishop Bergrav, on the other hand was remarkably adroit, knowing just when and how to speak. A disturbed young priest—and underground agent—sought the bishop's advice. "A priest should never lie," the distressed cleric stated, as he wondered if he should tell the truth if questioned by the Gestapo. "The truth," responded Bergrav, "is too valuable to be given to that type of person."

Scharffenberg provided help to the fledgling movement in a different form. As prison physician at *Botsfengslet* he treated criminals with many skills. When the underground needed access to secret documents in various government or German offices to search for important directives or discover impending Nazi actions, Scharffenberg provided one of his "qualified" prisoners to carry out the task in the dead of the night. The "locksmith" would be brought back to his cell once the mission was accomplished.[11]

As the German military poured troops into Norway to meet the threat of an anticipated Allied invasion, small, local underground fighting units were formed, with the intent of assisting the invasion forces. At the outset, and nearly to the end of the war, most of these units were without weapons and trained with wooden facsimiles. Two former Norwegian Army officers, Major Olaf Helset and Captain John Rognes, began work with these small groups. They advised young Norwegians to form units of four to six men without reporting to any central command. In time, however, the necessity of coordination became apparent. Dr. Johan Holst, professor of surgery at the University of Oslo, and Lieutenant-Colonel Ole Berg then formed the Military Council for that purpose. Since Berg was too conspicuous as a military figure, responsibility for the day-to-day operations of *Milorg*, the new coordinated organization, fell to Holst.

Norwegian inexperience with underground operation was costly, for they had not yet learned the importance of silence, nor had they reckoned with the efficient ruthlessness of the Gestapo. *Agent provocateurs* were recruited by the Nazis to infiltrate the fledgling units. Group after group was "rolled up" and the captured Norsemen tortured to force revelation of their fellows in the Resistance movement. In the summer of 1941 the unit in Stavanger under the direction of Dr. Carl Johan Oftedal was infiltrated by an *agent provocateur* and twenty young Norwegians were arrested. Eleven, including Dr. Oftedal were executed. Additional arrests followed and the leaders became exposed. In the autumn of 1941, Dr. Johan Holst was forced to flee to London. His assistant in *Milorg*, the surgeon Carl Semb, then stepped into Professor Holst's resistance shoes.[12]

13. The Underground Organizes

From its inception at the home of Professor Werner Werenskjold on November 7, 1940, the R-Group devoted its attention to coordinating Home Front activities and strengthening the people's will to resist both the Nazi invaders and Vidkun Quisling's *Nasjonal Samling* sycophants. Overt acts of violence were shunned and sabotage was discouraged. The communications section, led by Dr. Jan Jansen, and the information service were entrusted with the R-Group's most vital activities. *Bulletinen* (The Bulletin) and *Fri Fag Bevegelse* (Free Trade Union Movement) served as both spokesmen for the Resistance movement and moral support in the most trying of times. Dr. Jansen, as warden of the residence hall of the University of Oslo, maintained a position of intimate contact with university students, and held their confidence and trust. Jansen's information service was responsible for distribution of the two clandestine journals and for the countrywide dissemination of information gathered by the R-Group. For that second and most hazardous task couriers were employed—bus drivers, crewmen on coastal steamships, railway workers, traveling businessmen, and of course, Jansen's students.

The dangers of transporting forbidden material extended far beyond the courier—for Gestapo savagery often exposed others as well when any messenger was apprehended. Many were unable to withstand the heinous torture. No matter the patriotic determination, names important to continuing underground function were often revealed, and the informants were held blameless by their understanding colleagues. Widespread arrest would follow and the revelation process would begin anew. Plunging underground whenever a courier was arrested soon became standard for Resistance operatives about whom the captive had information. Several key members, including Bjørn Helland-Hansen, were arrested, forcing others who faced exposure to flee. As ranks of the R-Group were depleted to near nothingness, it passed out of existence.

With each act of resistance *Reichskommissar* Joseph Terboven's ruthlessness toward the captive nation increased. On September 8, 1941, milk rationing was introduced. For Norwegian workers milk was an expected necessity accompanying the *smørbrod* (open-face sandwiches) constituting their traditional noontime meal. When shipyard and steelmill workers failed to receive their supply at the same time milk was provided to Germans engaged in identical labor, Norwegians walked out in protest. Shop stewards and labor leaders recognized the fearful consequences and urged their countrymen to return to their jobs. The workmen remained defiant, however. By the next day other industries closed down in a gesture of solidarity as over twenty thousand Norwegian workers joined in the strike.[1]

Joseph Terboven struck violently at all who opposed him. At dawn on September 10 the Gestapo swept through Oslo, arresting leaders of labor unions, shop stewards, signatories of the protest of the previous May 17, the chief of police, and Rector Didrik Seip of the University of Oslo. Editors and journalists were seized or were dismissed from their positions. The Boy Scout movement was declared illegal and humanitarian organizations were placed under the control of the *Nasjonal Samling*. Vigo Hansteen, the Trade Union's principal legal counsel, and Rolf Wikstrom, a shop steward, had recognized the dangers of intransigence against an amoral foe and strongly advised against the strike. Their own position notwithstanding the two were summarily executed in reprisal.

One week after his infamous day of terror, Joseph Terboven made "disturbance of economic life or peaceful conditions of work" punishable by prison or execution. Other severe restrictions and penalties were subsequently imposed by the Nazis. Jews were already forbidden the use of radios, and later in the autumn all Norwegians' radios were ordered confiscated. Attempting escape to Britain, reading underground publications, or even listening to British broadcasts on clandestine radio receivers became offenses punishable by death.

New organizations and new systems became crucial to the Home Front's survival, if Nazi incursions into the lives of the Norwegians were to be resisted. Gestapo terrorism only stiffened Norse determination. Aside from the minute numbers of native Nazis and the handful of opportunists who joined them, Norwegians remained loyal to king and country.

State Commissioner of Health Andreas Diesen led the first secret group of physicians to oppose the Nazi Occupation. Jan Jansen sat as a member of that committee with Drs. Carl Semb, Leif Poulsson, Gunnar Johnson, and Hans Jacob Ustvedt, chairman of the Young Physicians Association and a chief physician at Ullevaal Hospital. On June 18

Ustvedt was given the specific task of forming an Action Committee and he recruited Dr. Ole Jacob Malm to join him in the effort. In the autumn, Dr. Ustvedt's committee was superseded by the *Koordinasjonskomitteen*[2] (The Coordinating Committee) which, more than any other group, would direct freedom-loving Norwegian people in their daily struggles with the Nazis.

Under the impetus of attorney Tor Skjonsberg the smaller, but exceedingly important and prestigious "Circle" was formed on June 20, 1941. The Circle soon replaced an R-Group that had ceased to function as its members fled or were arrested.[3] Among the ten constituting the new organization's nucleus were important survivors of the R-Group—Justice Paal Berg, Gunnar Jahn, Bishop Eivind Bergrav and the ever-involved *Prosektor* Jan Jansen.

The Circle's primary mission was to maintain communication with the government-in-exile in London and to promote cooperation among factions of differing political persuasion within the Resistance movement—with particular attention to the Norwegian Communist Party.

In the first fourteen months of the occupation the Communists had been staunch advocates of cooperation with the Occupying forces and the New Order—looking back to the Soviet-German Non-Aggression Pact of 1939. Once the Nazis had invaded Russia in June 1941, however, the Norse Communists became aggressively anti-Fascist, and turned to sabotage and armed attacks on the Germans. By that time, Terboven had loosed terrorism on the country. Each act of sabotage provoked torture of prisoners and execution of hostages. *Reichskommissar* Terboven decreed that assassination of a single German soldier would be followed by execution of fifty to one hundred Norwegian hostages.

In the early summer of 1942 the Circle along with others in the Home Front leadership recognized that sabotage and espionage would bring death and barbarism out of proportion to the advantages obtained. They agreed that such operations would be launched only from abroad by Norway's government-in-exile in concert with its British ally—preferably by Britons or by special units of the Norwegian Armed Forces—whenever possible in full military uniform. The Communist Party was loath to heed the interdiction, and an effective liaison was essential to maintaining control over underground activities that were of such potential danger.

In October of 1941, when Hans Jacob Ustvedt merged the Physicians Action Committee with what would become the Coordination Committee (the *KK*), he invited representatives of the teachers, engineers, lawyers, doctors, civil servants, and the church to meet in his home to form the new and vital organization. Dr. Ole Jacob Malm was given the crucial position of secretary-general. Most important he was entrusted with establishing and maintaining the countrywide communication network that was critical in civil opposition to Nazi demands.[4]

Malm's new responsibility was all-consuming and to it he gave every bit of his energy. He was ideally suited for the task, having forebears who had long been consumed with Norway's independence of any form of foreign domination. At the end of the last century his father had delayed a legal education to enter the military academy in preparation for an anticipated showdown with Sweden. Professor Worm-Müller, among the original leaders in developing resistance strategy, was his maternal uncle.

Malm was unemployed in October 1941, having already resigned his position at Aker Hospital. His chief of service, Axel Christensen, had been appointed leader of the Nazified but impotent Medical Society, and Ole Jacob found it intolerable to continue medical duties under a disloyal superior. As Dr. Malm announced his resignation Christensen questioned, "You are quitting because of my political view?" After Malm responded affirmatively, Christensen continued: "I will tell you why I see things differently than you. I have hated Englishmen since the Boer War. They were the first to put concentration camps in place in the Transvaal that killed women and children by the thousands through dysentery and other epidemics. That broke the Boers' morale in the field. England must be crushed, and only the Germans can manage that."

Unmarried as well as unemployed, Ole Jacob Malm entered into what he would later call his busiest and most sleepless year. Malm had no need himself for Johannes Heimbeck's financial wizardry, for he was economically independent. His strong-willed mother left the legacy that permitted him to commit his entire being to the Resistance. Thirteen months before Ole Jacob's birth his older sister had been delivered on an obstetrical service. The twenty-one-year-old mother insisted her next child be born at home. Against her husband's desire she engaged a midwife, a woman who had become a deptheria carrier following the 1908 epidemic and was forbidden to practice her trade. To maintain herself she continued secretly to deliver newborns whenever the opportunity arose.

Ole Jacob's birth went smoothly on December 21, 1910, but within two months his mother was dead. She had contracted a fatal diphtheritic endometritis from her attendant. When he had reached the age of twenty-one, Ole Jacob Malm received the inheritance that freed him to serve the Home Front. He forever considered his mother's life a gift to her country.

The crucial system of *paroles* had already been instituted when Malm took over his underground role. These directives issued by the Home Front leadership instructed loyal Norwegians on actions to take in the face of Nazi demands or pressures. Magnus Jensen, the extraordinary creator of the *paroles* system, described their significance: "*Paroles* created within the individual organizations at a very early time gave the feeling of solidarity that was an essential for the civil struggle."[5]

Couriers had proven not only dangerous but relatively inefficient in distributing the *paroles*, so Dr. Malm set out to improve the method of communication. Ordinary Norwegian mail was unquestionably the simplest and most effective, but Nazi censors barred the way. From Ingvald Lid, chairman of the Postmen's Union, Malm obtained the formula German intelligence used to develop invisible ink. In Dr. Asbjorn Følling's glistening laboratory at the Veterinary School, Ole Jacob perfected his own formula—merely reversing the process. For ink, he employed the German developing solution. Dr. Malm's method withstood the acid test—his invisible ink was utilized undetected throughout the Occupation. As an added precaution he instituted cut outs—pages with open spaces that would allow an underground message to stand out from an otherwise innocuous communication.

Lid also provided means of shunting *KK* mail around the Nazi censors. Following routine Nazi surveillance in Oslo's central post office, outgoing mail was placed on a conveyer belt to be unloaded on the floor below for delivery. After the postal official had drilled an opening into the wall beyond the censors' post, underground communications were secretly placed on the belt at that point and sent on their way. Couriers were then no longer necessary. Malm's inflexible rule, strictly minimizing the number of contacts for each individual in his underground network, diminished the danger of disclosure of Resistance operatives through torture of those apprehended by the Gestapo.

Once the system was perfected Ole Jacob Malm organized twenty prime contacts throughout the country. *Paroles* and other communications were to be given first to these contacts, who would then disseminate that information. Physicians, operating through the Medical Society network, constituted a large proportion of the most critical contacts. For most effective action it was necessary that *KK* contacts be individuals of authority, and for this the more senior physicians were ideal. Most were established in positions of authority in local hospitals and had earned the trust of both colleagues and community. When physicians were unavailable, other selections were made after careful consultation with trusted members of the teachers, lawyers, or other professional groups in Oslo.

Ole Jacob Malm traveled incessantly and throughout the entire of Norway—to Bodø, Narvik, and Tromsø in the north; Trondheim, Bergen, and Ålesund in the west; and Kristiansand and Larvik in the south. To counteract suspicions of the Gestapo, or other Nazis who might stop to question him, he traveled always with a sheaf of X rays at his side. He was working on a doctoral thesis of bone disease, the story would go, and was searching for cases at the various community hospitals. Always he carried contrived correspondence to buttress his contention—and never traveled without having previously fabricated some convincing reason for that particular journey. Although he was stopped for questioning frequently, he easily escaped detection on every occasion.

For potential candidates as prime contacts who might not know him Dr. Malm sent advance instructions through a confidant in Oslo or leader of the local community. Mr. Hellum, the individual would be told, would be coming from Oslo to speak of an important service to the country. Under that pseudonym Ole Jacob would interview the candidate and lay out his rigid rules for maintaining security. He then based his decision to accept or reject the recruit on his own perception of trustworthiness and willingness to undertake the mission. Malm's judgement was invariably sound. Throughout the entire Occupation only his Trøndelag contact group was uncovered, and that through infiltration by an informer.

Perhaps fifty *paroles* of varying significance were issued while the Germans still controlled Norway. None were of greater importance in rebuffing Nazification attempts than the *parole* Malm sent out to all teachers in February 1942. Having failed to subject Norwegian physicians to the discipline of the *Nasjonal Samling*, quislings turned their attention to the teachers. In November 1940, they had prepared a set of demands requiring all students to be educated in accord with Nazi dogma. Furthermore, teachers were expected to support the new regime, and demonstrate that support with a pledge of loyalty.

Before the Nazi circular could reach its target, however, the R-Group had obtained a copy of the proofs, and Bishop Bergrav was notified. The *parole* he issued alerted all teachers and proposed a uniform reaction— each teacher would declare adherence to Norway's traditional teaching values. The teachers' overwhelming response was sufficient to delay the actual confrontation until February 1942, when Orvar Saether, leader of Quisling's *Hird*, was appointed as head of a new teachers' union. Membership in that organization was to be compulsory for all teachers and, as in Germany, they were to indoctrinate their students with Nazi ideology.

After repeated consultation with both the Circle and *KK* the Teachers' Action Committee agreed on the following letter of protest to be sent by each individual teacher to the department of church and education:

I find myself unable to cooperate in the education of Norway's youth
following the lines established by NSUF's Youth Service, since they are
contrary to my conscience.

Since membership in Norway's Teachers' Union, according to the
pronouncements of the National Leader, among other things places upon
me the duty for such education, and moreover places other demands that
are contrary to my conditions of employment, I find it necessary to inform
you that I can not consider myself as a member of the teacher's union.[6]

Quickly, Ole Jacob Malm had the document reproduced then distributed throughout his communication network. Thousands of letters
conforming to the *parole* reached the Nazi department of churches and
education soon to be followed by protests from Norway's bishops and
university faculty. In March, well over a hundred thousand protests from
parents flooded the department.

Vidkun Quisling, recently appointed as minister-president threatened
dismissal and forced labor, but the teachers stood firm. The traitor
delayed, declaring the schools closed for a month due to a "fuel holiday,"
but when that period ended the teachers still would not yield. The
Germans, accustomed to Quisling failures, took charge and dispatched
more than a thousand teachers to prison camps. Johannes Heimbeck was
called upon to provide funds to support the teachers' families during the
"holiday" and throughout their imprisonment.

The imprisoned Norwegians were repeatedly and ferociously abused
as their captors demanded retraction of their refusals, but few acceded.
Quisling was unable to maintain the standoff. The schools reopened in
March, and teachers resumed their usual duties, after once more reading
aloud the contents of their declaration of protest.

The collective action of the teachers, mediated by the *KK parole*
not only prevented Nazification of Norway's youth, but solidified the
determination to resist and fortified other groups as well. Both the clergy
and the legal profession faced similar pressures by the *Nasjonal Samling*
and, following the teachers' example, they too stood firm.

Hans Jacob Ustvedt, Ole Jacob Malm, and their *paroles* were also
instrumental in setting the course for Norway's cultural life during the
Occupation. Both young physicians were performing musicians and as
such, were readily accepted in Oslo's musical circles. Malm was an accomplished pianist, and Ustvedt a sought after singer. The noted composer,
Monrad Johansen, turned to Ustvedt for the premier performance of his
"Petter Dass" song cycle, "Nordland Trumpet," in the University *Aula*,
then Oslo's major concert hall.

Early in 1942 performing vocalists and instrumentalists were under
increasing pressure by the *Nasjonal Samling* to Nazify their organization,
and perform in accord with Nazi principles. Music by gifted Russian
or Jewish composers was strictly forbidden and Germanic compositions
encouraged. The first of the three *paroles* dispatched to individual per-
formers in the summer of 1942, just before the first concerts of the new
season, ended with: "No concerts, no appearances with orchestras."
Public performances came to a halt.

Heimbeck's resourcefulness was called upon once more for now musicians required assistance, some with very special problems. A soprano
had recently acquired a mink coat on credit. She could not break the
contract without losing her furs. Since Ole Jacob Malm was unknown to
the singer, the young doctor paid her a visit, using his code name, and
carrying 15,000 kroner from Heimbeck's stores in his pocket from which
he supplied 10,000 kroner to the singer.

On August 21, 1942, an officer in the National Police entered his office
on Henrik Ibsen's Street to find his records stolen. The policeman lifted
the telephone receiver to report the theft, only to be thrown into the air by
a violent explosion. The operation bore the trademark of the Communist
sabotage group led by Asbjørn Sunde, better known by the code name
"Oswald." The enraged Nazis sought Sunde and his helper, Petter Bruun,
throughout Oslo, covering the city with placards offering 100,000 kroner
for information about the fugitives. Despite their differences with the
Communists, *Milorg*'s central leadership recognized that "Oswald's" capture could have a devastating effect on the entire Resistance movement.
Not only would morale plunge, but the Communist saboteur's widespread
knowledge of the underground membership would force many of those
most important to the Home Front to flee the country. They turned
to their linchpin in the *KK*, Ole Jacob Malm. The saboteur's face must
become unrecognizable, and the distinctive tattoo—A.S.—on the back
of his left hand must disappear.

Dr. Malm first enlisted the aid of *Rikshospital* otolaryngologist and
Home Front operative, Hans Fredrik Fabritius, who had employed an
injectable paraffin compound capable of altering facial features. The
material's low melting point allowed warming and injection beneath the
skin without damage to the tissue—then while still warm the paraffin
could be molded to the desired configuration. Sufficient hardening would
result at body temperature to maintain the newly acquired appearance.

Some evenings later Malm brought the fugitive from his hiding place.
With characteristic caution, Ole Jacob blindfolded the patient to maintain
the secrecy of their destination and drove to his appointment. There was

little problem injecting paraffin beneath the saboteur's skin. Fabritius eliminated a cleft in his chin, and the paraffin filled out the tissues about his nose and eyes. Sunde's appearance had been radically changed. His features had become unrecognizable, though not improved, for the "unparaffinned" young Communist had been a handsome man.

When the two doctors injected a local anesthetic, then began removal of the damning tattoo, the saboteur fainted. He had no problem shedding the blood of others, but the sight of his own was more than he could tolerate.

The operation completed, Sunde was blindfolded once again, and returned to his underground refuge. The Home Front planned to export the disguised Communist once the intensive search had eased; however, "Oswald" had plans of his own. He was already an experienced guerilla and dedicated Soviet-style Communist before the Nazi attack on Norway, having fought in the Dimitrov Battalion during the Spanish Civil War. He had expert guidance, as he learned the arts of assassination and sabotage in Spain, and he resurrected those skills when his own country was invaded. It was to "Oswald" that the Home Front turned whenever an informer was to be liquidated. Asbjørn Sunde was bound only loosely to the Norwegian Communist Party, but maintained his original and closer connection with the Soviet Communists in Moscow. He was not to be deterred from his mission, especially as he now had a new face. As soon as the coast had cleared Sunde slipped away from his underground refuge, and continued his operations in Southern Norway—undetected throughout the remaining years of the Occupation.

14. The Campaign Against the Jews

Leo Eitinger had hardly completed preparations for departure to Bodø and the Rønvik Mental Hospital when the Nazis marched into Oslo. Caring Norwegians—Christians and Jews alike—feared for the safety of the country's tiny Jewish community. Eitinger's newfound friends warned that all those rescued by Nansen Relief—once thought safe—were imperiled anew. Marie Lous Mohr came to Shua's aid, offering her isolated mountain cabin in the valley of Gudbrandsdal in central Norway. There, Eitinger was told, he and his friends would be "as safe as in Adam's shirt," that is to say, as in paradise.[1]

On April 11, just two days after the Germans had swarmed into Oslo, Eitinger boarded the last train leaving the city—with Robert Weinstein, Nora Lustig, one of her two sons, and Hugo Eisler with his wife Helene and brother Otto. Panic surged to the surface as German troops passed along the train, but the soldiers paid the fugitive Czechs little more heed than they did the crowds of Norwegians fleeing the occupied city.

For a week Leo Eitinger and his friends lived in complete tranquility in the small cabin, set on a peninsula jutting into the still-frozen Lake of Lesja Woods. The idyll ended as a roar of engines reverberated from the skies, then one after the other, a flight of British planes touched down on the thick ice covering the waters before their cabin. The lake was to become a base for attacks on Nazi troops in the north. The warming sun of the long spring day and the weight of the planes liquified ice beneath the wheels then, as the temperature dropped during the short night, the surface froze firm again, gripping the aircraft in an unyielding vise. The immobilized squadron was easy prey for German bombers winging overhead, and the captive British planes were destroyed as they sat helpless on the ice.

The peaceful haven was transformed into a valley of danger, forcing the seven Czech refugees to reconsider their future. Nora Lustig chose to

130

rejoin the second of her twins who had remained on a Norwegian farm. The men sought out the commander of a small group of Norwegian soldiers encamped in nearby Lesja, searching for transport to England where they planned to enlist in British forces and play their own part in the battle against the Nazis. The Norse captain wondered of what possible concern the war could be for the refugees. It was not their war he told them, but the Englishmens' war. Three were Czechoslovakian officers, they protested and Eitinger himself a military physician. The fugitives should return to the hut, the captain pronounced. If need arose, they would be summoned.

Dissatisfied with helpless waiting, five of the seven Czechs separated from the Lustigs and started off toward the highway—hoping to find passage to Åndalsnes, where they would seek transport to England on British ships then lying moored in the harbor. Sometime later, aboard an open lorry in a military convoy on the final night of April, the tiny band of fugitives rolled toward their goal.

By April's end, days had lengthened in the north, bringing brief nights that were little more than dusk. Forest shadows and stark outlines of towering mountains patterned the enchanted landscape as light shimmered from snow that everywhere covered the rocky terrain. Never had Eitinger seen nature so magnificent.

The snow-lit scene, however, provided more than enchantment to the German bombers that rained explosives on the Norse convoy. The attack unnerved Helene Eisler, who pleaded to be sent back. Despite Nazi harassment the transport reached the harbor at Åndalsnes, where clusters of British troops were seen dashing back toward the moorings. The lorries had not yet reached their own goal and rolled onward without pausing to discharge the five fugitives.

When the fleeing Czechs finally alighted from their lorry at Åfarnes, far beyond their goal, they could discover no immediate transport to Åndalsnes. On arrival in the port city the following morning, however, the fugitives found the quay emptied. The British flotilla had departed during the night, leaving the downcast refugees to shift for themselves.

The new arrivals appeared a suspicious lot to local Norwegians. Unshaven, in unkempt clothing, rough-looking and speaking with foreign accents, the five were taken for spies, and questioned by the authorities. Once officially cleared of suspicion and despite the fears and doubts of some, the fugitives found temporary havens on farms and in the nearby village of Nesjestranda. On May 24, however, when the Allies began to evacuate Norway, German forces appeared in the village streets. Leo Eitinger and his friends once more felt endangered.

Again the Czechs went into hiding. The Gestapo had not followed on the heels of the soldiers, however; and the troops had little interest in the village. By the end of May telephone communication had been reestablished with Oslo, and Eitinger contacted Jørgen Berner, secretary-general of the Norwegian Medical Association. "Why are you not in Bodø?" the astonished Czech physician was asked over the phone. "But there is a war, and the occupation," Eitinger replied. "Yes," responded the secretary, "that is not your business, it was our war, and not your war. You are a doctor in Bodø, that is your position, so try to go there."

Travel to Bodø was just then out of the question. Together with the small refugee group, Eitinger returned to Nesjestranda. He found work in the Malos lumber mill, while attempting to obtain the transportation that would allow him to resume his profession. The occupying Nazis had restricted civilian movement and required permits for all who traveled. Determined to reach his goal, Eitinger first returned to Oslo then journeyed to Trondheim in his quest. Despite the danger in identifying himself as a Jew, he contacted the Gestapo who were only contemptuous of his attempts, telling him the trip could never be made without a permit, then adamantly refusing to issue the necessary document.

Finally, by joining a group of students, Dr. Eitinger was able to board a coastal steamer for Bodø. He shuffled about the deck for hours until a decision was made to allow the vessel to depart Trondheim. For three days the ship hugged the coastline then docked at Bodø in the early morning, just after 3:00 A.M. to be greeted by an emptied and devastated city. Bodø was completely without military value, yet Nazi terror bombing had left the buildings in smoking ruins and had littered the streets with shattered glass. The local hospital had been destroyed, and fires smoldered in still-standing structures.

The young physician disembarked with a group of students who sought a glimpse of the deserted city. When the students strode back up the gangplank to resume their journey to Finnmark, Leo Eitinger was left standing alone on the quay. As long as the vessel lay moored to the pier he remained alongside, chatting with passengers gathered at the railing. Once the ship had departed, he was alone on the dock with his small suitcase—solitary, with no idea as to how to proceed. The local hospital existed no more, but Eitinger's destination was the Rønvik Mental Hospital somewhere outside town. He knew not where, and he had no means of making the trip.

In time a plain-clothed figure appeared, a local citizen and volunteer policeman, who questioned Eitinger as to his mission in Bodø. With his foreign accent and disheveled condition the young Czech recognized that none would believe him a physician so he merely replied that his goal was Rønvik Hospital. The Norwegian understandably assumed Eitinger to be a prospective patient, and in alarm instructed him to remain on the quay and be certain to move nowhere.

Shortly, the police assistant returned with a car and drove the three kilometers to the hospital, the only structure in the environs of Bodø to remain unbombed. Before arriving at Rønvik after 4 A.M., Eitinger revealed that he was indeed a physician. At their destination his skeptical escort roused the porter, declaring he had a passenger claiming to be a physician—but he doubted the claim.

The porter was unconvinced as well, as he called the physician on duty, reporting that a man had arrived announcing himself to be a doctor. Left waiting until morning, Leo Eitinger dozed fitfully in the waiting room. At the breakfast hour he appeared in the dining room. He repeated his story—that he was to be an assistant physician in the hospital—only to be challenged by a young Norwegian. There was only one position for an assistant, Eitinger was firmly informed, and that position was already filled by the speaker.

Eitinger sought out the superintendent, whose recollection was dimmed by the catastrophic events of the past two months. Eventually Dr. Eitinger's situation was clarified, however, and he began his medical duties.

Chaos reigned about the Rønvik asylum. The remains of the Bodø hospital had moved out to Rønvik, with the entire administration, the pharmacy, and even the bakery. With battles ended on Norwegian soil in early June the Army that had fled into the north was disbanded, and troops were slowly making their own way home. The shattered town of Bodø lay astride the homeward path, and as a natural course, all military physicians turned into the hospital for temporary shelter—filling every possible sleeping space. Most were compelled to settle for a mattress on the floor. As a staff member, Leo Eitinger was entitled to a bed. He was, however, forced to sleep sitting up—his cot was only half the normal length.

For the first time since graduation from medical school, Dr. Eitinger was able to practice his profession completely and openly. He was appointed to the northern mental hospital, not because of competence in psychiatry, but merely because of the availability of an open position. The appointment was a good fit for Shua Eitinger, however. The young Czech physician had long maintained an interest in human behavior. He had begun his university studies in the philosophical faculty, emphasizing courses in foreign languages and psychology. His fluency in English,

French, and German had already been important to survival and would prove life-saving in the future.

Despite his religion, his foreign background, and his heavily accented Norwegian, the Czech refugee was readily accepted by his colleagues, but not so readily by the natives. Rønvik's physicians habitually patronized a local shop and were able to obtain small quantities of cigarettes or chocolate when available. Shua, however, was continually unsuccessful until the cause was uncovered. The proprietress reported that a German doctor in civilian clothes appeared repeatedly, but was always turned away empty-handed. Once the truth became known, Eitinger not only purchased goods freely, but became steadfast friends with the owners.

For the most part the 280 patients in Rønvik Mental Hospital had been in custodial care for years, diagnosed as chronic schizophrenics. Shock therapy had made its entrance into Norway only recently and was then in its crudest form. Electroshock was not yet standard, and metrazol injections sent patients into toxic convulsions. The primitive therapy was trying for both patient and physician. Patients approached each coming treatment with intense fear, and therapists were apprehensive about resulting fractures and other possible complications. But the change was at times miraculous. Patients who had been doomed to a lifetime of confinement often improved, and even returned home. Within months of beginning convulsive-shock therapy the hospital turnover rate had doubled.

Leo Eitinger read voraciously at Rønvik, and soon established a small reputation for himself. Shortly after he had studied a paper describing acute hyperparathyroidism a patient exhibiting symptoms of that rare malady appeared at the hospital, puzzling all but Eitinger. The young refugee's scientific reputation was made when his diagnosis was confirmed. The patient's behavior returned to normal after surgical removal of the overactive parathyroid gland. The article Eitinger then published was to prove helpful if not life-saving in the year to come.

Terboven's edict of September 25, 1940, bringing ascendance to the *Nasjonal Samling* terminated Eitinger's employment at Rønvik. Jews were forbidden the practice of any profession. In December Dr. Eitinger's work permit was revoked and he was forced to leave the hospital.

Leo Eitinger rejoined his friends at Nesjestranda—Nora Lustig, then with both her twins, Robert Weinstein, and the three Eislers. The small band was to be increased by the later arrival of eleven-year-old Vera Taglicht from the orphanage in Oslo. Shua then resumed his old work in the Malos lumber mill. The village was doctorless, however; the closest district physician was some thirty kilometers away in Molde. Whenever a local medical emergency surfaced in Nesjestranda, the young doctor resumed his professional role, to be paid by barter. He lectured to the village volunteer health aides, and taught a first aid course. "I did not believe I could ever come to feel such joy in my work as I did just here," he wrote at the time.

From the first days of the Nazi aggression Sigrid Helliesen Lund had searched throughout Norway for Nansen Relief's charges to provide whatever aid was still possible. Once she located the Nesjestranda group of Czech refugees Mrs. Lund counseled them to remain in place. The village was still free of Germans, and far less dangerous than Oslo. For a time, at least, she was right.

The entire village was warm and accepting. A woman was said to have volunteered, "They have had so much stress and pain when they must live hidden away, without the work they want and are accustomed to, I must now try to do them a little good." The local Lutheran pastor, Aksel Kragset, who became foster father to Vera Taglicht, was humane and supportive of the small fugitive group. When Eitinger commented on the kindness of Norwegians to the refugees the clergyman responded: "What do you want? If we have guests in our home we wish them to feel at home. If we have guests in our country we wish them to feel at home in our country." In a letter to a friend, Leo Eitinger wrote, "If in the days of my radical youth someone had told me that I would be a good friend of a clergyman at some time I would have laughed in his face. He is my best friend in the village. All small differences disappear when life is really at stake."[2]

Throughout 1941, the small band of Jews continued to receive the hospitality of the country. They did so without the three Eislers, who were confirmed urban dwellers unused to the quiet of village life. Hugo, Helene, and Otto Eisler returned to Oslo late in 1941.

Outside the rural refuge foreboding signs scrawled by Quisling's hooligans, the *Hird*, appeared on Jewish shop windows—"Palestine Calls," "Jews out of Norway."[3] In May 1940 Jews were forced to deliver their radios to the Nazis. On Thursday, January 16, 1941, Ernst Glaser, concertmaster of the Oslo Philharmonic Orchestra, prepared to perform Sinding's violin concerto in Bergen's concert hall. The local *Nasjonal Samling* began a violent demonstration against "the Jew" first outside then moving into the hall—preventing the performance.[4] January 10, 1942, brought the infamous order by Jonas Lie, the quisling minister of justice, forcing all Jews to be registered and have the red "J" stamped on passports or identification papers. On March 7, 1942, four Jews were executed in Trondheim, falsely accused of spreading propaganda on behalf of a hostile foreign power.[5]

By early 1942 Nazi pressure on Norway's Jews caused growing panic in homes that had accepted Jewish children through Nansen Relief. The benevolent Norwegians feared for their own safety as well as that of their wards. Sigrid Helliesen Lund then combed the land in search of havens for the threatened children. Her act of charity toward the two Taglicht children she dispatched to Nesjestranda was to bring disaster to the Czech refugees.

Pastor Aksel Kragset had a large family of his own, but had generously offered shelter first to Vera Taglicht then to the fourteen-year-old Tibor whose foster family in Trondheim feared to keep him longer. Tibor was dispatched by bus to Molde to arrive on March 14, just two days after Vidkun Quisling reinvoked the bigotry-stained Article 2 of the Norwegian Constitution, forbidding Jews entry to the country. When Leo Eitinger and Robert Weinstein arrived in Molde to meet the young refugee the Gestapo was well entrenched in the city. The two Czechs looked "different" and were identified as Jews.

On the following day the *lensmann* (a local official) called Eitinger to the village for an important conversation. After considerable "hemming and hawing" the Czech refugee was informed he must accompany the *lensmann* to Ålesund for a hearing. On March 16, when Leo Eitinger arrived at dockside with Robert Weinstein, Nora Lustig and her twins, he found a worried group of villagers clustered about the quay. As the Czechs prepared to board the vessel that was to carry them to the Gestapo, a villager whose son Eitinger had treated without charge pressed five kroner into the doctor's palm—a large sum for a man of small means, but a sum he felt Eitinger had "honestly deserved."

Initially Leo Eitinger was imprisoned in solitary confinement in Ålesund, then he shared a cell with Weinstein. The two Czechs were forbidden every diversion. The Bible that had been left in the cell was flung out in anger. Vicious guards destroyed the makeshift chess set the two had molded from bread crumbs and carved from soap, and Weinstein was even forbidden to sing in his lyrical voice. They did have the stump of a pencil and scribbled thoughts and letters on purloined toilet paper—one blocking the peephole in the door with his body while the other wrote. Through a single sympathetic Norwegian prison guard, Stein, the toilet paper missives were smuggled out of the prison, and the news from London passed in. Their benefactor was also able to report that Aksel Kragset had approached the Gestapo to plead the Czechs' cause—but was booted out.

Each day the prisoners were marched out into Ålesund to shovel snow. Even the watchful eyes of Norwegian guards did not prevent the townspeople from encouraging the captives and passing them food and chocolate—"Hold out," one woman told them, "the news from London is good." After fifty days Eitinger and Weinstein were ordered to Gestapo headquarters in Trondheim.

The four Norwegians guarding the twelve prisoners en route to Trondheim were kind and undemanding. The captives were kept below deck as the vessel approached land. Somehow news of the ship's passengers had preceded them, and they were met at each stop with gifts of cakes, flowers, and cigarettes.

Among the prisoners was the "American," an elderly farmer who had lived long in the United States, and had fought for his adopted country in the First World War. In later years he had returned to northern Norway and purchased a small farm. The veteran decided to wear his aged U. S. Army uniform as he journeyed into Ålesund for dental care and was observed by a Nazi trooper on disembarking.

The German fled to his barracks, announcing in alarm, "The Americans are coming." All Ålesund laughed at the uproar that followed. The humorless Nazis thought otherwise, and the unfortunate Norwegian-American was delivered to the Gestapo.

At Vollan prison in Trondheim Leo Eitinger quickly learned the difference between their former Norwegian jailers and the Nazis who now held him captive. Five prisoners were crowded into a one-man cell. Instead of "the doctor" he was now "the Jew." Blows and the usual maltreatment heaped on political prisoners was doubled for the Jews. Shua soon feared for his life. Three prisoners had escaped, clearly with help from the inside. Should no one admit to complicity, the commandant announced, "five men will be executed each day until the 'guilty' one is identified—or the prison is empty." No one stepped forward, and no one denounced his comrade. On the following evening Trondheim's Gestapo chief arrived and Eitinger heard the following conversation just outside his cell.

"These are the two Jews from Nesjestranda."

"Why have they not been taken to Falstad?"

"There is no car to Falstad before tomorrow. We will certainly send them there tomorrow."

The two prisoners knew not what Falstad held, but at least they were not to be shot.

Thirty German guards controlled every move of Falstad's 120 inmates —political prisoners of every hue and Jews. Brutality was the Nazi order of the day. Leo Eitinger was singled out for particularly harsh treatment merely because he was a physician. His captors were anti-intellectual and especially brutal to educated Jews. He was beaten and tortured until he collapsed. Dr. Øverlid, himself a political prisoner who was permitted to treat fellow inmates, came to Shua's aid—diagnosing cardiac dilatation. The Norse physician reported his patient's condition to be critical, requiring immediate hospitalization.

On discovering the episode the camp commandant was furious. It was unheard of he said, to hospitalize a Jew after "normal treatment" and Dr. Eitinger was returned immediately to the camp. He reappeared at the hospital in a short time with a diagnosis of scarlet fever. The Nazis lived in mortal fear of contagious disease, a fear that served the Home Front as a weapon many times during the Occupation. Leo Eitinger was hospitalized and it was then his article on hyper-parathyroidism came to his aid. Published at just that time, it came to the attention of a German non-commissioned sanitary officer. The sergeant could neither read the Norwegian nor understand the contents, but he was impressed. When the illness had passed the non-com kept the young doctor officially a "patient" throughout the summer and spared him further barbarism. By September, the ruse was no longer possible. Eitinger was returned to remain at Falstad—subjected continually to Nazi bestiality. His Jewish comrades, however, took comfort from his presence. Secretly and "illegally" in the loft during the evening he treated their wounds and gave solace to their spirits.

From the first days of their presence the Nazi occupiers had begun harassment of the country's tiny Jewish Community. Jews had been slow to enter once the restrictive Article 2 of the Constitution was rescinded. They trickled in over the last years of the nineteenth century as peddlers and small merchants. Numbering about fifteen hundred in a nation of three and a half million at the outset of the Second World War, Jews had yet to join in the intellectual or political life of the country. The very few who had managed to enter the professions were quickly forced out by Nazi edict, and passports of all were stamped with the red "J." Together with all foreign Jews, Dr. Eitinger and his Czech comrades were imprisoned. Yet the early persecutions fell short of the Jewish community's fearful expectation. A number of those who had fled to Sweden even returned to Norway in the mistaken belief they could survive the war.

The Norwegian police were in a difficult position throughout the Occupation. Kristian Wellhaven, Oslo's chief of police was dismissed directly after Terboven's edict of September 25, 1940, and Quisling henchman Jonas Lie was named the *Nasjonal Samling* minister of police.[6] Under the new minister's combination of threat and prodding, nearly half of Oslo's police force signed on as members of the Norwegian Nazi party. Although a number of new party recruits already had Nazi dispositions, others joined in the belief that by doing so they prevented their replacements by hard core adherents of the *Nasjonal Samling*. Many who acceded to Lie's urging used their positions to aid the underground movement. Throughout the following years of Occupation loyal policemen passed on advance information of impending Nazi actions to the Home Front. Many clandestine workers escaped arrest in those actions.

On October 7, 1942, all male Jews from the Trondheim community and the north of Norway were hunted down and sent to join Eitinger and Weinstein in Falstad Prison, where they were brutally abused and lived under the most despicable conditions.[7] Three were executed after becoming ill during Nazi "normal treatment." Five days later death was decreed for any Norwegian sheltering Jews or assisting their escape. Norwegian "border pilots" remained busy, however, escorting Jews across the frontier to Sweden, usually travelling across rugged terrain that made detection difficult. Half of Norway's Jewish population found refuge in Sweden by the end of 1942.

On Saturday, October 24, quisling Chief of State Police Karl A. Marthinsen sent out the order to arrest all male Jews from the ages of fifteen to sixty-five—a week after Vidkun Quisling had announced confiscation of all Jewish property.[8] The roundup was to begin on Monday the 26th. Early the same morning Sigrid Helliesen Lund answered her telephone to hear an unfamiliar voice announce simply, "There will be a great party tonight. We shall only have the large packages."[9] To the women in Mrs. Lund's humanitarian circle, large packages were adult male Jews. The women spent the day and night covering Oslo, warning every Jew they could find to go into hiding.

Arrests were carried out entirely by Norwegians under Vidkun Quisling's control. More than a hundred groups of three—one policeman and two helpers—fanned out over Norway in their detestable task. Many of the still-loyal police used their knowledge to warn the endangered. *Lensmann* Anders Gut in Trøndelag telephoned those he was to apprehend.[10] "An arrest order was issued for you," he would say. "I will come for you *tomorrow*."

In their zeal the state police emptied the mental asylums and old age homes of male Jews. Patients were dragged from hospital beds, although compassionate physicians managed to save some. At Lovisenberg Hospital, Jews were safely hidden in the cellar and attic.

Indignation was widespread, none more vigorous and pointed than that of the State Lutheran Church. Bishop Eivind Bergrav and six other leaders of church, who had already been deposed by the Nazis, expressed their protest in a letter to Vidkun Quisling on November 11. As a part of their message they wrote:

> By remaining silent about this legalized injustice against the Jews we make ourselves co-guilty in this injustice. If we are to be true to God's Word and to the Church's Confession we must speak out. . . .
>
>   . . . With the power of this, our calling, we therefore admonish the secular authority in the name of Jesus Christ: Stop the persecution of the Jews and stop the racial hatred that spreads through the press in our land![11]

On the following two Sundays prayers were said for the Jews in churches throughout the land and the letter was read in its entirety from many pulpits. The text was read over the BBC and was reprinted in the Swedish press.

Tove Filseth and the refugees she continued to aid profited through her relationship with Oslo's police. She had managed to keep the Nansen Relief office open for well over two years of Nazi Occupation with considerable assistance from certain police officers. They notified her of expected "visits" by the police or the *Nasjonal Samling*, illegally provided her with passes to allow her refugee charges to reach the Swedish frontier in safety, and kept her out of the Gestapo's hands.

Toward the end of October 1942, loyal members of the police arrived at Tove Filseth's secret living quarters, warning her to stay clear of the Nansen Relief office.[12] The Nazis had learned of her direct assistance to Jews and were searching for her. They had already ransacked her mother's home in Lillehammer as well as the Nansen office. Her protectors kept her from any contact—even preventing her from using the telephone as a warning to others. Any signal of her presence in Oslo was too dangerous. With police "protection" she was spirited out of Norway to safety in Sweden.

The Gestapo raid that closed the Nansen Relief office for the duration of the Occupation found twenty Norwegians seated on the benches awaiting assistance in evacuating endangered persons from Norway. The twenty waited throughout the day and into the evening—and patience led to their arrests.

Among those taken by the police was Dr. Haakon Natvig, then with the Oslo department of health, who had come seeking aid for a Jewish refugee physician.[13] The refugee had fled Germany with his daughter, and like all Jews, was forbidden to practice his profession. The fugitive survived on whatever small jobs he could obtain, principally translations. He had lived with a Norwegian woman whom he could not marry under

Nazi law. She had since become pregnant—a death sentence for the doctor. Fathering a Norwegian child was also denied to Jews under the penalty of immediate execution. The frantic doctor had been translating a thesis for Natvig into German, the language then the most frequently used internationally in medical science. He appealed to Haakon Natvig who first arranged an abortion, then later sought Tove Filseth to fix passage to Sweden. At the very moment of the Gestapo raid on Nansen Relief the German physician and his daughter were in hiding in Natvig's home. They were rescued later by the underground; the daughter was placed in the Jewish orphanage, and the father hidden for two weeks, then transported to Sweden.

Fourteen hours before the October 26th roundup of all Norway's male Jews, Ole Jacob Malm was brought the news of the impending disaster by Robert Riefling, the country's leading pianist.[14] The distraught Riefling insisted some action must be taken. Riefling, like all Malm's friends, was completely ignorant of the doctor's *KK* activities, approaching him only as a comrade and individual of conscience who could have no other alternative but to help countrymen who were on the verge of destruction. Time and again throughout his tenure as secretary-general of the *Koordinasjonskomite* loyal but unaware Norwegians requested Ole Jacob's assistance in one or another underground task. Malm always demurred, for he could not risk exposure of his more critical function. At such times his own loyalty and concern for his fellows was questioned. Nazi persecution of innocent people had become so horrendous that Malm put aside his doubts and agreed to meet with the pianist.

A few hours later Ole Jacob was horrified to enter the designated meeting place and find more than twenty Norwegians gathered. During all underground activities he had permitted himself the company of only a few at any one time—security risk with a larger number was too great. Nevertheless, Malm remained, for he risked even greater disclosure by leaving the meeting. After a brief but intensive discussion, each attendant was given responsibility for a number of Jews. Ole Jacob Malm's quota was twelve. Temporary hiding places were to be found, and the imperiled were then to be escorted to Sweden by the underground at a later date.

By 2:00 A.M. in the morning Ole Jacob had secured concealment for ten of the twelve, leaving only an old Czech physician, Dr. Wilhelm Israel Jaroschy, and his wife, Marianne Katarina, without safe shelter. As a last resort he brought the fugitives to his father's villa. Erling Malm quickly agreed, and for the next six days kept the fugitive pair hidden, awaiting safe transport.

On the last day of October Malm's two charges set out toward safety in Sweden in a group of some forty refugees. It was necessary, however to cross rugged forest terrain at the frontier on foot and by night. The seventy-year-old Jaroschy felt unable to manage. The underground guide warned of the risk, but Jaroschy had prepared. He carried a fatal dose of morphine should he be accosted by the Germans.

The two refugees set out along the road toward the border and before long blundered directly into the path of a German patrol. The doctor swallowed the morphine on seeing the enemy and quickly fell into a stupor. The Nazis carried their unconscious captive to a nearby hospital where they ordered a young physician to resuscitate Dr. Jaroschy. Using artificial resuscitation, and all his art and skill, the Norwegian doctor brought his patient back from the point of death.

Ole Jacob Malm was never to forgive this "young idiot of a colleague" for his stupid and insensitive act. Once the elderly doctor was revived he was transported to Gestapo headquarters on Victoria Terrasse in Oslo. There he was tortured into revealing his place of concealment. Two Gestapo details set out immediately, one seeking Erling Malm and the second intent on capturing his son.

The older man was easily arrested, but Ole Jacob had learned all the wiles of underground existence. His experience and his Home Front connection kept him safe from the Gestapo. No longer did he live at home, but spent every night away, switching secret sleeping quarters frequently. After the Home Front had warned Malm of the Gestapo's interest, the young doctor easily evaded the Nazis.

As he moved from one place of concealment to the other Ole Jacob spent two weeks tying up loose ends and passing his responsibilities to his successor, the teacher Kaare Norum. Hans Jacob Ustvedt was also exposed, so on November 3, 1942, the two key doctors in the *KK* fled to Sweden. Norway's physicians were then represented in the *KK* by Dr. Peter M. Holst until January 1945 and Dr. Olaf Bang until the end of the war.

The elder Malm was brutally tortured on two separate occasions at Victoria Terrasse, but remained silent. He was removed to Grini Prison on the southern outskirts of Oslo, where he expected to be subjected again to characteristic Gestapo treatment.

Dr. Haakon Natvig was awakened in fear in the middle of the night in early November. In those dark hours torture and questioning by the Gestapo usually took place. He was called for another purpose—to look after a prisoner who had just hung himself with drapery cords. It was Erling Malm, who feared he might no longer withstand Gestapo torture and continue to keep his son's involvement from his tormentors. He had first attempted slashing his wrists and groin without achieving the desired result before successfully turning to the cord.

Later that very day German guards removed all drapes from prisoners' quarters. Natvig was never certain that Ole Jacob Malm learned the truth about his father's death, and never related the events of that fatal night.

On the morning of November 25 Sigrid Helliesen Lund responded to a ring of her doorbell. An unknown man delivered his brief message: "There will be still another party tonight, and it is the small packages that shall be fetched this time." Mrs. Lund never discovered the identity of the messenger, but she had little doubt the information came from the police.[15]

The message needed no further interpretation; women and children were to be the next victims. Her circle of women spent the day in warning and placing those threatened in "safe" homes.

At 9:00 P.M. on the night of November 25th the air raid sirens shrieked through Oslo, clearing the streets in anticipation of the early morning *razzia* (raid). Dr. Caroline "Nic" Waal ignored the warning wail and wheeled her small auto toward the Jewish orphanage. Dr. Waal had been involved in social and political action since her university days as a member of the left-leaning *Mot Dag* (Toward Day) student group. When war came to Norway she was on the staff of Gaustad Psychiatric Hospital, and like Leo Eitinger, she became involved in the early use of convulsive-shock therapy. "Nic" Waal underwent shock treatment with metrazol herself to better understand what effects the drug might have on her patients.[16]

Dr. Waal had been immersed in underground activities from the very beginning of the Resistance. She functioned particularly in the illegal press and as a courier since, as a physician, she was allowed to keep her car. She also contributed to developing the system transporting fugitives to Sweden. "Nic" Waal's Home Front functions earned her interrogation by the Nazis. She had remained silent despite the brutality, then used her experience when released, to teach other women in the Resistance methods to tolerate Gestapo brutality.

Once at the orphanage "Nic" Waal found the children already in bed.[17] Dr. Waal aided Nina Hasvold, director of the Children's Home to prepare her young charges for the clandestine journey. The children were dressed, provided with food, then piled into the auto lying atop one another on the back seat and the floor, then covered with a tarpaulin. In two trips the young fugitives were spirited to hiding places and friendly homes, although Dr. Waal was halted once by the Gestapo. Her papers allowing bypass of the curfew were in order, and without a complete search the loaded vehicle was allowed to pass. Within weeks the Jewish children were safe in Sweden—among them Berthold Gründfeld, one of the refugee children rescued from Czechoslovakia by Sigrid Helliesen Lund.

There was scanty knowledge of the outside among the captives in Falstad Prison. Leo Eitinger and his Jewish friends had little concept of what awaited when they were awakened at night in late November and ordered to shed their prison garb for civilian clothes. One by one they were summoned by the commandant and their valuables were returned. In the dark of the northern morning they were driven to Vollan Prison, and in the evening to the railway station. Soon three buses arrived—filled with the prisoners' wives and children who had been swept up in the *razzia* of the 25th. Among the women was Falstad's only female prisoner, Nora Lustig. Any joys at reunion were short-lived. The thirty-four men were quickly separated from the thirty-eight women and children and, in separate railroad cars, sent on to Oslo.[18]

The trainmen had little doubt of the travelers' destination—the steamship *Donau* docked in Oslo and filled with the "catch" of Oslo's *razzia*. Deliberately, loyal Norwegians delayed the train's progress. When the captives arrived in Oslo, more than a day later, the *Donau* had departed, carrying 530 doomed Jews toward Stettin, on the way to Auschwitz.

The seventy-two travelers from Trondheim were trucked to Bredtvedt Women's Prison where they settled in to await their own transport. Within the prison walls the small band of Jews set about placing their lives in some semblance of order—for their warders were Norwegian, not German Gestapo. Children from the ages of six to fifteen gathered together in a "school," to be taught by nineteen-year-olds, still *gymnasium* students themselves. Dr. Eitinger cared for the ills of his companions and lectured on health and hygiene.

In the early days at Bredtvedt Nansen Relief provided clothing for those in the greatest need. The visits were short-lived, for Nansen Relief itself had been closed down by the Nazis.[19]

In mid-winter Leo Eitinger was shocked to be reunited with Vera and Tibor Taglicht. Aksel Kragset had managed to keep the two children safe for months. In January 1943, however, they were no longer thought to be safe in Nesjestranda and were brought south and hidden near Lillestrøm. Betrayed by an informer, the young fugitives were then to share in the prisoners' fate.

The near "idyll" ended on February 24, 1943. The Bredtvedt contingent and a group of Jews that had been held in Grini Prison—the last vestige of the Jewish community in Norway—boarded the deportation ship *Gotenland* to follow in the path of the *Donau*.

Like Haakon Natvig, the humanitarian pianist Robert Riefling was imprisoned for his assistance to the Jews.[20] Dr. Natvig, however, spent little time in Grini. Shortly after his incarceration a minor epidemic of typhoid broke out in Oslo. The Nazis, constantly fearful of infectious disease, approached Dr. Andreas Diesen, state commissioner of health. He could provide no assistance himself, Diesen responded. The one best qualified to handle the epidemic, he insisted, was his assistant Dr. Natvig, who was then unfortunately incarcerated at Grini. Dr. Diesen's straight-faced ploy won Haakon Natvig's immediate release.

Neither Ole Jacob Malm nor Hans Jacob Ustvedt gave up their efforts to be of use in Norway's struggle for freedom. Dr. Ustvedt took over the direction of the medical section of the Norwegian Refugee Office in Stockholm, while Norway's government-in-exile summoned Malm to London.[21]

By the time of Ole Jacob's journey, travel was extensive between Stockholm and London as well as between Stockholm and Newcastle on the regular Norwegian Air Service operated by Colonel Bernt Balchen. Malm's December passage called for the DC-3 aircraft to pass Rorås near the Swedish border, then cross central Norway to overfly Ålesund, where the Germans had placed powerful anti-aircraft batteries. The plane was primitively equipped—lacking oxygen masks, a pressurized cabin, or even heat. The aircraft flew at its maximum altitude of about eleven thousand feet to avoid anti-aircraft fire—sending Malm into paroxysms of shivering. As shells exploded beneath the aircraft, Malm's chills were obliterated by excitement. Actual danger was minimal, however, for the skies were obscured by the dark of the Norwegian winter, and the moving target was completely invisible to the German gunners. The plane soon arrived safely in Newcastle.

Ole Jacob Malm's underground experience was invaluable to the government-in-exile, and he spent his earliest days in England in military intelligence. Even after he had turned to medical matters Norwegian ministers approached him for frequent consultation on the operation of the Resistance on their native soil.

Dr. Malm's first medical assignment was the eradication of venereal disease from the Norwegian armed forces in both Great Britain and Canada. Systematically, he made contact with each camp, and with every seaport through which Norwegian personnel passed, then established and maintained a registry of all those known to have contracted a venereal disease. His meticulous study paid dividends, for every infected Norseman received treatment before being allowed to return to his homeland.

15. The Destruction of Telavåg

The year 1942 was catastrophic for Norway's Home Front. The notorious Henry Oliver Rinnan and his corps of native *agent provocateurs* had infiltrated a number of *Milorg* groups; a wave of arrests and scores of wanton executions followed in the wake of their treachery. In the spring, the Nazis perpetrated their most heinous of crimes against the Norwegian people— the destruction of Telavåg.[1] The full force of the Gestapo's vengeful act on the valiant villagers was blunted—at least for the women, the children, and the elderly—through the intervention of Konrad Birkhaug.

Birkhaug's distinguished career in medicine, immunology, and microbiology at the University of Rochester had led to his appointment to the famed Pasteur Institute in Paris, and then to an invitation to return to his native city. In June 1935, still an American citizen, he had accepted a position in research at the Christian Michelsen Institute in Bergen.

The Third International Congress of Microbiology that Birkhaug attended in New York in September 1939 as the Norwegian delegate was filled with acrimony between participants who abhorred Fascism and those who represented the Nazi Regime. Tensions continued on the return voyage aboard the *Oslofjord*. Despite Norway's still neutral status a British submarine sent a party aboard the vessel in search of contraband and took prisoner a number of German citizens who were returning to their warring country via Norway. Before reaching the safety of Bergen on October 26, the *Oslofjord* was closely inspected by a flight of British bombers.

With the same humanitarian concerns that had prompted his relief efforts in Russia and France during the First World War Konrad Birkhaug again became involved with the human problems resulting from German aggression. As chairman of the Red Cross of Western Norway he toured the coastal area appealing for aid to Finland in the Winter War with the

146

Soviets, and locating foster homes for three thousand Finnish children should the need for evacuation arise.

As he left home on the morning of April 9, 1940, Birkhaug was accosted by an armed and uniformed German with the challenge, *"Sind Sie ein Fiend, oder ein Freund?"* (Are you an enemy or a friend?). Disguising his American identity, Konrad replied, *"Gott sei dank, Ich bin Norweger!"* (Thank God I'm Norwegian).[2] The Nazi trooper, first slapped Birkhaug in the face then searched him for arms and let him go on. At the Geophysical Institute Konrad saw the entire staff held helpless while the invaders destroyed all radio, telephone, and telegraphy equipment in the meteorology division.

The Red Cross activities that occupied the major portion of Birkhaug's efforts during the German Occupation gave him little time to pursue his own investigations at the Christian Michelsen Institute. He placed the bulk of his scientific studies in the hands of trusted assistants. Repeatedly, Birkhaug was summoned to Gestapo headquarters to account for his challenging acts and incisive comments about the Nazi aggressors and their violations of the provisions of the Geneva Convention. The motion picture film of the New York World Fair of 1939 that he had shown at a meeting of the Odda Red Cross was confiscated—Polish and Czech flags had been shown flying at half-mast in sympathy for their conquered nations. Remarks about his 35-mm Kodachrome slides at a meeting of the Bergen Red Cross similarly cost him his entire collection. "Such was the food situation in the good old days," Birkhaug had commented as a slide showed a market overflowing with food before the German arrival, and "Such foreign guests we are happy to have among us," as another slide displayed a flock of wild ducks skimming a Bergen pond.[3]

The Swedish border was inviting and easily crossed by Norwegians living in the easternmost part of their country. From the western coast along the North Sea, however, the problem was far greater. The occupying Nazis had divided the country into zones, issuing identification cards to Norway's citizens in characteristic colors that specified their zones of residence. Travel outside one's zone was forbidden without special permit, and was carefully monitored. Escape from Bergen and the west was virtually limited to passage across the storm-swept waters of the North Sea to the British Isles nearly two hundred miles away. Patrolling German ships and aircraft made that voyage extraordinarily hazardous. Despite the perils, an almost regular service developed to ferry escaping Norwegians westward to the Shetland Isles and return agents, saboteurs, and supplies from Britain and Norway's government-in-exile.

The North Sea Bus, or Shetland Bus,[4] as the service affectionately came to be known, was developed after hardy Norse mariners made their way across the hazardous waters on their own. From that intrepid group some one hundred volunteers were collected to man the route from Lunna, and later Scalloway, on the Shetland Isles to various points on the west coast of Norway. The traditional Norwegian fishing craft that were the mainstay of the route were fifty to seventy feet long and slowly but reliably propelled by one-cylinder engines at a maximum speed of seven to eight knots. The sturdy, double-frame, wooden construction gave the vessels the extraordinary seaworthiness required to withstand the most violent North Sea weather. Stormy days and nights that grounded enemy aircraft and beached their ships added to the security of the Shetland Bus. Although they remained civilians, the volunteer seamen were outfitted with Norwegian naval uniforms and assigned appropriate ranks.

Despite the occasional capture and even execution of patriots seeking escape to Britain to take up their country's cause, traffic was brisk in both directions across the North Sea. By April 1942 more than five hundred Norwegians had made the hazardous voyage successfully, and numerous missions had been carried out by agents traveling in the opposite direction.

The isolated fishing village of Telavåg to the south of Bergen was an ideal transit point for the Shetland Bus. Small houses lined the rocky sides of the small, isolated bay that connected to the sea through a wide passage dotted with tiny islands. The continual flow of fishing vessels through the bay allowed the Bus to slip in and out undetected. The fierce loyalty of the fishermen and their families gave the government-in-exile the necessary feeling of trust to establish agents among the villagers.

Telavåg served the nation diligently and faithfully until its very survival was threatened by an informer's betrayal.

Early in the morning of Sunday, April 26, twelve "Gestapists" burst into the home of Telavåg's postmaster, Laurits Telle, and sprang up the stairs to the second floor where they found Arne Vaerum and Emil Hvaal, two Norwegian agents from Britain, sound asleep. The young operatives were dragged from their beds and ordered to dress while ringed by the Gestapo. As he reached downward to draw up his trousers, Arne Vaerum suddenly threw *Sturmbandführer* Behrens, the Gestapo chief in Bergen, to the floor, seized the Nazi's pistol, and shot him through the head. Hvaal reached for his own gun and before the shooting had ended, Behren's second in command, *SS-Führer* Bertram, and Vaerum were dead as well. Hvaal and another German were severely wounded.

Incensed, particularly by the death of his personal friend, Behrens, *Reichskommissar* Joseph Terboven traveled to Telavåg himself on April 30 to wreak his vengeance on the entire village. First he ordered all males between the ages of sixteen and sixty assembled before the Telle house—to watch as the Nazis blew it to bits. Next the entire village was systematically destroyed—all livestock slaughtered and entire fleet of fishing vessels sunk. Seventy-one Telavåg men, virtually the entire male population between sixteen and sixty, were initially imprisoned in Bergen then dispatched to Sachsenhausen Concentration Camp in Germany. The remaining 268 women, children, and elderly males were held in Telavåg's chapel.

Dr. Arnljot Gjeldstein telephoned Konrad Birkhaug for help. Gjeldstein feared the chapel had been mined and Terboven intended to wipe out the entire village in reprisal. At Bergen's Gestapo headquarters, Birkhaug pleaded the villagers' case, and requested permission to transfer the women, children, and the older men to the high school in Fana, just outside Bergen, while they were interrogated for "guilt or innocence."

The negotiations were lengthy, and filled with "squabbling and bickering" and telephone calls to Gestapo headquarters in Oslo. Finally, Bergen's Gestapo relented. In the dark of night the terrified villagers were herded like cattle and transported to the Fana High School. Instead of a voyage heading toward a German concentration camp, the Gestapo victims found the people of Fana had prepared well for them. Alfhild Utne Riisoen, a nurse and head of the local Red Cross, had mobilized Fana's population to provide beds, food, and every need for the villagers' continuing confinement. In the meantime Emil Hvaal had been tortured and later executed. Lars Telle, one of Marte and Laurits Telle's sons, was put to death for his assistance to Allied intelligence agents and fugitives.

The interrogations continued for weeks, until the Gestapo tired of the effort and decided to send the entire group of women, children, and the elderly to a German concentration camp as well. Infectious disease once again came to aid of the Norwegians, as a number of the youngest fell ill with diphtheria. Playing on Nazi fears of infection, the Red Cross managed to convince the Germans to transport the incarcerated villagers to a vacant boarding school on a peninsula in Hardanger, where they remained for the duration of the Occupation.

In the aftermath of the Telavåg disaster *Milorg* units were "rolled up" in Stavanger, Sunnfjord, Bergen, and in the Oslo area. Key leaders in the Home Front were forced to flee as their names were revealed through torture. The Home Front readily learned from their costly lesson. Captured Resistance workers began to speak freely and provided mountains of unimportant information. They readily revealed names of their fellows in the Resistance to the Gestapo—but only those who had already fled the country.

16. The Norwegian "Reserve Police" in Sweden

In the summer of 1940 Drs. Carl Semb and Kristian Kristiansen recognized that medical services adequate to sustain any form of military action no longer existed. Should the hoped-for invasion materialize, medical support for both *Milorg* fighters and invading Allied troops would become essential.

Semb, head of the department of surgery at the Oslo City Hospital (Ullevaal Hospital), had been deeply involved with the Home Front from its inception, and had succeeded Professor Johan Holst in *Milorg*'s Council with Holst's enforced departure to England. Kristiansen was resident in neurosurgery at *Rikshospitalet* and had also served as consultant for head injuries in Semb's department. Determined to secretly reconstitute military medical services, the two surgeons recruited their colleagues—Sten Florelius, chief of medical services of the Norwegian Civil Defense; Hans Fredrik Fabritius, an otolaryngologist; and Herman Dohlen, one of Semb's assistants—to help lay the groundwork for *Sanorg* (medical service for the Home Front Military) and fulfill the need for crucial medical services should Norwegian forces return to their native soil with the invading Allies.

Sanorg's organizers knew where to turn for those materials essential to the new venture—Christian Plesner, director of Norway's largest medical supply firm. Even before the outbreak of war, when Nazi-fomented crises had threatened the flow of medical and surgical supplies to non-involved countries, Plesner had been engaged to stock Norwegian medical installations with scarce and vital equipment. Plesner was already firmly entrenched with Sweden's leading manufacturers and thus had access to the critical materials. Swedish surgical instruments were unquestionably the world's finest and Norway's Nazi occupiers also competed in the marketplace for the Swedish products. Since the occupying Germans had also turned to Plesner, he found it simple to disguise his activities on behalf of *Sanorg*.

Between 1940 and 1943 Semb, Kristiansen, and the *Sanorg* forces gathered enough materiel to equip forty 100-bed field hospitals and sixty smaller units containing forty beds each. Funds from the Norwegian government-in-exile, Johannes Heimbeck's acquisitive genius, and other sources allowed Christian Plesner and his son Teleph to procure the necessary equipment and supplies in Sweden.

Kristiansen never really knew the exact source of the money, only that funds were always available. He recalled meeting with Heimbeck in the small, private Red Cross Hospital in Oslo, coming away carrying twenty thousand kroner, then delivering the cash to underground workers in an Oslo suburb.

Swedish medical supply firms were well aware of Plesner's cause from the outset and cooperated fully. They provided first choice for even the most sophisticated equipment then available and supplied everything from medication and simple surgical instruments to efficient x-ray units. Refrigerators were dismantled, and the space between the walls filled with messages for the Resistance back in Norway. The Norwegian State Railway was used as much as possible. Erling Föien, director of transportation in a government ministry, and Sten Florelius then managed the distribution. As head of the Civil Defense medical services, Florelius controlled a fleet of ambulances that he freely employed for *Sanorg* transport, often with patients in the same vehicle.

By 1943 the hundred field hospitals were distributed throughout the country—from Kristiansand in the south to Norway's northernmost reaches in Finnmark. The physicians' network secreted the medical chests away from prying Nazi eyes. Well over six thousand beds were stored in the various community hospitals without arousing a shred of suspicion. Several structures were selected for possible use as emergency hospitals, and larger cases were stored in various buildings—the agricultural school south of Kragero, other smaller schools and institutions, and local hospitals. In hours the chests could be unpacked, and the equipment readied for use. Each hospital would begin operation completely equipped, from beds, medication, and nursing paraphernalia, to functional operating rooms. The hundred bed hospitals would have x-ray units as well. No matter the civilian need *Sanorg*'s secret stores were to remain untouched until invasion or Nazi capitulation. The system worked. The Germans discovered only a single cache during the five years of *Sanorg*'s existence.

One evening in February 1943, while enjoying a party at the home of a friend, Kristian Kristiansen received an urgent telephone call. In

November 1942, a *Milorg* section in southern Norway had been broken up by the Gestapo. A young member from Kristiansand had been taken and subjected repeatedly to the usual barbaric interrogation by the Gestapo. Having erroneous information that Dr. Kristiansen had already left for Sweden the captive had yielded Kristian's name. There was no alternative—the Kristiansens must go under cover. Without even returning home Kristian and his wife Brit went directly to the home of Dr. Fabritius at Vindern. Kristiansen and Fabritius then put through a telephone call to Carl Semb.

The three men talked long into the night, but there could be only one solution. Kristiansen and Semb must go into hiding then leave Norway at the earliest possible moment. The two doctors changed quarters quickly and moved to Olav Torgersen's apartment. Dr. Torgersen, a pathologist at the Institute of Pathology with Leiv Kreyberg, was involved in Resistance activities, mostly in the publication of underground papers. He was quick to offer his home and for the following few days the two fugitives occupied the Torgersen's double bed. They dared not go abroad in daylight, leaving the apartment only in the dark winter nights. In the meantime, Carl Semb's wife Helga had moved with her five children into an apartment near Ullevaal Hospital until all was in readiness for the escape to Sweden.

Brit Kristiansen returned home briefly to her two young daughters, who were being cared for by a young woman living in the Kristiansen home. Brit was extremely cautious, for she had every reason to suspect her maid—who had taken up with a Nazi friend. Before long Brit was off to the home of another physician, Dr. Haakon Rasmussen, in the suburb of Sogn. Meanwhile, Teleph Plesner and the transport arm of the Underground selected the safest export route. The Sembs and Kristiansens were to leave immediately for Sweden.

The Kristiansen family was reunited as planned at the East Railway Station late in February 1943. They boarded the train for Halden on the narrow Iddefjord, the border with Sweden, to meet up with Carl Semb and his family. Their underground contact in Halden had been arranged—they would be met at the station, they were told, by a man with a walking stick.

All went as planned. The four Kristiansens and the seven Sembs were taken to safe quarters for the night. In the morning the two families walked along the railroad tracks to the fjord. There they found a boat and eight additional fugitives. Carl Semb then rowed the nineteen across the fjord to safety in Sweden.

The two doctors and their families arrived penniless, passportless, with nothing but the clothes on their backs. Their passports, money, and any possessions that could be of use to the underground were left for fellow workers in the Resistance. The Norwegians were taken to the nearby town of Strømstad, then provided with a small amount of money, the first of which was used to purchase toothbrushes. The refugees then traveled the well-worn path from Strømstad to Gothenburg, and on the following day went to the Norwegian Central Reception Station at Kjesaeter in central Sweden. The two families slept only a single night at the refugee center. After a day of heavy telephoning to Norwegian authorities in Stockholm, the entire group set out for Sweden's capital city.

Aboard the train from Gothenburg to Kjesaeter, Carl Semb and Kristian Kristiansen had begun to discuss what they might accomplish in Sweden. The time had come for a plan that had, in part, been considered by several other Norwegian physicians. The earliest suggestion had come from Dr. Gunnar Johnson in a letter to Defense Minister Oscar Torp on March 3, 1942. By that time thousands of young Norsemen had flocked across the border into Sweden, many of whom hoped to travel on to Britain to join Norwegian forces in training abroad. For more than a year Norwegians had journeyed on from Sweden, crossing the Soviet Union to the Siberian port of Vladivostock then making their way to England or Canada. Once Hitler attacked Russia, that path was closed. The opportunity to leave Sweden by air became limited to those who, like Ole Jacob Malm, had important services to provide the government-in-exile.

There was little employment opportunity in the cities for the thousands of young Norwegian refugees who had flooded into Sweden. There was, however, great demand for lumberjacks in the north, and Norsemen without special qualifications were sent there in droves. Life was hard in the lumber camps, and refugees often expressed their bitterness in antisocial behavior that led to jail. They had fled their own country to escape Nazi concentration camps, only to end up in Swedish prisons.

Johnson proposed that young Norwegians be screened medically to identify those available for military service.[1] In September 1942, Dr. Emanuel Buchman elaborated on the plan, suggesting that medical examination, vaccination, and blood typing be carried out on all young, male Norwegians in Sweden. Shortly thereafter Leiv Kreyberg made similar recommendations to Dr. Karl Evang, director of medical services with the government-in-exile.[2] Hans Jacob Ustvedt, in his position as director of medical services for Norwegian refugees in Sweden, journeyed to London in the first days of 1943.[3] On January 20 he met with Evang, representatives of the minister of defense, the foreign minister, and the minister of social affairs and of the military high command. All agreed that the plan for health examinations as a preliminary to military preparation was desirable, but political and practical considerations must first be overcome.

Implementation of the "health programs" among young Norwegian refugees was not yet appropriate in late 1942. From the very moment of the Nazi attack on Norway, Swedish attitudes toward their Scandinavian neighbor were ambivalent. Swedes in the west were intensely pro-Norse, particularly in Gothenburg where ringing editorials castigated the Germans and supported the Norwegians. In Stockholm, the seat of the Swedish government, the reaction differed.

The intellectual and commercial connection between Sweden and Germany had flourished for centuries. The might of the victorious German military convinced many Swedes that Nazi successes would continue until England was vanquished as well, and the war would end in a German triumph. Then too, some officials feared that the Nazis might overrun Sweden, should too much assistance be offered to runaway Norwegians.

Considerable acrimony expressed toward the Swedes on the part of Norwegians did little to ease the situation. Norwegians were incensed by Sweden's acquiescence to the railway transport of German troops across Swedish soil and bitter about movement limitations imposed on them in Sweden.

After several weeks in Stockholm, Carl Semb and Kristian Kristiansen completed the details of their health camp proposal they had begun aboard the train to Kjesaeter. By that time, the string of Nazi defeats had begun. Success after Allied success had taken place in Africa, and the battered remnants of a defeated German Army had surrendered at Stalingrad. The Swedes, becoming confident of an Allied victory, were more responsive to Norwegian desires. The Norwegian Refugee Organization in Stockholm accepted the new proposal. The two doctors were commissioned in the Norwegian Army, and provided an office through the efforts of the military attaché in the Norwegian Embassy, Ingvald Smith-Kielland. In early May Carl Semb journeyed aboard a Mosquito bomber to England where he won approval of the health camp plan from the Norwegian government-in-exile.

Norway already had powerful friends in Swedish governmental service who provided critical support for the health camp proposal: Dr. Axel Höyer, director of the Swedish Social and Health Service, and Harry Söderman, chief of the Criminal Institute in Stockholm. Höyer had long been active in support of Norway and was chief of the Action Committee for Swedish Help to Norway. Söderman was particularly well situated politically. In addition to his police duties he was a close friend of Swedish Prime Minister Per Albin Hansson. Looking to the end of the war,

Söderman had already organized a camp for training Norwegian police in Sweden. A number of the policemen in Norway had been recruited from local Nazis, so it would be necessary to provide replacements with the return to peacetime. Some two hundred Norwegians were undergoing training—all in a legally acceptable manner at the time. Höyer was, of course, concerned with the health aspects of the proposal, and Söderman's interests were in the military possibilities.

While Carl Semb was still in England, Kristian Kristiansen, accompanied by Arnt Brodtkorb, deputy chief of the Norwegian Registration Office in Stockholm began rounds in Sweden, armed with a letter of recommendation and support from Höyer.

Invariably the two Norwegians were met with good will and understanding, particularly by teachers and the directors of schools. Kristiansen and Brodtkorb arranged rental of spacious sites for the health camps at farms, schools, estates, and at least one chateau.

Assisted ably by two young Norwegians, Nils Heldal and Erik Juel, Semb and Kristiansen opened the first of the camps on Midsummer Day—when daylight never leaves the north and nights in the south are no more than dusk. Traditionally, it was a time of great festivity in Sweden. In 1943, Norwegians enthusiastically joined in the celebration.

Thirty health camps were established in the first round. In each an administrator was appointed, usually an officer in the Norwegian army—himself a refugee. All Norwegian males from ages eighteen to forty-five throughout Sweden were called in for "examination and inoculation." The plan called for registration, blood typing, and inoculation against tetanus and diphtheria. Semb and Kristiansen considered it important to add immunization against typhoid—serving a double purpose. Not only did Norwegian youths obtain their needed protection, but more importantly initiation of military training could begin. Two injections, three weeks apart, were required to confer immunity. Reactions to the first could be severe, and observation was necessary to make certain no one contracted the disease from improperly prepared vaccines. The young men could receive military indoctrination while being held in camp for "medical reasons."

By November 1943, the first phase of health camp operations had ended well. More than eight thousand young Norwegians had been examined. Over 90 percent were found fit, and had begun military preparation. The time had come for full scale military training—with the aid of Harry Söderman.

Carl Semb had met with Söderman (later to be known among Norwegians as "Revolver Harry") on September 17, 1943, proposing establishment of ten large installations for the military training of Norwegian refugees. In the end sixteen permanent camps were formed. Another camp, *Stralenbo*, was established for training medical corps personnel to support the activities of the Norwegian youths who had been enigmatically designated as "Reserve Police." Operations were directed by Hans Fredrik Fabritius, who was forced to flee Norway in November 1943 and Sten Florelius, who was called to Sweden in September 1944.

With a war in progress, time was too short for Carl Semb to await official approval for purchases to establish and equip the camps. He applied to the Norwegian government-in-exile for funds and for Swedish building permits, but began construction of the necessary barracks before either had arrived. Paul Hartmann, Norway's minister of finance, was incredulous. "What kind of person is this Semb?" he asked Ole Jacob Malm. "He sends me bills for a million Swedish crowns."[4] Malm described Semb as resourceful, reliable, and knowing how to get the job done.

In the more advanced camps troops were gradually allowed to train with heavier arms, including mortars. In the beginning Söderman saw that weapons were supplied from Swedish sources. Later in the war, Sweden permitted access to U. S. military aircraft for transport to Finnmark— the northernmost region of Norway that had been liberated by Soviet troops in October 1944.

The health camp phase proceeded rather smoothly. Once military training had begun, however, other problems arose. Some young Norwegians, unhappy about their living conditions and prospects for the future, just disappeared. Communist infiltrators, though few, fomented their usual disproportionate degree of unrest. A strike of cooks throughout the system in 1944 produced the most severe crisis. The refugees' pay was small at best and the "Reserve Police" protested. Semb and Kristiansen successfully applied to the Norwegian government for a salary increase. Cooks, somehow, were excluded from the increase.

The bypassed cooks responded to the humiliating treatment by striking —with the full support of their comrades. The entire personnel in several camps struck in sympathy. The protesters added to the turmoil by threatening to pack their gear and take to the roads. Had they done so, the strikers were subject to immediate arrest and internment in one of the several Swedish "collection camps."

Prompt intervention by Söderman, Kristiansen, Semb, and Norway's military attaché Ole Berg prevented a debacle. In the end cooks too shared in the increase.

By the time the Germans capitulated in 1945 a force of fourteen thousand Norwegian "Reserve Police" had held large-scale military maneuvers in Sweden and were prepared to cross over into Norway. The purpose of the health camps had been well concealed throughout. Advanced training was well under way before the higher echelon of Sweden's military were aware of the camps' real intent. General Swedlund, chief of the Swedish armed forces, told Carl Semb afterwards, "How you fooled us with those health camps!" The enterprise initiated by two Norwegian physicians set a historic precedent for modern times. Never before had a belligerent army been trained on sovereign territory of a neutral nation.

When the health camps had completed their mission in November 1943, and were converted to Reserve Police Camps the Royal Norwegian Health Office of which Carl Semb was chief and Kristian Kristiansen deputy chief, was reorganized, renamed the *Forvaltningskontor* (Administrative Office), and added to the gradually increasing bureaucracy headed by Ole Berg. Semb continued his responsibilities in Sweden until the spring of 1945 when he was appointed chief medical officer of Norwegian forces. Kristian Kristiansen was called to London in September 1944 where he was assigned the responsibility of arranging medical supplies for postwar Norway.

17. The Power of the Press

From the moment their government had fled to London, Norwegians hungered for word from abroad. Buoyed by King Haakon's determination to struggle side-by-side with the Allies until the Nazi's defeat, every loyal household turned to Norwegian language broadcasts over the BBC for news from the battlefront and for moral sustenance from their government-in-exile. The Germans had first censored then closed down Norway's independent newspapers—permitting only the *Nasjonal Samling* organ *Fritt Folk* (Free People) to be published and circulated. From the very first days of the Occupation Quisling's henchmen were in command of Norway's broadcasting system. For Norsemen, the BBC was their lifeline to truth.

Before 1940 ended the occupying Nazis had made their first attempt to overcome the BBC effect. On December 13, broadcasts from Britain, the United States, and Canada were forbidden in Norway's gathering places—the restaurants, cafés, hotels, and other sites of entertainment. The major blow, however, fell in August 1941. After Norwegians were compelled to deliver all radios to the occupying authorities, listening to BBC broadcasts, whether in Norwegian, English, or even German, became a serious crime. Seven months later, the first executions were carried out for listening to, then spreading information about BBC broadcast news. Five Norwegian citizens, four of whom were Jews, were executed in Trondheim.

Despite all threats and atrocities, the Nazis were unable to deny Norwegians their sustaining news. Clandestine private radios became a new part of the underground apparatus, and the information garnered was funneled to "illegal" newspapers. The Resistance press that had begun with such publications as *Nitten Titten* out of *Møllergata 19* swelled in response to repression. Ten new papers were formed in October, seventy in September, and another fifteen in November. Some were hardly more than crudely typewritten and stenciled sheets, while others were formally typeset and numbered up to a dozen pages. In 1943 as many as five hundred thousand copies from the "illegal press" were distributed each month.

Newspapers such as *London Nytt* (London News) and *London Radio* reproduced BBC broadcasts and had enormous circulation. Others embellished the news with interpretation and editorial comment. The most important of those was the voice of the trade unions, *Fri Fagbevegelse* (Free Labor Movement) and *Bulletinen* (The Bulletin), which soon became the quasi-official organ of the Home Front leadership. Announcements from the Home Front appeared regularly in *Bulletinen* as did certain *paroles* requiring widespread circulation.

Norwegians became devoted to their clandestine press, and over the years of Occupation thousands became involved as publishers, editors, news-gatherers and distributors. All lived hazardous lives, for hundreds were taken by the Nazis and imprisoned at Grini or in concentration camps in Germany. Survival of the majority of underground publications was transitory, ending with the arrest of publishers and distributors. *Bulletinen,* however, exerted its powerful influence until the German capitulation.

Few loyal Norwegians, if any, contributed more to their country's underground efforts than did Dr. Jan Jansen—yet even those closest to him in the Home Front were oblivious to the full extent of his involvement. Jansen served as policymaker, advisor to his fellows in the Resistance, political and military analyst, shaper of opinion, and linchpin of the clandestine press—all in the quiet, unassuming manner that was both characteristic of him and critical to keeping his activities undetected.

When he had completed his year of required military service in 1925, Jansen chose a life in academic medicine. He spent several periods of study and research abroad—in The Netherlands, England, and Germany. None were more significant to his career than the period of 1927 to 1928 when he worked together with C. Judson Herrick in Chicago. His investigations at that time served as the basis of the doctoral dissertation he defended in 1931.

By the summer of 1942 Jansen was immersed in his clandestine activities. He had survived the demise of every early underground leadership group, and maintained a central position in each succeeding organization. Jansen had not only been a member of the R-Group since its inception, but had remained undetected as one after another of the principals were apprehended or fled. With the collapse of the R-Group Jansen became a key member of both The Circle, and the Coordination Committee. The geologist, Tore Gjelsvik, Ole Jacob Malm's successor as secretary-general of *KK*, not only worked closely with Jansen in distribution of

Bulletinen, but met him almost daily seeking counsel on other Home Front responsibilities.[1] Through it all Jansen continued his university duties in anatomy, and as master of the student residence at Blindern.

When Jansen returned to Oslo after a brief holiday in the summer of 1942 he found the editor of *Bulletinen* and all his colleagues in the clandestine publication arrested. Quietly, and without the knowledge of even his closest associates, Jansen took over the responsibility of editing and publishing the paper himself.[2] Throughout the remaining years of the Occupation it was *Bulletinen* in which the Norwegians placed their final trust. Through couriers from Sweden and liberal use of the BBC, Jansen always had access to the most accurate sources of news. Although lacking in any military background his analyses of the war's progress were sound, perceptive, and reassuring to his countrymen. His editorial comments sagely interspersed moral support with caution, and realism with optimism. The February 1944 issue of *Bulletinen* carried Jansen's insightful and influential article, *Åndelig balans* (spiritual balance):

> The stress has long been great among us, our nervous strength has been drained through nearly four years, so it is not at all strange that our equanimity may become somewhat labile. It is understandable, but it is unfortunate, and we must work against it. . . . The swings are exceptionally distinct when optimism and pessimism over the war's events are involved, not when it concerns the outcome, for there has never been any doubt as to that, but when it concerns the question of the war's duration. After a couple of exciting events at the Front people are inclined to believe that all will end within two to three months, but when fourteen days pass without any special sensational occurrences, suddenly there appears to be no end to the misery. . . . The Home Front is not served by such uncontrolled, unrestrained fluctuations. We have need for a steady course and balanced people.[3]

Bulletinen was reproduced in the office of Erling Malm at that time, with only staff member Sigrid Steinnes and office worker Erik Bratsberg to support the editor. Steinnes, under the code name "Elisabeth" had been indispensable to Ole Jacob Malm and his successor, Kaare Norum, in the *KK* since the end of 1941. Ole Jacob spoke of her as "amazing," and Norum described her as "doing the most dangerous things with the same nonchalance as if she were dusting."[4]

Jansen prepared his clandestine text at home, then bicycled to Malm's office with the manuscript. One day, as he pedaled along Drammensveien with the contents of the upcoming issue of *Bulletinen* bulging from his pocket, his way was barred by a column of Nazi troops marching in front of the University Library. Jansen could ill disguise his disgust as the enemy passed before him. He spat upon the ground, muttering "*Fie Fanden*" (Fie, the devil), Norway's traditional expression of disdain. He had been observed, however, by two quislings in a nearby auto. They alighted and charged the doctor with an act of disrespect for German troops. Jansen was ordered to accompany the two Norwegian Nazis to Gestapo headquarters.

The "crime" of disrespect with which he was to be charged was insignificant compared to that of participation in the underground press. The manuscript in Jansen's pocket—if discovered—would be his undoing. Jansen assumed the mask of practicing physician—insisting he was unable to follow the order immediately. He was hurrying along to the nearby Red Cross Hospital to care for an emergency patient.

Jansen's colleagues at the hospital played their roles as convincingly as he did, and grudgingly the quislings yielded. Jansen was permitted to continue his "patient care," but ordered to report for further questioning and a subsequent hearing.

At trial Jansen appeared innocently incredulous. He had been, he claimed, merely responding to the recurring discomforts of his chronic ailment. He had indeed suffered from a gastric ulcer since before the war, and spitting, he said, was only an attempt to relieve his acid discomfort. Dr. Jansen's lawyer then produced a bottle of dilute hydrochloric acid—mimicking the acidic stomach contents—and challenged the prosecutor to sample the solution. The *Nasjonal Samling* attorney declined the invitation. The judge was satisfied no gain could come by further prosecution. Jansen was released, with a warning against any repetition.

January 1944 began the year of crisis for the "illegal" press. Near the end of 1943, a Gestapo deserter had informed the Norwegian Legation in Stockholm that the Nazis had been gathering information on Norway's underground publications, and had prepared for widespread action. Forewarned, Norwegians set about changing sites of the "illegal" print shops in January 1944, but that was not to be enough.

Dr. Reidar Eker and the two lawyers who worked together in the publication of *Svart på hvit* received information through contact with a Home Front operative whom they knew only as "Uncle Andreas." When Dr. Eker attended a meeting of the underground press at the Deichman Library in the beginning of February he carried the manuscript for a lecture on the organization of sabotage. The Gestapo, however, had wrung advance information of the meeting through torture of a captured editor of *Svart på hvit*, and swooped down on the library. Quickly and quietly, Eker let his manuscript fall to the floor. When the questioning began, however, he admitted to ownership of the incriminating document. Reidar Eker well knew the entire group would be tortured until the true source was discovered.[5]

None of the participants escaped jailing. On February 2, a roundup of editors, printers, and distributors of the "illegal" newspapers in Oslo began. Dr. Olav Torgersen, who had sheltered Kristian Kristiansen and Carl Semb as they awaited passage to Sweden, was among those hunted.

Professor Olav Torgersen, of the Department of Pathology at *Riks-hospital*, had felt powerless at the outset of the Occupation, but as small clandestine newspapers appeared he became active in publication and distribution.[6] Once radios were confiscated he sold his rowboat, and with the proceeds purchased a powerful receiver from a member of the underground. He mounted the radio to the underside of a laboratory table then monitored BBC broadcasts for news to be used in the "illegal" press.

The apparatus was discovered by a washerwoman who, unlike the usual close-mouthed, loyal Norwegian, began to question the pathologist. Torgersen turned to his supplier, who followed the woman to her home, then threatened her life should she reveal her knowledge. Although they were confident the shaken woman would remain silent, a better location was clearly necessary. A still more powerful receiver was supplied and placed just beneath the roof. Whenever the underground passed word of an imminent search the radio was concealed in the abdomen of cadaver.

As time passed, bodies of Norwegians who had spied against their countrymen and were "liquidated" by the underground were brought into the department of pathology for autopsy. At first Olav Torgersen was repelled by the violence, but he began to feel a certain satisfaction at observing the informers' fate. He recognized how violence springs up so easily, and how dedication to a cause "can turn good people into beasts."

Once committed to the Resistance, Torgersen forsook sleeping at home, for the Gestapo unerringly chose the night for their arrests. Each evening he left his apartment for a secret room. When Professor Torgersen heard his name had been revealed through torture, he abandoned his home entirely. There were, however, important and incriminating documents in his apartment. Mrs. Torgersen, recognizing the danger, called Dr. Viktor Gaustad, saying only there were some medical books he should have, and "How would 11:00 A.M. be?" At the appointed time on the following morning two young women of about eighteen, dressed in work clothes and looking "very ordinary," appeared with a truck and drove away with the dangerous material.

Torgersen readily eluded Gestapo pursuit but soon became bored with an underground existence. In the end, boredom would have been preferable. After some days he elected to return to work at the Institute of Pathology. In the open he was easily apprehended, and he spent the remaining fifteen months of the war in prison.

The Gestapo action against clandestine publications peaked on February 16, when the printing press for even *Fri Fagbevegelse* was closed down. Only Jansen's *Bulletinen* remained to cooperate with the Home Front in printing announcements and *paroles*, but Jansen's own time was soon to come. Late in April 1944, he received word that a University colleague, no longer able to withstand torture, had implicated Jansen in the Home Front leadership. The efficient underground information system functioned well, however, and the prisoner managed to pass along the damning disclosure to Jansen.

On the eve of his departure Jansen confided in *KK* Secretary-General Tore Gjelsvik, his closest underground associate of the past four years. Gjelsvik was aware of Jansen's crucial function as a member of "The Circle" and of some mysterious connection with the editor of *Bulletinen*. He had met with Jansen virtually daily, and continually sought his advice. Yet he was astounded to learn that it was the quiet, modest, and unassuming Jansen himself who had been solely responsible for the editing and publication of the morale-sustaining *Bulletinen*. Jansen asked Gjelsvik to assume editorship of the paper and informed him only that Sigrid Steinnes would see that the manuscripts reached the proper hands for printing. Jansen then took the underground route himself, crossing over to Sweden. Gjelsvik recruited journalist C. A. R. Christensen and another colleague in the Resistance, Tore Sund,[7] to aid in continuing what Jan Jansen, to everyone's amazement, had managed single-handedly for almost two years.

18. The University Is Closed

The spontaneous acclaim given Johan Scharffenberg by University of Oslo students following his ringing address on September 21, 1940, provoked their first confrontation with the Norwegian Nazis whom *Reichskommissar* Joseph Terboven had given authority over University affairs. Scharffenberg's challenge brought not only his own arrest and imprisonment, but also that of John Sanness, chairman of the Students' Association.[1] Scharffenberg's oratory sparked the interruption of studies for many students who were propelled into the Resistance. For others both studies and lives were ended. Many who continued with their educations used the University as a base for underground activities, as did a number of the faculty. For all remaining in the university, harassment by the *Nasjonal Samling* was flagrant and persistent.

On October 14, 1940, the Norwegian Nazis suddenly introduced a new regulation governing appointments to the University faculty.[2] The ministry of churches and education was authorized to appoint professors without regard to qualifications and without the customary search and selection by a committee appointed through royal mandate. Shortly thereafter, Minister Ragnar Skancke designated three professors, bypassing both Rector Didrik Seip and the University faculty. Later, in the aftermath of the disastrous milk strike, Skancke replaced Seip as rector, substituting the quisling professor Adolf Hoel. Two other professors were also removed from their posts. Rector Seip was imprisoned at Grini for seven months then spent the remaining years of the war in German concentration camps.

Skancke called all students to a convocation in the University's *Aula* on November 12, 1941, threatening immediate and permanent expulsion for all failing to attend. To a packed auditorium, he announced that students would be named rather than elected to committees—an easily recognizable ploy to Nazify those committees. When the quisling minister relinquished the podium to the leader of the *Nasjonal Samling* student organization every student, except the few Nazis and members of the superseded committees, rose and left the hall. On November 14, they struck in protest of the new ruling.

The faculty and student body split badly over the proper course to follow. One group opted for some attempt at practical coexistence. The second felt the uniform opposition the teachers had employed so successfully to be the better course of action. The majority voted to keep the University open. Mindful of the experiences of the catastrophic ending of the milk strike, the consequences of a continued strike appeared far greater than the gains. The strike was ended after a single day. The uneasy truce lasted less than a year.

Choices had been difficult for Dean Georg Monrad-Krohn in the face of *Nasjonal Samling* attempts to Nazify both Norwegian medicine and the University of Oslo. Throughout the Occupation he trod a fine line in his efforts to keep the medical school and *Rikshospitalet* operating without yielding unduly to the pressures of the new regime.

Dr. Monrad-Krohn's ancestors had been distinguished leaders of Bergen's communal life for generations. As a professor he left a mark on neurology that extended far beyond his native city and even his own country. A gifted linguist, the young Monrad-Krohn was able to make the most of the months he spent in post-graduate study in Berlin and in Paris. It was London, however, where he matured after six years of study and neurological practice at the National Hospital for Paralysed and Epileptic—Queen Square, Maida Vale Hospital, and the Bexley Mental Asylum. On January 1, 1922, Georg Monrad-Krohn was appointed professor of neurology at the University of Oslo and chief neurologist in the University Clinics at Rikshospital. With that appointment he became the most junior of the sixteen professors who headed medical school departments.[3]

Deanship of the faculty of medicine rotated at three-year intervals among the professors. In February 1941, ten months after the fateful invasion it became Georg Monrad-Krohn's turn to assume the mantle. Well aware of the wartime problems of that office, his colleagues inquired if he were willing to accept the responsibility. Monrad-Krohn did so, feeling it unworthy to refuse the "difficult assignment in such a difficult and dangerous situation."[4] Witty, urbane, and dexterous in every social circumstance, the newly appointed dean needed all his skills in dealing with the Nazis on one hand and the Resistance on the other. The Home Front had ordered "No cooperation with the Nazi commissars," yet without some semblance of rapprochement the medical school would have passed out of existence and *Rikshospitalet* would have been taken over by the Nazis.

In September 1942 Professor Monrad-Krohn, as dean of the medical faculty, together with the dean of the faculty for mathematics and natural sciences, faced off with Ragnar Skancke over the *Nasjonal Samling*'s latest attempt to influence University policy. Sixteen extra medical students and two additional pharmacy students were to be selected by Minister Skancke's department and admitted for study. The two deans stood adamant—all selections must be made on academic qualification alone. Skancke was forced to back off—largely, but not completely. Students he proposed to add would be allowed to attend certain open lectures, but were to be excluded from the more important compulsory courses.

Skancke's capitulation provided only temporary respite—even more severe measures were on their way. On February 22, 1943, Vidkun Quisling announced still another new law.[5] All males between the ages of eighteen and fifty-five and all females from twenty-one to forty were required to register for a National Labor Service. On the following day the *Nasjonal Samling* student organization called an assembly of the student body. Such a call ordinarily would have evoked no response whatsoever, but Quisling's edict aroused considerable anxiety. About four hundred loyal students attended the meeting—at least to formulate the most effective response.

Following the assembly Nazi newspapers announced that for the first time students at the University of Oslo had accepted the leadership of Quisling's student association, and had unanimously approved mobilizing for national labor. Students responded with immediate protest. Over twenty-five hundred of the twenty-seven hundred mailed letters to university authorities, clearly stating they would they recognize the Nazi organization as their representative under *no* circumstances.

February's successful repelling of quisling attempts to subjugate the University was only a temporary victory. On August 31 Skancke declared the *artium*—the student comprehensive examination—would no longer be the sole determinant of admission to the University. Other factors related to "existing conditions" would also be given weight. It was obvious that "other factors" meant membership in or support of the *Nasjonal Samling*.

Once more the faculty rejected Skancke's directive. Although his minister was prepared for further discussion, Vidkun Quisling had no patience for negotiation with the recalcitrant faculty. On October 15 his police arrested ten faculty members and fifty to sixty students, then imprisoned them at Bredtvedt Penitentiary.[6] Each was asked to sign a statement accepting the new entrance rules. The alternative would be a six-month sentence to prison. Not a single student or instructor accepted the terms. Protests from deans and faculty followed once again, with only small effect. Between ten and twenty of the medical students were freed. The final blow against the University was then close at hand.

On November 28, 1943, a group of saboteurs unassociated with the University set a small and easily extinguished fire in the *Aula*. Josef Terboven—infuriated at the Underground's temerity—used the event to serve his own purpose, learning from Nazi pretexts after the infamous *Reichstag* Fire in Berlin. On the following day, Terboven decided to close the University of Oslo for the duration of the Occupation.

On the evening of Terboven's decision, the Coordination Committee learned of the impending action. Lieutenant Colonel Theodor Steltzer of the German Transport Service, who headed a group of anti-Nazi officers in the *Wehrmacht*, had been passing on secret information from the German command to a sociologist, Arvild Brodersen, for some time. Brodersen, in turn, informed the *KK* of all significant developments.

Immediately on learning of the Terboven's intention, Steltzer notified Brodersen that the Nazis would move at 11:00 A.M. on November 30, round up all students, and ship them off to concentration camps in Germany.[7] After receiving the information from Brodersen, Tore Gjelsvik, secretary of the *KK* quickly dispatched a general warning that reached the students in the new buildings at Blindern as well as in the older campus in the city's center.

The three hundred German troops who had set out on their mission at 11:00 A.M. found few students in Blindern. Forewarned, the majority had melted away. At the city center, however, the Nazis were far more successful. Many students had fled at the first notice, but others were doubters. Frequent false alarms lulled several hundred into a false sense of security. The nonbelievers were taken in the classrooms and reading rooms. Since preclinical teaching for the medical school took place on the main campus on Karl Johansgate, many of the captured were medical students.

The Nazis had planned thoroughly, and moved to *Rikshospitalet* to arrest medical students in their clinical years. Norway's state hospital, and center of medical student teaching, lay at the junction of *Pilestredet* and *Nordahl Brunsgate* just a five-minute walk from the central campus. The hospital's gray stuccoed buildings were closely surrounded by a high wall. All traffic entered and left through the single main gate on *Nordahl Brunsgate*.

On the morning of November 30th, after donating blood, student Wilhelm Harkmark was intercepted on his way to Professor Olav Hansen's class in internal medicine at *Rikshospitalet*.[8] An agitated student hurriedly gave Wilhelm two notices, one for Hansen's class and a second for Professor Salvesen's. Harkmark quickly passed the notice for his own class to a fellow student then stood outside Salvesen's lecture hall awaiting the end of the class. Harkmark's warning message confused the students as they filed out of the classroom. Most felt the communication to be little more than a provocation—too fantastic to be true—the Germans must be circulating rumors to goad the students into reactions that could justify closing the University.

Two young women marched into Monrad-Krohn's office brandishing the warning message. The dean and professor of neurology counseled the students to behave as if nothing were amiss while he spoke with the Germans. Students clustered about, discussing alternatives when Monrad-Krohn arrived at the room Salvesen had just vacated, prepared to deliver his own lecture in neurology.

As Monrad-Krohn began to speak, one youth, finally realizing the potential seriousness of the matter rose to leave. The professor looked up, sternly saying, *"Ingen inkoordinerter bevegelser, unge man"* (No uncoordinated movements, young man). The student disregarded the interdiction.

Wilhelm Harkmark and Martin Sensay decided escape was prudent, and moved toward the main gate on *Nordahl Brunsgate*. They found the wide opening cordoned off by autos and large trucks. Four massive SS soldiers stood menacingly at the gate, allowing none but women and children to pass. The two students were ordered brusquely, *"Dere må gå tilbakke"* (You must go back). Harkmark and Sensay turned, walked nonchalantly together around the corner of the building, then sprinted toward the only possible escape—a small locked door that opened out into *Pilestredet*.

The two fugitives reached their goal just as a third fled the adjoining Institute of Pathology. Harkmark and Sensay felt blessed, for the new arrival worked in the institute and had the "key to freedom." The three managed to slip through the door only seconds before Nazi troops arrived to seal off the exit. Harkmark scurried from the scene before Nazi troops appeared. His newest companion crossed the street, and pausing momentarily, saw the pursuing Germans. At that very moment an ancient street car swung around the curve on *Pilestredet* allowing the escaping student to fling himself to safety aboard the open rear platform as the trolley car rolled past.

Only one other medical student avoided the Nazi net at *Rikshospitalet*. Emerging from the outpatient clinic at the precise moment of German arrival, he darted immediately into the otolaryngology clinic where his brother was a physician. The doctor flung the fleeing student onto a bed, then covered him with a blanket. Nazi troops searched the entire area, but the bogus patient remained undiscovered.

Striding up the hill overlooking the University campus Wilhelm Harkmark set out toward his quarters near the West Railroad Station. On the hilltop he came upon a group of young men cautiously peering down on the proceedings below. Although heeding the warnings to avoid classrooms and reading rooms, curiosity kept them in the vicinity to observe the German action. Nazi troops had already cordoned off Oslo's center entrapping both the fleeing and the curious.

Harkmark, finding the observers to indeed be students, advised them of the peril. Nazi pursuit was vigorous and intense. German troops arrested even more young Norwegians as they searched student lodgings thoroughly. In all twelve hundred were collected, almost half the entire student body. For all others, the advance warning had been effective; the evading students disappeared underground. More than a thousand were later evacuated to Sweden by special transports organized by the Home Front.

Returning to his room barely long enough to collect the few belongings he could carry Wilhelm boarded the tram for his sister's home. Quickly depositing his spare clothing he too went into hiding while considering his options. Although escape to Sweden was possible, Harkmark chose to return to his family home in Mandal. His identity card then became his enemy. Not only was he branded a student, but the card was valid only about Oslo; Mandal lay far to the west.

Harkmark described the problem in a letter to his brother in Mandal, enlisting his aid. A cooperative government official issued a western zone pass identifying the young student as a *"Prosektor Minor."* The title— an assistant in the teaching of anatomy—would be meaningless to any German.

The fugitive medical student encountered little difficulty on his southward rail journey to Kristiansand. Traveling west by bus to his native village, Wilhelm found his brother at the busstop—behind a horse and atop a wagon. His vehicle like virtually all of those owned by Norwegians, had been requisitioned by the Germans.

Harkmark's brother brought disturbing news—a young friend who had suggested Wilhelm join him in escape to Sweden was quickly taken by the Nazis. Wilhelm Harkmark spent the Christmas holidays at home, then arranged to work as assistant to a local physician, Dr. Gullafson. He became too visible in that occupation, however. The fugitive student decided to return to Oslo and arrange underground transport to Sweden. It was then late in the Occupation, and passage that had once been secure and simple had become difficult and dangerous. Forged identity cards for the eastern border zone no longer provided safety. That area was well patrolled and a newly constructed frontier within Norway itself barred the approaches to the Swedish border.

On February 24, 1944, bearing a two-day supply of food and a pair of skis, Wilhelm Harkmark met with an unidentified Resistance operative, as instructed. The fugitive student was handed a sealed envelope that was to remain unopened until he was safely aboard the train. Inside Harkmark found a railroad ticket and instructions. He was to leave the train at Eidsvoll and remain in the station café until he recognized a specific Resistance agent from Oslo. He was then to leave the café and meet his contact in the dark outside. After the successful meeting the two young men were transported by car to the edge of a wood, through which they then skied. Emerging safely from the trees, they were brought by a second vehicle to another forest. Led by two guides Harkmark skied through the entire night and safely crossed the Nazi boundary into the eastern border zone. The final ski journey brought Wilhelm into Sweden, where he was reunited with fellow students who had escaped the Nazi net. Together they entered the reserve police training program that Carl Semb and Kristian Kristiansen had spawned in the guise of health camps.

On November 30, 1943, the very day of student roundup by the Nazis, the faculty of medicine reappointed Georg Monrad-Krohn as dean for the coming three-year period. At that time his colleagues offered him no choice. Although he had lost all his students, Monrad-Krohn was successful in maintaining the administration of *Rikshospitalet* in Norwegian hands for the duration of the Occupation and keeping the staff free of Nazi physicians—in marked contrast to other Oslo hospitals that were forced to yield to the occupier's demands.[9]

19. An Underground Refuge

As Germany's military position disintegrated in Western Europe, local Resistance operatives were called upon to impede transfer of fresh Nazi troops from Norway to bolster German forces at the front. In these actions and in the occasional armed clashes of underground members with the occupying military, clandestine sources of medical care were required for the wounded. Norway's physicians, among them Dr. Per Giertson,[1] rose to every occasion.

Giertson was no stranger to the Gestapo. Just after Easter of 1942 while seated before his fireplace, reading the illegal *London Nytt*, he heard a car braking before his home—then through the window he saw the Gestapo alight. Before answering their summons Per Giertson added the underground publication to the flames in the fireplace. He was already a recognized target for his well-known opposition to the Nazis, and the Gestapo had arrived to take him hostage. A German soldier had been shot as a Norwegian prisoner escaped from Grini. Giertson was one of thirty dissidents taken. If the soldier died, fifteen were to be executed in reprisal. Fortunately, the soldier survived, and after an only moderately unpleasant incarceration Giertson was released.

Until the Nazis denied Norway's Jews their right to work Per Giertson had had a Jewish physician as his assistant. For several years the Norwegian doctor had provided medical services to employees of the Fred Olsen Line. Thomas Olsen, the line's owner, had long used Dr. Hirschberg, a distinguished Jewish internist in Berlin, as his private physician. After Hitler had initiated his atrocities against German Jews, Olsen ransomed Hirschberg and brought him to Oslo. There the noted refugee was licensed and practiced as assistant to Per Giertson—until that too was forbidden by the Nazis. When Norway's Jews were rounded up and shipped off to their destruction in 1942 Hirschberg remained hidden in Giertson's home until the Norwegian physician could arrange both safe transport and maintenance of his colleague in Sweden.

Giertson's reputation in Norwegian shipping circles led sailors in plight to approach him frequently for aid. One evening after returning from a professional call he observed a figure in a German military uniform standing in his doorway. The man's face, however, was Norwegian and familiar. Dr. Giertson had examined him before the seaman had shipped out in Norway's merchant marine. He had been taken in Kristiansand by the Nazis, the mariner reported—his documents confiscated and he himself impressed into the German military. Now he had deserted, the visitor claimed, and had come to one he trusted for aid and refuge. Giertson was appropriately suspicious, for too many Norwegians had fallen victim to *provocateurs* among their countrymen's turncoats. He did not dare believe what he had heard and would call the police, he told the soldier. The young seaman's fright was exactly the response Dr. Giertson had hoped to see. Reassured, he immediately took in the deserter, burnt the offensive uniform, provided money and clothing, then sent a "new man" off toward refuge in Sweden.

Scarcely two days had passed when a Norwegian presenting himself as a "farmer" appeared at the door with regards from Giertson's recent visitor. He would transport the fugitive to Sweden, the farmer reported, but he must have additional money. Dr. Giertson expressed his displeasure, but added three hundred kroner. When the same man appeared two days later with a similar request the doctor knew he'd been duped. The two men, both sailors, had been living high on Giertson's money, and planned to milk their source to the utmost. Giertson would have no more. He had contacts among the Germans, he told his visitor, and if the two sailors failed to depart for Sweden he would inform the Nazis, who would execute them as deserters. Furthermore, Dr. Giertson demanded, he expected a postal card from them by Christmas so he could be certain they had indeed fled across the frontier. At the appropriate time the card arrived in the mail.

Giertson's medical facilities were on the ground floor of his apartment home on a quiet street close by the famed Gustav Vigeland Museum. His office and outpatient surgery lay at the end of the hall and the glass doors at the office rear opened into a garden that was shared with the adjacent apartment. A small trap door, concealed beneath the carpet of his office, led to a basement room the doctor had outfitted as a refuge.

Once underground actions increased late in 1944 the secret quarters were in frequent use. In October three young men, with a fourth on guard, had set about removing gasoline from German stores at the Westdam

School, a short way from Giertson's home and office. The operation was proceeding well when a German guard emerged from the building. The Norwegians had no alternative but to shoot the soldier. Others quickly appeared and fired after the fleeing young men. One was struck five times, yet the four reached the spot where they had left their bicycles, evaded both their pursuers and Nazi sentries in the street, then separated. The wounded man found refuge at the home of his aunt, and early the following morning appeared at Dr. Giertson's surgery.

With a plastic surgeon friend and accomplice, Per Giertson removed the five bullets. He then took the young man into his home to recuperate. The convalescent had the freedom of the house, but at each knock on the door he descended through the trap door until any possibility of discovery passed. For Dr. Giertson it was like having a young son in the house.

As happened so often throughout the Occupation Per Giertson's next confinement to Grini followed the Gestapo's interest in someone else. His neighbor in the adjoining apartment possessed an "illegal" radio receiver and served as active contact for underground agents who were often dispatched on missions of liquidation by Norwegian authorities in Sweden. Giertson was invited repeatedly by his neighbor to listen to the "London News," but he felt the radio was too poorly concealed. When Giertson offered his hidden basement, the set was then moved to safety.

To both Norwegians' misfortune, however, Per Giertson's neighbor employed a housemaid who was friendly with a German soldier—freely sharing her knowledge of activities in the household. Her report that her employer had housed agents from Sweden and had provided an illicit wireless set to his neighbor brought the Gestapo three times to the adjoining Giertson household. The trap door remained undiscovered and twice the Nazis left empty-handed. On the third visit, however, the Gestapo arrived in an armored car, surrounded the apartment at night, and entered the two adjoining abodes simultaneously, surprising Giertson, the neighbor, and his underground visitor from Sweden.

Per Giertson heard gunfire from the rear garden as the two men next door attempted escape. Both fell wounded in the snow, and were taken. The Gestapo next turned to Giertson, and during the questioning the doctor saw two hands on the glass of a garden door. A patient, arriving by chance at just that moment, was signalling for entry. The new arrival was taken for interrogation as well. While the German turned to place a telephone call, the patient suddenly shoved his wallet and a sheaf of illegal papers into Giertson's pocket—incriminating evidence that the doctor barely managed to conceal before he was taken to Gestapo headquarters at *Viktoria Terrasse*. Per Giertson was interrogated throughout the night, but his earlier stretch at Grini had taught him how to respond. The Nazis learned nothing. From *Viktoria Terrasse* he was transferred to *Møllergata 19*, and finally to Grini. Per Giertson had joined the Grini Society, and was not to see Oslo again until after German capitulation.

20. Inside Nazi Prisons

In war as in peace, hospitals are in many respects like prisons. Both treat their occupants remarkably alike—abolishing personal freedom, restricting movement, and setting limits of behavior through some higher authority. In times of peace, however, a single difference is clear—prisons restrict transgressors against society and hospital confine the ill. In wartime Norway the distinction became muddied—jails overflowed with the country's worthiest citizens while the greatest criminals in the nation's history roamed free. At the same time hospital beds often protected healthy "patients" from the tyranny of the criminals controlling the nation. Throughout Norway hospitals departed from traditional peacetime functions by serving the Home Front in the most diverse fashions.

For many Norwegians the threat to life and freedom began with the terrifying process at *Viktoria Terrasse*. The fortunate endured no more than intense questioning, reinforced with threats and blows—then were released with ominous warnings. More commonly, victims were beaten and tortured as the first step of a harrowing experience that led to further imprisonment or even to execution.

Before the fateful Nazi invasion only ordinary criminals were led manacled through the doors of the long, low Victorian buildings strung the length of *Viktoria Terrasse* just across *Drammensveien* from the grounds of the Royal Palace. Once the Germans had abandoned their fruitless wooing of the Norwegians, a parade of Norway's most prominent and respected citizens crossed the foreboding threshold of the structure the Gestapo had requisitioned as their headquarters. There under the direction of *Kriminalrat* (Criminal counsel) Siegfried Fehmer "routine" initial questioning took place for all suspected of any role, no matter how minor, in the Resistance movement: editors, printers, and distributors of underground publications; possessors of prohibited radios or newspapers; members of *Milorg*; union leaders; saboteurs; noncooperating civil servants; teachers; clergymen; and University professors. Any individual

175

aiding, or suspected of abetting, escaping Norwegian or Jewish fugitives—
or any family member, friend, or contact of anyone under suspicion of
the various "crimes against the Occupation Forces"—was subject to the
Gestapo's "routine" interrogation.

"Routine" included every method Gestapo torturers could conceive
to extract information from reluctant captives. As their wartime position
deteriorated the Nazis became almost hysterical in their pursuit of Home
Front members, and "routine interrogation" knew virtually no bounds.
When the Allied net tightened still further in 1945, Dr. Viktor Gaustad
was arrested and brought to Gestapo headquarters in *Viktoria Terrasse* for
such an interrogation.[1]

Immediately following the Nazi march into Oslo, Gaustad, after sending his family to his parental home in Hamar, set out to join still resisting
Norwegian forces as an officer in the Army Reserve. With his brother-in-
law he skied across the rugged mountain terrain of *Nordmarka*, the nature
preserve bordering Oslo to the north and west. Two days later he joined
the government contingent at Hamar. Gaustad then crossed Norway
with the Royal Party to reach the sea at Ålesund and board the cruiser
Glasgow that bore them to Tromsø. When Norway's forces abandoned
the battle on its home soil in June and the government sailed for England
Dr. Gaustad started off for Oslo by foot. He was first among Norway's
defeated forces to cross the German lines stretching between Narvik and
Tromsø. By the end of the month Viktor Gaustad had reached Oslo.

In autumn of 1940, at his own request, Gaustad was dispatched back
to Tromsø by the State Department of Health to establish a microbiology
laboratory. In the process he visited medical installations in a number of
northern Norway's coastal cities and sowed the seeds for the information
network Ole Jacob Malm would bring into full flower. Gaustad's laboratory was primitive, even by standards of the day, and remained only
briefly under his direction. It performed some simple serologic testing and
bacteriologic studies, including sputum examinations for tuberculosis.
Before the laboratory could develop further the Nazis took command of
the State Department of Health. Dr. Gaustad then resigned his position
and left Tromsø in March 1941.

Over the next four years Viktor Gaustad merged his medical efforts in
the department of infectious disease at Ullevål Hospital with underground
activities. Ullevål, as a city hospital of some two thousand beds, served all
Oslo, thus required an enormous infectious disease service.[2] Antibiotic
medications now in common use were still unknown, and only the
sulfonamides were available for therapy—a therapy with little effect on
the infectious and contagious diseases that Gaustad and his colleagues

faced daily. Severe epidemics of diphtheria, scarlet fever, meningitis, and poliomyelitis taxed the four hundred-bed capacity of the service to overflowing and sent patients into the reserve hospital outside Oslo itself. Smaller epidemics of paratyphoid and typhoid fever resulted from the war-induced breakdown in sanitation.

Before long the prison ward, which had replaced the dermatology service on the fourth floor of Ullevaal Hospital, came to occupy an important position in the resisting nation's underground activities. A number of loyal Norwegians injured in sabotage efforts or in other confrontations with the Gestapo were treated on that ward, and others were transferred in from Oslo jails. A total of five hundred passed through the prison ward during the Occupation. Viktor Gaustad became a conduit between those patients and the still free underground and functioned as an operative on the transport network to Sweden.

An underground contact regularly delivered bundles of forged passports to Gaustad to aid fugitives in their flight. He kept those life-giving documents in his desk drawer, for hospitals, and particularly infectious disease wards, were threatening to the Nazis and virtually immune from search. Fleeing Norwegians were supplied the false passports, delivered to Dr. Immerslund, then concealed in small groups until "border pilots" took over. Fifty thousand Norwegians, among them seven hundred Jews, used Gaustad's, Immerslund's, and other underground routes to escape to Sweden. In later years, however, the transport became riskier. In 1944, along with many other links in the network, Immerslund was arrested.

After four years of safety, Viktor Gaustad's turn came in March 1945. One of his principal contacts, a young woman with a code name of "Vera," was arrested. Gaustad was informed, but expected no danger to himself, for "Vera" could be depended upon to keep her silence, no matter the brutality of the "examination." Another underground agent, one who had functioned as a member of the Norwegian Nazi State Police until discovered, was found with a note in "Vera's" handwriting. The bogus policeman nurtured an almost hysterical fear of drowning as a result of a near fatal episode during childhood. Under Nazi water torture he revealed Dr. Gaustad's name.

On the day of his arrest Gaustad sat calmly and unsuspectingly in the dining room at Ullevål Hospital. When the Gestapo arrived at his office, frantic colleagues began a search. Had he been located in time he could have easily disappeared into the enormous hospital.

The Gestapo first isolated Gaustad in a corner of a reception area in *Viktoria Terrasse*. As he awaited his captors' next move, one Nazi after another filed into the room, took a cigarette, pointed to him, then whispered furtively to his guards. Gaustad paid little heed, considering this merely psychological pressure, a softening-up procedure for the steps to follow. In time, the door swung open again. A German soldier beckoned, saying, "*Kommen Sie Mit* (Come with me)." As he followed through the open doorway a pair of huge hands grasped him about the throat. The Norwegian owner of the massive hands began to beat him ferociously.

Viktor Gaustad's strongest reaction was surprise at the degree of punishment he was able to tolerate. Suddenly his attacker ended the blows, asking in Norwegian, "Do you know Vera?" Taken off guard, Gaustad responded honestly. Of course he knew Vera. That was, however, the last bit of information the doctor offered. The thrashing continued, and finally Fehmer himself appeared to carry on the questioning—accompanied by threat after threat. The examination finally ended with no more than beatings, and the battered doctor was placed in a cell.

Two days later, Dr. Gaustad experienced the infamous "water treatment." He was placed before a tub of ice-cold water, hands manacled behind his back, and ankles bound together. With the words, *"Nun fahren Sie zum Himmel"* (Now you go to heaven), he was seized and his head and upper body thrust forcibly beneath the frigid water. As unconsciousness closed in, Gaustad was lifted from the water until he recovered. Then he was questioned. When the Nazi torturers received no answer, the process was repeated again and again. The torture ended finally when the inquisitors conceded they would get no answer. Gaustad, still silent, was returned to his cell where, frozen, he was barely able to dress himself with cold-stiffened fingers.

The Gestapo had too many victims to dwell long on a prisoner unlikely to reveal names or information. Dr. Viktor Gaustad was dispatched to the next step of imprisonment.

From outside, the Oslo City Jail at *Møllergata 19* is hardly impressive. The prison gates overlook a large square, filled during the day with the carts of street merchants and flower vendors. Across the open square is a block of stores and an arcade leading to what is now Oslo's Opera Theater. It was to *Møllergata 19* that Dr. Gaustad was transferred when Nazi barbarism failed to jar loose any of his closely guarded secret information. In the five years of Nazi Occupation *Møllergata 19* had become both a place of terror and a way station in the Resistance movement.

Many wartime inmates, like Dr. Johan Scharffenberg, were deeply respected in their communities. Still others had distinguished themselves through service to the Home Front. As a consequence *Møllergata 19* became an important conduit for the transfer of vital information to free and active members of the Resistance movement on the outside. Message routes beyond the prison walls were varied and plentiful, including German officers and underground agents who had infiltrated the *Nasjonal Samling* Police itself.

As Dr. Viktor Gaustad was placed facing the prison wall along with other new arrivals at *Møllergata 19* he was warned to look only straight ahead. He turned his head slightly, however, just as the prisoner beside him did the same, and they recognized each other as participants in the same cause. From the moment of his arrival in his cell, Gaustad was in frequent communication with other imprisoned members of the Home Front.

As Nazi paranoia mounted in the late years of the war the smallest suspicion could lead to imprisonment. Cells that had been constructed for single or double occupancy then housed up to five prisoners, and most slept bunched together on the floor. Even the smallest fragment of information was passed between inmates, then at night from cell to cell by tapping with coins in Morse code on the separating walls.

Gaustad's presence in *Møllergata 19* was made known to his medical colleagues by an officer in the Occupation forces. Lieutenant Colonel Alois Hauer, who directed the German medical unit at Ullevål Hospital, was an Austrian pulmonary disease specialist with no love for the Nazis who had forced him into their service. He was friendly to Norwegian physicians in the hospital, and in the course of examining another prisoner in *Møllergata 19* with tuberculosis recognized Viktor Gaustad. When the Austrian turned his head toward his Norwegian colleague and whispered, "Ullevål Hospital," Gaustad knew the information on his whereabouts would be passed on to his countrymen. By that time the end of the war was little more than a month away, as was the end of Gaustad's confinement.

As a result of his own "stupidity", Olav Torgerson's imprisonment in *Møllergata 19* just preceded that of Gaustad.[3] The University of Oslo pathologist shared his cell with three other patriots at *Møllergata 19* for three months before transfer to Grini, the larger prison that became a permanent home for so many Norwegians during the Occupation.

Unlike Professor Torgerson, Dr. Reidar Eker's sojourn at *Møllergata* was extended throughout the remainder of the war.[4] As had all Norwegian political prisoners, he endured his ration of torture, but he survived and maintained his morale by teaching and learning. For two hours each day he was instructed in the law by an attorney cellmate, in return for his own lectures in medicine. By night he used Morse code to exchange with the philologist in the adjoining cell. For communication with the outside through cell windows a series of hand signals was developed—signals that one day reported to Dr. Eker that he was targeted for execution. The inmates then began their own propaganda counter offensive, circulating the fiction that Eker had given aid to a German soldier. The anticipated execution never took place.

After months in *Møllergata 19*, Dr. Eker attempted to arrange a transfer to Grini. Living, he understood, was better in the larger prison and prisoners were even said to have some tobacco. Since *Møllergata 19* inmates were taken to Grini for dental care by imprisoned Norwegian dentists, Eker feigned a toothache. His ploy failed, however, as the transport vehicle had broken down on its previous trip. Instead, the inmate-dentist was brought to *Møllergata 19*. In the course of the dental "treatment" he tapped information in Morse code on his patient's teeth—information that was in turn relayed throughout the prison and to the Home Front beyond the walls. Eker, however, continued as a "lodger" in *Møllergata 19*.

21. The Infamous Grini Prison

Odd Nansen had every reason to find himself in prison once the Germans mastered Norway. His rescue of the persecuted through Nansen Relief, his position in Norway as son of national hero Fridtjof Nansen, his role as spokesman for loyal Norwegians confronting the Nazis at Fornebu Airport, and his opposition to Vidkun Quisling made him a prime target for the occupying forces and the *Nasjonal Samling* alike.

Despite his own vulnerability Odd Nansen felt the need to confront Vidkun Quisling directly. The Norwegian traitor had not only declared himself his country's *Fører*, but pictured himself as philosophical successor to Fridtjof Nansen. From the earliest publications in 1936, *Fritt Folk* (Free People), the official organ of the *Nasjonal Samling*, repeatedly claimed Norway's national hero as a supporter of Quisling policies. Fragments of his speeches, articles, and lectures were torn out of context and distorted to suggest that the dead humanitarian and statesman supported the Norwegian Nazi ideology.

Fritt Folk's continual attacks on Nansen Relief for its unremitting support of Jewish victims of Nazi tyranny added to the younger Nansen's simmering indignation. The Fascist tabloid, however, refused to reprint any of Odd Nansen's angry responses. He resolved, therefore, to meet with the self-appointed *Fører*. Even though he hardly expected the *Nasjonal Samling* leader to receive him, Nansen telephoned for an appointment barely three months after the Nazi invasion.

Odd Nansen was mistaken. Vidkun Quisling readily agreed to a meeting on the following day, July 8, 1940 at 11:30 A.M. in the *Nasjonal Samling* headquarters in downtown Oslo.[1]

Odd was led into Quisling's private office at the appointed hour by a young member of the *Hird* in a *Nasjonal Samling* uniform. The Norwegian traitor failed to rise to greet his visitor, but from behind his desk motioned Nansen to be seated.

"Quisling appeared tired and worn. His eyes were bloodshot and protruding. His gaze—as usual—was shifty and his entire physiognomy gave the appearance of a beaten man. Certainly those must have been difficult and nerve-racking days that he had just lived through—and the blow he had suffered [Quisling's removal from power by *Reichskommissar* Terboven] must have gone hard with him," noted Nansen.

Odd Nansen reconstructed the conversation that followed as fully as possible in his diary. Quisling was often incoherent, rambled frequently, and failed to respond in any manner to the most searching questions. Nansen began the discussion saying:

> I come to you, Quisling, not because I believe you will pay particular attention to what I have to say, and what I will ask, but because it is a matter of conscience for me to speak. . . . I ask you first to let my father's name rest in peace. You know full well, Quisling, that you cheat when you use Fridtjof Nansen's name in support of your politics.
>
> Vidkun Quisling stood erect and slammed his fist so hard that the desk shook—thundering his denial and claiming the sacrifices he had made gave him full right to use Fridtjof's revered name.

When the irate Norwegian Nazi became calm, Odd launched a query.

> Were Fridtjof Nansen alive do you believe he would have stood with you today and welcomed the Germans to Norway?
>
> Immediately Quisling resorted to digression, claiming Germany had acted in accord with international law.

After considerable discussion Odd Nansen directed a second question to Quisling.

> Do you think Fridtjof Nansen would have joined in urging persecution of the Jews and creating an atmosphere of a pogrom here in the country—as you are in the process of doing?
>
> Quisling denied the charge—claiming a duty to warn "against the great danger that threatens us through Jews and international Jewry."

As time went on Odd Nansen noted:

> Quisling had become noticeably more tired. His anger had slipped away, and he spoke more calmly, but all the same in an irritated and "sulking" manner. . . . "I think it is unworthy of you and your newspaper, Quisling," [Odd persisted] "at this time when free speech is gagged in our country, to come forth with so coarse and so obviously untruthful accusations against

people who cannot defend themselves. You claim innocence when I lump you together with *Fritt Folk*, but as the situation is, you can not possibly feel free of responsibility for what is printed there—especially when such slanderous and serious accusations are involved. You yourself must see that it is cowardly and despicable, Quisling."

"The same applies to parading my father's name, but I can assure you, Quisling—that his name and his deeds are so deeply and safely entrenched in the consciousness of the Norwegian people that you cannot budge it with coarse and clumsy attempts to use him as support for a politics and a view of society that he stood against with all his life and all his deeds! Therefore my mission to you is to ask you to discontinue that practice. . . . That you who carried out such marvelous work together with my father, in Russia, Armenia, and the Balkans, to save human beings in the utmost need, regardless of race, nationality and political opinions, can today condemn that type of work, and at the same time acclaim that man who has set in motion and carried out the most inhuman persecution known to history, is to me completely incomprehensible.

Can you seriously believe that to be in the spirit of Fridtjof Nansen?"

Quisling remained silent—and Nansen continued.

"All your work in the service of humanity and charity for which you have received recognition, from my father as well, cannot justify what you are now in the course of doing. Exactly the opposite! It makes it all the more terrible and incomprehensible! That a Norwegian like you could degrade himself so deeply is tragic. Deeply tragic."

Quisling appeared mentally exhausted now. He was not angry about my profoundly insulting pronouncements, only irritated, then with a movement of his arm that seemed to signify that he was not offended by what I had said or thought, answered:

"I am a good Norwegian, I am! I could only wish that you were such a good Norwegian as I!"

That was the end of a conversation that had taken over an hour.

Quisling and all he stood for, no longer occupies one's mind. The coming generation scarcely knows who he was. His tragic legacy is that his name has become synonymous with traitor, in all the countries of the west . . . he presented a sorry sight. I no longer considered him a danger. He gave the impression of a man already doomed to death.[2]

Odd Nansen's own time came eighteen months later. At 7:30 A.M. in the northern dark of the morning of January 13, 1942, the East Gausdal *Lensmann* (local official) arrived at the Nansen cottage, along with two men in German uniform, one of whom turned out to be a Norwegian traitor. As a friend of the Royal Family Odd Nansen was to be held hostage. The two tranquil nights Odd spent in Lillehammer's county jail stretched into more than three years of harsher imprisonment. Once he had reached *Møllergata 19* in Oslo, Nansen began to understand the reality of captivity by the Nazis, the ferocious bellows and savage blows of the guards, and the rations that previously would have filled him with disgust. Odd Nansen was transferred to Grini Penitentiary on January 16, 1942.

Looking down upon the serene valley on the outskirts of Hosle about twenty kilometers from the center of Oslo, and seeing the heavy walls surrounding the infamous Grini Prison, it is difficult today to imagine the turbulence and the pain that incarceration brought to the lives of thousands of loyal Norwegians—from the simplest to the most distinguished—and the intimate society they formed to help them survive and strengthen their resistance to Nazi oppression.

A compulsive diarist, Odd Nansen preserved the agonies and the reliefs of life under German warders at Grini. His journals of the "Grini experience" were published as a portion of *Fra Dag til Dag* in 1947 (subsequently slightly reduced and translated into English as *From Day to Day*).[3] Nansen maintained his daily record despite the enormous penalties discovery could bring—savage beatings, deportation to a concentration camp in Germany, or even execution. It became the avenue of communicating his innermost thoughts to his wife Kari, and the very foundation of his psychological sustenance. "As time went by inside the barbed wire, writing became a great help to me," Odd Nansen later wrote. "It was like confiding in a close friend and relieving my mind of all that weighed—it became a private manner of forgetting."

The danger peaked during the actual writing, for chance appearance of a Nazi or an informer was his greatest peril. Once he finished writing, however, the threat was ended, for hiding or sending on any document had already been simplified by inmate ingenuity. Nansen wrote in the smallest of hands on the thinnest of paper then secreted each day's work in one of the myriad storage spaces Grini's inmates had skillfully located about the prison—in the main drain opening into the furnace room; in pipe shafts; in hollowed-out table tops, legs, and shelves; and in floors, ceilings, and walls of all buildings in the prison camp. None of the periodic searches uncovered the diary or any other important document stored by prisoners during Nansen's confinement in Grini.

Transport of diary entries from the prison to Kari Nansen was also simple, for the Grini underground had organized a plethora of avenues able to accommodate slender sheets of tiny writing—whether a page or two of Odd Nansen's diary or an urgent message to the Home Front.

Concealment in the double bottom of a match-box, within a rolled cigarette paper, or surrounded by the piping being taken into Oslo for repair kept the precious papers from Nazi eyes. Mail and parcels flowed in both directions, as key inmates among the "builders" accompanied their warders into Oslo to collect construction materials for the prison.

Norwegians from all walks of life were thrust into the large dark barracks that added to Grini's capacity during the Occupation, criminals and political prisoners alike. Criminals were quickly outnumbered by loyal Norwegians, for felons were released on completing their sentences. Few of those imprisoned for any role in the Resistance regained their freedom as long as the Nazis held sway. Captives who departed were usually dispatched to concentration camps in Germany—the fate of all Jews as well as those who earned their captors' displeasure for any reason. Some were transferred from the makeshift prison dispensary to Ullevål Hospital in Oslo for more sophisticated medical treatment. Occasional suicides or natural deaths cast an air of depression about the prison camp, but when one or more of their Norwegian comrades was driven through the gates in a closely guarded van in the darkness of night to face the execution squad at Akershus or Trandum, comrades left behind only stiffened their resolve to continue to oppose the Nazis.

Lauritz Sand, "Norway's most tortured man," was an ever-present symbol. Still today, Norwegians repeat with admiration that every bone in his body was broken, yet he would not yield. Between torture sessions Sand would lie in pain, covered with bandages, yet calmly puff at his pipe, and await his next encounter with Gestapo barbarians. His spirit was never broken, his resolve never faltered, and his humor persisted. Sand was moved to tears, however, when Lord Chamberlain Broch—like Nansen, held hostage in the prison—thanked him in King Haakon's name, assuring the tortured patriot that what he had done would never be forgotten.

Although barbarism was the rule at Grini, the brutality of *Møllergata 19* was unparalleled. Odd Nansen described the arrival of Martin Strandli:

> He has been seven weeks in *Møllergata*. He came here along with thirty-five others from the same place. He has had a hideous time, has been whipped and tortured and looks deplorable. When he caught sight of me he was quite agitated; he had to come up and put his arms round me, and the tears stood in his eyes. It was easy to see how strongly it affected him to come here and suddenly find himself among comrades. He wouldn't tell a great deal, but by degrees one got enough out of him to form a picture of all he has gone through. They whipped him with steel springs until he

could neither stand nor walk. They did it time after time to make him
speak. But he didn't speak. Now they must have given it up. To him Grini
seems a mountain sanatorium pure and simple. We are looking after him
as well as we can. He had got a job as building foreman here in the office,
and yesterday he moved into our hut to take the place of Hofmo, who was
sent to Germany. In a while we shall get him back in trim all right, and
make him forget some of the deviltry.[4]

Communication, the lifeblood of the Resistance, flourished within
Grini, nourished by the resourcefulness of the patriot prisoners. Word
of mouth was easily passed within single barracks rooms, but reaching
between floors and into the seclusion of the *Einzelhaft*, the string of
solitary confinement cells, required ingenuity. Odd Nansen, together with
an old friend, Fridtjof Legvamb, and a young student, Ola Bonnevie,
formed their "illicit company" in order to communicate throughout the
prison during the dark of night. Using the Grini hospital as a base, with the
complicity of the hospital physician, Dr. Halvorsen, a prisoner himself,
they created a system of "string mail" to penetrate throughout the prison,
even into the *Einzelhaft*.

The prison hospital, or *Revier*, occupied the second floor of the center
block as well as the entire third floor of the north wing. Strings were
stretched over the prison facade from the *Revier* to connect every level
of the building, down to *Einzelhaft* on the lower floor. The system
worked smoothly and undetected for "Germans are the stupidest of God's
creatures," according to Odd Nansen. He wrote:

> At this moment they're rushing about the square and through the passages
> with tommy guns and all kinds of murderous equipment, God knows
> on what account, while we, "the illicit company," sit here in the "closet,"
> silently and behind locked doors, writing our dispatches to the south and
> north wing and out into the world, undisturbed and in complete security.
> Moreover our "consignments" have been going undisturbed up and down
> the facade and on all our inscrutable paths, while the Germans bluster and
> carry on and "see and hear everything."[5]

Within the *Einzelhaft* communication was still simpler, for a small
hole at floor level led into the ventilation channels. By lying on the floor
and either speaking into or placing the ear beside the air hole, clearly
audible conversations could be carried on between cells.

The cells in the *Einzelhaft*—originally intended for solitary confinement—were kept to overflowing with "misbehaving" Norwegians, individuals considered most dangerous, and unfortunates awaiting execution.

Odd Nansen shared a cell with his friends, Alf Erikstad and Dr. Leif Poulsson, as they awaited transport to the concentration camp at Sachsenhausen for their "indiscretion."

Grini's residents developed a camaraderie and a cohesiveness that sustained them throughout the five years of the Occupation. For a nation's capital, Oslo was a relatively small city with an extraordinarily stable population of less than four hundred thousand. Many prisoners had shared friendships even before confinement, and others were well known by reputation. The inmates learned quickly who was reliable.

The Grini "Society" centered upon individual barracks, but on Sundays and special occasions, it spread out into "entertainments," the unofficial gatherings that took place in the chapel—or in very unusual circumstances, out-of-doors. Political discussions had little place, but the prisoners avidly awaited whatever news of the war that could be collected from underground newspapers. Lectures occupied virtually every night in Odd Nansen's barracks. At times Nansen spoke of architecture, the painter Per Krogh of art, and Norway's eminent pianist, Robert Riefling, of music. Otherwise Francis Bull, professor of literature, was the speaker.

Evenings combined serious learning with light-heartedness—blending children's games with knowledge. In one such game every prisoner wrote a lecture topic on a slip of paper then each blindly drew a subject. After two minutes of concentration the speaker stood to deliver his address. To complicate the delivery, at times the lecturer was required to complete his presentation standing on one foot. It became a challenge to the small group to select a subject in literature, philosophy, or the arts that would stump Francis Bull. The challenge inevitably led to failure. No subject was found upon which the learned Bull could not speak fluently although balancing on one foot.

During holidays and those times ordinarily calling for national celebration, the entertainments held special significance—none more important than in March 1942, when Norway's teachers streamed into Grini following their refusal to join the Nazified Teachers' Union and teach their students the tenets of Nazism.

On Sunday, March 29, 1942, the prison commandant, *Obersturmführer* Koch, reminded the teachers of their families and, as Odd Nansen recorded, "uttered the most barefaced threats of what would happen to *them* if they didn't join. They were to do it singly. He would have no joint action, thank you. Now they could think it over, each for himself, until nine o'clock on Monday. After that it would be irrevocably too late."[6]

That Sunday evening the teachers were special guests at the traditional Sunday entertainment. The abundant program varied from uproarious humor to discussions of the utmost seriousness. As usual Francis Bull's lecture was climactic. When he spoke of Ibsen's *Brand* and *Peer Gynt*, listeners had not the slightest doubt that teachers were the target. Peer Gynt was not difficult to understand, Bull instructed his audience, for Ibsen's character deluded himself and lied to others. Brand, the driven, single-minded cleric was another matter, for Bull had never been able to endure him. He had always appeared hard, detestable, uncompromising, and uncooperative. He had treated his wife and the child who had died badly. "But *now* I understand him!," Francis Bull concluded. "Brand had to go through his difficulties—where Peer Gynt went around his."[7] Bull's meaning was crystal clear. He had made his point through literature, and the teachers followed Bull's "directive."

As effective as were the lectures and discussions, it was to music and poetry that the Grini Society turned for sustenance whenever prison stresses became intolerable and when special solace was needed. Robert Riefling was denied access to a piano, but song substituted until the noted violinist Robert Andersen was imprisoned in March 1942. "Also we had Robert Andersen on the program for the first time," Odd Nansen wrote:

> He has got his violin in, and he played superbly. It was an experience to hear good music again. The sight of that eminent musician in prison dress and slippers, standing there on the table before the world's most superb audience, and playing Norwegian melodies until there was not a dry eye, made it an experience never to be forgotten. Tired and worn, the prisoners sat there, after ten hours' hard labor in wood and fields, in ditches, quarries, and workshops, and they listened. That little time in the church became a tonic rest for mind and soul, and in the roar of applause that went up to the church roof there was genuine gratitude, a deep, unifying sense of the significance of the hour.[8]

Occasionally an entertainment could be held in the corridor of the *Revier* with patients placed outside their rooms. At one such performance the "stage" was set just outside Lauritz Sand's room. Looking through the doorway, Nansen perceived a figure propped up on pillows that more resembled Sand's ghost than the man himself.

> A white-haired, emaciated old man, staring in front of him and sucking mechanically at the pipe he could just hold onto with the hand that was free from bandages and plaster. . . .
>
> Thus I slowly recognized him, feature by feature. It was actually the Sand I knew, the Sand I had lunched with almost daily last spring and summer. Last summer he was going around brisk and springy. Now he

was a broken old man; his eyes sat deep in his skull; his cheeks had fallen
in; his neck and chin had dried up and contracted. I saw that he could not
move. The only living thing about him was the eyes, deep down in their
sockets. I don't know what the gangsters have done to him, and I don't
want to ask. It must be an atrocious thing that can change a man so. His
arm was broken in two places, all the fingers of his right hand were out of
joint, his whole body seemed one affliction. He got part of this treatment
at the "Terrasse," part of it here. And it is known who are guilty. I don't
know how I managed to perform this evening, only that I got up in my turn
and repeated "Norsk Sang," by Collett Vogt, to Sand and to Sand alone,
and tried to put into it all I felt he was a martyr for. I had such a desire
to tell him right out that I was burning with pride to be his countryman.
But there was a guard standing motionless outside his door, and I could
see that he understood Norwegian; he was following the program with his
face. When I had recited that poem, I moved; I couldn't sit any longer
facing Sand's door and looking at him. I was to sing some lively songs for
the patients, and how was I to get through them with Sand before my eyes?
The hell of the German concentration camps is no longer Germany alone.
It makes one shiver to think what may happen before this nightmare is
done with. It is said they told Sand that as soon as he recovers they will
smash him to bits again until he talks.[9]

Beneath the light-heartedness of the games, the frivolities of the
entertainments, and the preoccupation with learning, the specter of death
hung heavily over the Grini Society. Many would leave the prison only to
meet their executioners. Particularly painful were the murders of hostages
and those whose "crime" was attempted escape to England—when the
flight had been underway even before the death decree was official Nazi
policy.

The success of the "export groups"—west coast fishermen and mariners
who ferried fleeing Norwegians across the North Sea to Britain—stirred
the Gestapo to employ the most feared of their weapons: Henry Oliver
Rinnan and his corps of native informers. On February 22, 1942, the
fishing smack *Viggo* lay at anchor just east of Ålesund with a cargo of
twenty-nine loyal Norwegians preparing for escape across the North
Sea to the Shetland Isles. Two Rinnan informers had infiltrated the
export group, and the *Viggo* was ringed by Nazi naval vessels. The entire
group of loyalists was captured. Fifty other Norwegians were arrested for
complicity in the escape effort.

The Gestapo loaded the captured smack with dynamite, towed it to
sea, then detonated the cargo, littering the waters with the *Viggo*'s debris.
One escapee was killed during interrogation, and the others were interned

at Grini, where they became identified as the "Ålesund Group." Odd
Nansen's attachment to one survivor, a young Oslo lad named Jakob
Friis, became particularly strong.

The Ålesund Group had expected the worst—but the end came
suddenly and without trial. Two Gestapo men had been killed in the
west; in reprisal eighteen of the group had been taken from Grini to
Trandum and executed on April 30, 1942. "The name of every man had
been read out," Odd wrote,

> each was like a whiplash, like a stab in the heart, the names of comrades
> with whom we had been living for weeks, had shared food and tobacco, had
> joked and laughed. . . . Comrades we had grown attached to, a rare band
> of stout Norwegians, all between twenty and twenty-five years old. . . .
> Eighteen brave Norwegian lads are no more. Eighteen atrocious murders
> that cry for vengeance. Vengeance! I am afraid that one day vengeance will
> be executed and that no one can prevent its happening. No one can prevent
> it, God help us all.[10]

Odd Nansen was shattered as he thought of his young friend and the
many opportunities Jakob Friis had had for escape. Friis let his chances
pass, for *Obersturmführer* Koch had let it be known that ten to twelve
prisoners would be shot for a single escapee. Now Friis was dead.

Just two days after the foul murders, Odd Nansen was summoned to
the quarters of *Zugwachtmeister* Tauber. The distraught German, who
was not yet dressed, explained he had a message for Nansen, passed on
by Jakob Friis, just before his execution. Tauber had been ordered to the
Eastern Front, and felt compelled to deliver the message before leaving.

> Tears came to the man's eyes. . . . Jakob had known the last two hours he
> was going to be shot and had entrusted him the *Zugwachtmeister* with a
> message of thanks for everything and a radiant reassurance of the certainty
> they all felt that Norway would be free again. . . . It had been a good time
> among their friends at Grini. I was to tell them all and thank them. . . .
>   "I've felt this more than you realize," [Tauber] said, "but war is terri-
> ble . . . I hope too with all my heart that one day you'll set Norway free,
> and that you'll be free men again. Free Norwegians in a free Norway, just
> as he wished."[11]

Nansen did not remember the parting, for he had an overwhelming
need to be alone with his thoughts. He did recall, however, that the two
"enemies" had parted as friends.

In September 1941, eighteen young Norwegians from the West Coast
village of Jaeren had made two attempts to cross the North Sea to

Britain. On both occasions motor problems ended the journeys early. The story of the failed flights leaked out, however, and finally reached the ears of a Gestapo agent. As a result, one of the ringleaders, Arne Vigre, was arrested on October 16. His seventeen companions, along with seven youths who had helped with preparations, were soon taken as well. When Odd Nansen began his own imprisonment in January 1942, their sentences had not yet been determined.

Not until May did the twenty-six youths from Jaeren come to trial. The prosecution demanded death for the eighteen who had actually attempted the crossing. Ludicrously, death twice over was demanded for six of those. "They can only shoot us once," responded one of the accused. Fifteen years at hard labor was proposed for the seven who had aided the attempt. Leif Rode argued for the defense that the decree under which the Norwegians were tried had not yet been passed at the time of the offense. The guilty verdict and sentencing was preordained, no matter the logic and brilliance of the defense—prosecutor and judge were one and the same. One of the eighteen escaped the firing squad—to be sentenced only to prison on the basis of his youth.

At supper on May 8, Robert Andersen approached Odd Nansen. Anton Bø, one of the condemned, wished some words with him. Nansen was never to forget the conversation through the tiny opening in Anton's cell as he prepared for death.

> I only got out a word or two. It wasn't as if he needed anything; he was the one with something to give. And it wasn't the hectic speech of a doomed man, with nerves unstrung, and judgement disorganized nor a strained effusion got by heart. No, it was a sedate man's plain, tranquil thoughts, for which he found concise, good expressions. When I asked if there wasn't any message I could take from him or anything at all I could do for him he only said, "No, all of us have everything worked out and settled so just let them know the truth. We'll get through it fine! We won't so much as blink! Say that from us, Nansen!"
>
> Later that evening Bø wrote his thoughts on a scrap of paper: *To him that finds this. Please write a letter home to all my brothers and sisters and dad and mother and say the truth that I took it quite calm, and put what's right besides. The address home is Ole K. Bø. Naerbø, Jaeren*
>
> *And one to my dear lass, I have gone with her about three years so it's not good to part like this, so write the truth it was for Norway. The address is Frk. Berta Halland, Hognestad, Jaeren.*
> *Anton Bø*
>
> Anton had written on the opposite side: *For our liberty and laws for Norway's sake it was. That Norway will be free though we fall all of us in here*

are full sure of that, and a day of reckoning will come and we all hope them
that are left will settle up the right way where it's wanted. (an illegible word)
The worst I see these days is the women, they walk about in the court yonder,
they walk about and laugh at us as we sit waiting for our death sentence but
they are forgiven for my part, for you know the woman fell first in paradise and
yet was forgiven. Then we are sure and certain of our God and put all trust in
him. Good luck to all them that are coming over, tell them not to go to work like
these here.

                    Anton, Naerbø, born 29/9, 1922[12]

Robert Andersen had suggested he play the violin, and the victims'
comrades in prison sing outside the cells of the doomed men.

"After my conversation with Bø," Odd Nansen wrote,

> Robert began to play, and it was grand. I'm sure that none who were
> there will be able to forget that concert in the passage outside the con-
> demned mens' room. One behind another down both sides of the passage
> their comrades stood in silence. And there behind the door they were
> sitting, close together doubtless, to hear better, and still, dead still! I sang
> a couple of songs, for I had promised Anton. Now I was almost repenting;
> I felt I couldn't get through it, but the second song didn't go too badly; I
> recovered my strength and calm, which for a while had left me completely.
> For that was just after the conversation with Anton, and I could think of
> nothing else, But I was glad I sang all the same; perhaps it gave the men
> inside there a little pleasure at any rate, a reminder of their comrades and
> our evenings down in the church and of the time gone by, which after all
> had been bright and good.
>
> Robert played again: "Ola, Ola—I Lay Down So Late," then at the end
> "God Bless Thee, Norway, My Fair Land!" We stood bolt upright while
> Robert played through these verses. We dared not join in, it was forbidden,
> it could only spoil things for everyone, for the men inside as well, but the
> words burnt into our hearts just the same, and Norway can never have
> received a finer, more thrilling tribute than when the men in there struck
> up the national anthem.
>
> They were not singers, and they began too high, so that it went right up
> into falsetto, but never have I been more affected by that glorious hymn.
> It was as if I hadn't known it until then. Every time I hear it again I shall
> think of the stalwart young Norwegians who sang it in the death cell and
> who put their souls into it, all they had to live for.[13]

The sentence was carried out on May 21, 1942.

Three other Norse patriots—Birkevold, Svae, and Fraser—were even
more daring than passengers on the Shetland Bus. They made off with
a German motorboat at Jeløy and set their course for England. Luck

was against them, for the vessel ran aground off the coast of Denmark. Birkevold, who had led the escapade, was imprisoned at Grini, then became a patient in the *Revier* with a fever apparently induced by Dr. Sven Oftedal.

"Birkevold was lying out in the hospital corridor last night, listening to our entertainment," Nansen noted.

> I waved to him. He smiled back, but he was a different man from when I last saw him. His mates have been condemned to death. Svae managed to escape, indeed, but Fraser is sitting waiting, yonder in Akershus. And here lies Birkevold, waiting to be condemned in his turn. He is ill; he has a fever, and never surely has a fever that will not yield been more blessed than this one. May it only last both spring and summer, yes, and far into the autumn for safety's sake. This is his one chance. For it doesn't seem as though they condemn sick people, at all events not yet. One fine day they will probably discover that they can shoot a sick man just as well as a sound one. Birkevold must be lying thinking such thoughts too, poor lad.[14]

The infirmary at Grini was a refuge to Norwegians suffering from physical abuse, compounded by the malnutrition and the indignities of prison life under the brutal Nazis. The *Revier* gave respite to the tortured, rest to the exhausted, and healing to the ill, the undernourished, and the troubled. Norwegian physicians at Grini aided their country's cause by playing upon the ignorance of their captors, and the Nazis' irrational fear of infection that infested the Nazis. Jailers shunned the infirmary unless forced to enter, and then rushed in for the necessary business and out in the shortest possible time. The isolation building, where Dr. Leif Poulsson was in charge, struck particular terror into the guards.

Early in his imprisonment Nansen was provided a room adjoining the tuberculosis ward—known as *Tubben* (The Tub)—as an office for an architectural project he was assigned. Commonly he worked late, or stayed in the office to read away from the congested prison barracks. On one such occasion he telephoned the guard at half past ten, asking to be let out so he could return to his sleeping quarters. The German appeared two hours later—only to find he had brought the wrong key, one fitting the far door of the building, the entrance to the tuberculosis ward. The unhappy guard was forced to traverse the ward before unlocking the door to Nansen's office. The German, as Nansen described,

> came running down the middle corridor and unlocked the lobby door.
> "Hurry. For heaven's sake! At once. *Sacramento*! Aren't you ready yet?"

He was behaving like a madman. I did not realize why until we got outside; then in a gasping voice, he asked me if I thought it was dangerous to go through the tuberculosis ward. He was brushing himself all over and repeated his question when I asked what he meant. He was exasperated by my stupidity and roared. "Don't you understand anything man? Its tuberculosis ! Tuberculosis!" He was in deadly terror of catching it. He had held his breath as well as he could while he was in there, and was now busy brushing off all the germs. On my asking whether he was positive or negative, he disclosed that he had not the faintest idea of what that might be. He only knew that tuberculosis was something frightful, something one died slowly of. I gave up trying to explain anything to this bold warrior. He was too German and stupid.[15]

Despite the small dangers of contracting the disease, the most desirable job of all for any Norwegian inmate of Grini prison was "washing up" in "The Tub." The duties were light—mopping the floor in the small ward and a little dishwashing after the patients' mealtime. The remainder of the day was free, for panicky fears kept the guards away. When inspections were required two Germans would storm through the room, and if one happened to dawdle, the second would shout "*Los Mensch! Los! Achtung! Tuberculose Mensch! Los! Los!*" When Einar Skavlan, the incumbent attendant in *Tubben*, was transferred to Ullevål Hospital for treatment of his own illness, the position fell to the most senior of Grini's inmates, Francis Bull. For Professor Bull it was more than just respite from the rigors of prison labor; it was the opportunity to compose his Grini lectures for publication after the war ended.

In his earliest months Odd Nansen enjoyed favored treatment, such as it was at Grini. The Germans had need of architectural skills in planning and constructing quarters to house the growing numbers of Norwegians kept captive. With his architect friend, Frode Rinnan, Nansen provided those skills. He was assigned space for an "office," access to writing materials, and the opportunity for occasional travel into Oslo to obtain building supplies or supervise their unloading. Nansen despised the company of the *Nasjonal Samling* interpreter Møller on those trips. Although the quisling attempted to curry his favor, Nansen refused to ask anything of the Norwegian Nazi. He'd accept the presence of his warders for "a German guard is something quite different. It is somehow cleanlier to accept understanding from one of them. But when Møller, the 'Norwegian,' the *NS* man and traitor, winks understandingly and thinks himself very fine for 'allowing' me to have ten cigarettes, then I feel sick."[16]

Nansen managed to obtain a huge coat, which he stuffed with cigarettes and provisions from family and friends on each journey into Oslo.

The smuggling, though obvious, was overlooked by German drivers and guards as he returned to Grini. Whenever Møller was along, the "sick feeling" kept Nansen from even caring about smuggling. On May 11, 1942, prisoners were forbidden travel into Oslo for any purpose.

On May 21, 1942, the day of the execution of the young Norwegians from Jaeren, Nansen lost another segment of his favored status. He was summoned to the office of *Lagerkommandant* (camp commander) Denzer who shoved a paper with the following text before Odd's face:

Proud sons of Norway, met
　From the lathe, the plough, and the net,
　Mountain and sea and shore,
　Classroom, office, and store,
　High and low from shacks or stately homes, and yet
　Chips of the same block
　The same old tough Norwegian saga stock,
　All of the same strain,
　Of the same grain,
　The same clear faith in heart and brain,
　Here we are Norwegians with prison numbers all;
　None of us are grandees and none of us are small;
　Lofty and low, (Pot-bellies too),
　Young men and nimble and graybeards and all:
　Join the throng
　In a common song!
　Grini nursing home will crown
　With a halo of its own
　Norway's long renown.
　Norway let us sing!
　Let all voices ring
　For our liberty, our laws,
　Our mother-wit still as it was,
　For justice and its cause![17]

It was the poetry he had written as lyrics for another prisoner's composition, Harris Norman Olsen's "Grini March." Denzer questioned Nansen briefly, suggesting that both Odd and Fridtjof Nansen had been Communists. When Odd insisted the two had only been humanists and never Communists, the prison commandant began to read the poem as it had been translated into German, for Denzer had no command of Norwegian. Nansen thought it sounded splendid—far better than in Norwegian as he had tired of hearing it hummed about Grini. In a continuing tirade, Odd Nansen was informed he was "not worthy of the favors you've enjoyed in this camp." He was placed in solitary confinement while the Germans deliberated his fate.

Eight days later, Nansen was allowed back again into the mainstream of Grini life. The Germans needed his skills, and he was again provided with an architectural office.

When more than a year had passed all court hostages other than Odd Nansen had been released. He was still held, Nansen was certain, because of his ceaseless efforts on behalf of the Jews and because of Vidkun Quisling's animosity. More than once he overheard veiled references in German to both Quisling and Nansen Relief when he was about the prison office. The autumn of 1943 marked the end of Nansen's imprisonment in Norway, and the beginning of concentration camp life in Germany.

A practical joke in the prison infirmary was the undoing of Odd Nansen and Leif Poulsson at Grini. Johannes Seiersted Bødtker, a Norwegian prisoner who functioned as barracks chief in the infirmary, also censored the outgoing mail to be certain no "illegal" information or contraband was included. His Norse colleagues discovered that the censor amused himself in the evenings by reading the most intimate love letters sent by young prisoners to their sweethearts.

Led by Nansen and Poulsson, and aided by Dr. Fretheim and Alf Erikstad, a young architectural student, the inmates decided to make Bødtker pay for his voyeuristic curiosity. Lauritz Sand, though still a patient, had recovered sufficiently to take pleasure in a good prank, and joined in willingly. Sand had lived in Indonesia for forty years before the war, and the pranksters had him write a letter in Malay to his wife. Interspersed with the exotic language were the Norwegian words, "barracks-chief" and "Seiersted Bødtker," followed immediately by Malay script that could be colloquially translated as "who can, for that matter, kiss my arse." Shortly thereafter a paragraph in Norwegian reported that now it had become quiet comfortable in Grini. Most patients had hidden radio receivers in their pillows, and the prisoners had installed a short wave radio transmitter in the refrigerator with direct connections to London and Stockholm. Besides, many had rifles and machine pistols sewn into their mattresses. This shocking "disclosure" was followed by a long section in Malay to the effect that his mother had been a monkey in Batavia, and his father had been a tomcat in Havana of Siamese extraction, and was well versed in the jungle that surrounded us. The letter concluded with salutations in an admixture of Norwegian and Malay.[18]

Bødtker was marvelously amused at the letter, so much so that he had concealed it in the drawer of his nightstand. The prank would long have been the source of amusement among Norwegian prisoners had it not been for the Nazi practice of infiltrating Grini's ranks with informers like the German "prisoner" Fischermann. The "Zebra," as Fischermann was nicknamed by the Norwegian inmates, had free run of the prison and pried everywhere. He rummaged through Bødtker's night-stand and became completely crazed after being taken in by Sand's letter. He overturned every chest and cabinet in the infirmary and emptied every drawer to find more contraband. These were caricatures of the "master race"—the German prison officials in Grini. The sketches had been ordered from Odd Nansen by the Nazis themselves for use in the *Kameradenschaftabend* (fellowship evening) when they ate, drank, and as Odd Nansen wrote, "amused themselves by making bloody fools of one another."

From his havoc in the infirmary, Fischermann passed on to the tuberculosis ward, where he threw out Dr. Poulsson and Francis Bull before discovering all Bull's manuscripts. Odd Nansen attempted to reassure his distraught friend, reminding him that the manuscripts were purely literary lectures, of which the Germans would certainly understand very little.

"Yes, but you understand," Bull replied, "I had written a foreword also, and there I had explained everything!"

Nansen could not help but exclaim, "But Good God, Francis, why couldn't you have waited for the foreword until later? Did you not think, perhaps, that you would not remember everything—exactly as you remember it today?"

"Yes, perhaps," Bull responded cheerfully, "But they can do no worse than kill me."[19]

Francis Bull's "cheerful" prediction never materialized, but disaster descended upon Odd Nansen, Leif Poulsson, and Alf Erikstad.

The informer's discovery was passed upward, treating Sand's spoof as fact, until it reached *Reichskommissar* Joseph Terboven himself. On the following day the inmates assembled on the parade grounds saw Terboven arrive in his gleaming Mercedes. He was accompanied by *Obergruppenführer* Wilhelm Redeiss, chief of the SS in Oslo, and Heinrich Fehlis, chief of the German security police in Norway. They were followed by assorted Gestapo and SS officers, several hundred troops, and finally an armed execution squad.

While the prisoners stood at attention on the parade grounds the Nazi soldiers searched from the lowest cellar floor to the topmost rafter without finding so much as an empty cartridge shell.

The presumed "ringleaders," including Odd Nansen, Francis Bull, Alf Erikstad, Bødtker, Dr. Poulsson, and Dr. Fretheim, were arrested. They were placed standing with their faces to the wall in the corridor outside Denzer's office, in preparation for the military trial to follow when all the material was assembled. Lauritz Sand, still too crippled to leave his bed, was questioned by Redeiss and a military judge. Redeiss threatened Sand with execution if he failed to reveal the entire truth. Of course, Redeiss said, they would not find it difficult to translate the Arabic in which Sand had written. They knew all languages!

"But, it is written in Malay, perhaps it would be simplest and most practical if I translated it myself," the amused Sand replied.[20] Thereupon, gravely serious, Lauritz Sand translated, while equally seriously, the judge transcribed the account that the cautious barracks-chief, Seiersted Bødtker, who didn't dare kill a fly, could kiss his arse. Further that his mother had been a monkey in Batavia and his father a tomcat in Havana . . .

At that point the door to the room where the "miscreants" were standing opened with a crash, an orderly entered, and with the clicking of heels announced that the *Reichskommissar* would depart. The comedy had ended, but Denzer's insane fury had just begun. He had been made a laughingstock in front of his superiors as well as German troops and prisoners. His days as commandant were numbered, but his revenge was immediate. Francis Bull, as a non-participant, was sentenced only to fourteen days on the "stone gang," then deprived of his job in Tubben. Nansen, Poulsson, and Erikstad as ringleaders received the bulk of the Nazi commander's ire. Nansen would no longer be treated as a hostage, but rather as an ordinary political prisoner, as he was he would be sent to a place from which he would never come back. He should only ask his friends to raise his tombstone at once.

In the meantime Nansen, Poulsson, and Erikstad were to share a cell in the *Einzelhaft*, as Nansen described in his diary:

> There the two (guards) had some private fun using Leif's head as a "punching ball." Until they were quite sated they had gone on taking turns to punch his face and head, the form and color of which were gradually modified by this Germanic pastime. They then handed him over to Porky, who promptly dispatched him in to me. And here we were sitting and laughing on the floor of the dark cell. But there was nothing to laugh at really. Our trip to Germany was assured, and Denzer's dark threats and prophecies did not exactly hold a cheerful prospect for the future.
>
> However, before we had sunk very deep in contemplation heavy foot-steps were again heard out in the corridor, and immediately afterward the rattling of keys in the lock.
>
> This time it was Erikstad who was shot in as we had been. Poor lad, he was quite bewildered with the doing he had had. His arms flew mechanically up to his face, as though to guard it from further depredations

when Porky, not omitting the usual ceremonies, shut the door with a crash. And indeed his face could not have stood much more if it was to go on reminding one of Alf Erikstad. . . .

As we sat gaping at each other, there came a rap on the wall from the next cell. I put my ear to the wall and heard a faint, faraway voice calling something about the air hole. The air hole? What on earth did he mean? Suddenly I remembered that of course the air holes and ventilation channel were the Einzelhaft's telephone system, and I got down onto the floor and laid my head against the air hole. A voice sounded clearly and distinctly, as though it were in the same room.

"Hullo?"

"Hullo!"

"Is that Fredrik? This is Harald! Who are you?"

I explained who we were and why we were there. The voice explained, "The cell you are in is called Fredrik, mine is Harald. Are you on bread and water?" I was able to say we were, for Denzer had pronounced so.

"Well," came Harald's voice again, "then we'll collect on the house front at eleven tonight." He got no further for the contact was interrupted by heavy steps and key-rattling far down the corridor. We looked at each other in astonishment. What on earth did he mean by "collecting on the house front?" What did he mean to collect? We were mystified, and eager for the night which was to solve the riddle. . . .

. . . It wasn't long before there came a rap on the wall, and we hastened to the air hole. "Hullo, Hullo!" It was Harald calling Fredrik, with the following instructions: "When I give two raps on the wall, go to the window, climb up and stand on the ledge. You raise the top window and stretch out your left arm as far as you can along the wall in our direction, then you'll just be able to reach a pole with a sock hanging from it, which we'll reach out to you. In the sock you'll find bread and potatoes, collected from all the cells on this side of the floor. Be cautious and put everything off if you hear the danger signal. The danger signal is three knocks on the wall. Good night and good appetite."

Such, in all simplicity, was the collection on the house front. The stick with the sock began its wanderings in the far cell nearest the center block and passed from cell to cell. Notice had been given in advance that there were three comrades in Fredrik on bread and water who needed food, and then all were ready to give their mite. Fredrik was the last cell but one in the wing, and when we heard the two raps on the wall and the instructions had been successfully carried out, we had a well-filled sock to help ourselves from. We woke Erikstad, and I can tell you we enjoyed the meal. None of us had had any dinner, and we blessed our new and unknown friends as their benefaction of sandwiches and potatoes vanished quickly into our lean stomachs.[21]

22. Through the Hospitals to Safety

No matter the closeness and the ingenuity of the Grini Society, attempts to escape the prison were close to nonexistent. Resistance operatives under threat of execution, and those carrying information vital to the Home Front were guarded with extraordinary diligence. If prisoners outwitted their jailers, the Norwegians left behind were certain to face cruel and barbarous Nazi wrath, designed to escalate the price of escape far beyond the gain. Execution of a dozen was promised for the escape of one. In response the underground developed simple and effective means of passing vital information to the outside, and paved an efficient road to safety through Oslo's physicians and hospitals.

Dr. Bjørn Foss was a common conduit between prisoners and the Home Front, passing important knowledge in both directions.[1] Foss, well known to the Nazis through his role in the medical division of civil defense, was considered "dependable" by the occupying forces throughout the war. He was thus called upon to treat any significant ophthalmologic problem among the prisoners, for the Germans had very special concerns about the eyes. Foss's particular technique made certain those problems would occur. Mercury ointment smuggled into the prison produced a raging, but temporary ocular inflammation. When patients were brought into his office under heavy guard Foss claimed his dark room was essential for the examination, because equipment within just could not be moved.

That pretext provided Halvard Lange, a member of The Circle, his opportunity for a family visit. Lange's wife had just given birth, and he longed to see the beloved pair. As Lange entered Foss's office, under heavy guard, not only did he discover his wife and child in the waiting room, but his mother and sister as well.

The simple subterfuge could not endure forever. Dark room space was too cramped to accommodate patient, doctor, and guard, forcing German soldiers to stand sentinel at the doorway during every examination. The dark room window, small as it was, allowed lean and agile Norwegians to squeeze through. Foss, in apparent distress, convinced the inquisitors that he too was an innocent victim after a Home Front prisoner escaped as sentries stood patiently at their post. Office examinations of prison patients were allowed to continue—appointments, however, were made only through the Gestapo. Both the door and window to the dark room were then scrupulously guarded. Nevertheless, during an "examination" of Major Halfdan Haneborg Hansen, chief of *Milorg*'s eastern district, information on the Home Front's plan for the major's rescue was transmitted.

After Hansen's escape suspicion once again fell on Bjørn Foss, who was summoned by the Gestapo. As he said later, "God was good." Foss was released, but from that moment office visits were excluded and the ophthalmalogist was compelled to travel to the prisons to see his patients. There, ophthalmoscope in hand, he would still lean over, forehead to forehead with his patient, and exchange information.

Although Foss's office served only once as an escape route, hospitals provided pathways to safety again and again. Norway's doctors fabricated pretexts to transfer prisoners to the hospital, then often cooperated in further steps to freedom. The primitive bacteriology laboratory Dr. Haakon Natvig established during his brief tenure at Grini was intended by his Nazi captors to serve only the needs of the prison infirmary. Natvig had his own motives, however.[2] Carefully he propagated cultures of pathogenic organisms from prisoners with gastrointestinal complaints, from the mildest to those with typhoid or dysentery. He culled the organisms of diphtheria from the throats of the afflicted, and even cultured the dreaded botulinus in tubes devoid of oxygen. All were put to good use except botulinus—for the deadly toxin gave too little margin of error. Even minor illness was enough to send paroxysms of fear of infectious disease galloping through the Nazi jailers. The "afflicted" were hastily transferred to the prison ward at Ullevål Hospital. On occasion, after ox-blood was smuggled into the prison, the designated prisoner would drink, then regurgitate the blood before his startled captors. The solicitous prisoner-doctor would diagnose a bleeding ulcer. "Anxious over the patient's survival," he would recommend the hospitalization that would inevitably follow.

Hospital escape carried neither the risks nor the penalties involved in flight from prison. Rather than the fanatical SS or Gestapo that staffed *Viktoria Terrasse* and the jails, German conscripts policed the hospitals. They had little desire to endanger their own lives when confronted by armed Norwegians, and security was lax.

Well-planned escapes were at times ridiculously simple as in the case of Major Hansen.[3] With other district *Milorg* leaders, he was betrayed by an informer, and early in January 1942 was arrested and imprisoned. Interrogation took its toll, and his physical condition deteriorated. The major's wife received word through Bjørn Foss that Hansen would be transferred to *Rikshospitalet* and that his escape had been scrupulously planned. Hansen's freedom was of critical importance to the underground. Not only could he identify *Milorg* members of whom the Nazis were unaware, but he knew who had been identified and placed in immediate danger.

Shortly after the major's admission to *Rikshospitalet* a black limousine bearing the license plates of Gulbrand Lunde, the *Nasjonal Samling* chief of information and propaganda, drew near the hospital gates. The German sentinels had no way of knowing the vehicle was stolen, the license plates forged, and both the uniformed chauffeur and the young civilian seated in the back beside Mrs. Hansen were *Milorg* operatives. Within minutes, Hansen left his sick bed and walked quietly down the stairs, out the door, and over to the small rear gate in the high wall surrounding *Rikshospitalet.* He found the gate locked. Despite his physical state, he clambered over the barbed wire-topped barrier and strode to the waiting car. As the black vehicle drove southward Hansen revealed all he knew to the *Milorg* agent, who then alighted at Moss to warn all those he had learned were imperilled. The limosine carried the freed Major to safety.

Foss himself took part in the action that freed Peder Holst from Drammen Hospital, sixty miles south of Oslo. The young student, who had operated a clandestine wireless transmitter for the British Secret Service, had been shot in the leg during an encounter with the Gestapo. The underground supplied Foss with a Norwegian police car and aides. Foss then pulled up to the hospital with blue lights flashing. It was a simple matter to locate the prisoner. A cooperative nurse led Foss to find Holst in the bath. The unsuspicious guards were readily disarmed, then locked in a room. Blue lights flashing once more, the Norwegians fled to safety.

The infection ruse brought freedom to a member of Parliament, Carl Wright, and three other prisoners who became "ill" after swallowing bacterial cultures.[4] Underground operative Oivind Øwre had easy access to Ullevål, where his physician brother headed a clinical department. Through his brother, Oivind contacted Margit Holthe, chief nurse on the prison ward. Nurse Holthe had complete confidence in the Øwres and, without asking the intent, "borrowed" a Gestapo release order from which an accomplice made copies and prepared the "official" stamp.

Through judicious use of the Gestapo telephone line in the hospital the chief nurse learned how prisoners were transported. The underground then set about preparing false Gestapo license plates, and obtaining the necessary vehicles and Gestapo uniforms. The loyal hospital watchman was brought into the scheme to make certain the electrically operated doors to the prison ward would be open for both entry and exit.

Oivind Øwre and his fellows in the Underground had planned the escape for February 1, 1942, to "celebrate" the date on which Vidkun Quisling was to be named minister-president. It was not until the evening of February 2, however, that all was in readiness. Dr. Øwre then invited the prison ward commandant, Dr. Schenck to dinner, to guarantee his absence. The Austrian physician had been friendly to Norwegians, and the Resistance had no wish to compromise him unnecessarily.

During the dinner hour underground agent Jan Skappel slipped into a telephone kiosk at Bislett, about a quarter mile from Ulleval Hospital. In German he telephoned the prison ward, ordering Holthe to prepare the prisoners for removal by the Gestapo in half an hour. Holthe, still unaware of the plan, protested vigorously. The prisoners were in extremely poor condition, and it was most inadvisable to move them. Skappel ended the conversation, bellowing into the mouthpiece, *"Haben Sie nicht verstanden! Es ist ein Befehl!"* (Haven't you understood it is an order!) Within fifteen minutes two black cars bearing Gestapo license plates left Bislett. Oivind Øwre and Jan Skappel, armed with pistols, stood guard along the fence surrounding the hospital grounds where they cut an opening should the alarm sound and the gates be closed. At the same time Arne Molen, Roar Opsahl, Jan Brambabi, and Vidar Lunde, in full Gestapo regalia, showed their forged credentials and drove the two vehicles through the hospital gates.

As the conspirators reached the prison ward they heard the telephone ring. Although they feared the Gestapo headquarters at *Viktoria Terrasse* might be at the other end of the line, they had gone too far. Suppressing concerns, they reached the patients' room, outside of which an inexperienced guard had been posted. Opsahl's school German was again called into play. *"Es ist die Deutsche Sicherheitspolizei. Wir wollen vier Haftlinge erholen"* (It is the German Security Police. We want to fetch four prisoners). The guard accepted the papers, made "official" by the name of Dr. Schenck stamped at the bottom. The telephone call, the Norwegians discovered, was merely from the gate, announcing the Gestapo arrival. The Resistance agents remained undetected. The four prisoners were collected and ushered into the cars. They disappeared into secret underground lairs with their rescuers. Søster Holthe was summoned for questioning on the following day by three Gestapo agents, but released without harm.

Two hospital escapes had been planned for the day Vidkun Quisling was to be inaugurated as minister-president. Didrik Cappelen was to be freed from Akebergveien prison at the same time the four Norwegians were to be rescued from Ullevål Hospital. Cappelen's release was advanced to January 30, since the Home Front had received indication that Cappelen might be executed earlier than February 1. When both missions were successful and word was passed through the clandestine press, loyal Norwegians rejoiced. Morale that had sagged but a month earlier with the *Milorg* arrests was bolstered once again.

To the Gestapo the most notorious of Home Front agents and saboteurs was unquestionably Max Manus. His capture was to be considered a major coup; not only would a figure of great repute be removed, but Manus was a potential fountain of information on Underground operations and personnel. The Nazi opportunity to tap the fountain was frustrated by the combined action of Ullevål Hospital physicians and nurses with the underground.[5]

Following orders from London, Max Manus had set plans in motion to assassinate Albert Viljam Hagelin, *Nasjonal Samling* minister for domestic affairs. Hagelin, who had lived for many years in Germany as a businessman, had become Vidkun Quisling's advisor and closest confidant. Hagelin's destruction was calculated to strike fear into other cabinet members, and to raise morale among loyal Norwegians.

Manus's assassination plan was simple, but well laid. Manus and a companion would station themselves just within an attic window commanding a view of Gestapo headquarters at *Viktoria Terrasse* about sixty yards away. Hagelin was to be gunned down as he emerged from the doorway. The search for the gunman would be slowed by an accomplice—as if in panic—closing the gate to the building from which the shot had come. In the meantime Max Manus and his companion would vault the fence to the rear of the structure and escape. All Manus required was approval of the plan from London. He had been instructed to meet his contact to pass on the plan on January 17, 1941.

As he entered his apartment on January 16, however, six figures surrounded him, shouting as if in one voice, "State Police." Two rather lame attempts to approach the window in his bedroom or bathroom were unsuccessful. By that time Manus's captors had found his backpack stuffed with incriminating material, including the assassination plans. Manus had no illusions about his fate, so he boastfully pointed to a group of medals hanging on the wall. As the six briefly turned their eyes away, Manus suddenly crashed head-first through the heavy glass window, landing on the cement two floors below.

Max Manus awoke to find himself sitting manacled in a car—then vomited and passed out. He heard two voices as he was trundled along a corridor in Ullevål Hospital. The first insisted he be examined while still handcuffed. The second replied, "It matters very little. He will probably die very shortly."

The examining physician was heard to report the x rays showed a fractured shoulder and a broken back. In addition there was a serious cerebral concussion. The first gruff voice replied, "Very well, then, if he is as bad off as all that put him in a bed and we'll see how he is in the morning."[6]

As he was placed in bed Max Manus motioned his nurse to lean close, then whispered that he was important in the Resistance, and the Nazis should not get hold of him if Norway were ever to be free. The nurse stepped to the door, then returned quickly, saying, "I have sent for the doctor. You must tell him where it hurts. He will be able to help you." Manus understood the signal. When the doctor arrived Manus listed those who were endangered by his capture, and the names were passed on to the Underground. The physician also informed his patient that the injuries were not serious and he would recover in time. The sedatives and analgesics were doing their work, and Manus easily followed instructions to sleep.

When he awoke, Manus found two guards with pistols drawn seated on the edge of his bed. He did his best to vomit on them—but had nothing to bring up but bile. Soon a nurse arrived carrying a printed sign: "ADMISSION STRICTLY FORBIDDEN." The soldiers protested, for Siegfreid Fehmer, chief of the Gestapo in Oslo, had ordered a constant guard. "Fehmer has no authority here. Nor any policeman. I am the head nurse in this hospital and my orders are to be obeyed. This man is going to die. The doctor who examined him has said so. It is not likely he will give the police any more trouble," said the nurse. "Now he is a very sick man and must be treated as one. Since you want to kill him anyway you can at least let him die in peace."[7]

The guards retreated and took their stations outside the room—one on either side of the door. The head nurse blocked their view by covering the opening with a screen. Sentinels remained posted continuously throughout the twenty-seven days of Manus's hospitalization.

When the underground received word of Manus's capture they considered him lost. As did the Nazis they believed a broken back would ultimately prove fatal. Every act of Resistance until the point of his hospitalization was attributed to Max Manus. He became the king-pin of everything "illegal"—plans for assassinations, the underground press, espionage, communications with the government-in-exile, liqui-dation of informers, assisting escape to Sweden, collecting funds for the Home Front, and organizing a guerilla movement. Nothing was beyond his scope.

Once his faculties returned Max Manus found an avenue for escape. His window had been boarded closed as protection against British air strikes. There was, however, a hatch at the top which was opened daily. Manus became convinced he could squeeze through. He devised a scheme that required medical assistance.

Through his usual channel Max Manus sent word of the plan to a friend and underground colleague, Per Jacobsen. The action revolved around the loyal nurse in whom Manus had confided, and a fishing pole she brought into the sick room concealed beneath the full skirts of her nursing uniform. The time was set for 3:00 A.M. the following day.

Manus's doctor suspected some plan was afoot. On surgical rounds, just before noon, he warned his patient, "The police are getting impatient about you. They have been in to tell me that they do not intend to wait until you are well to try you."

At 3:00 A.M. in the dense darkness of the winter night, Max Manus cast his line through the open hatch. No one was there to take his bait. Shaken and "clammy with sweat" Manus waited until the day nurse arrived to inform him what went astray—Jacobsen had been unable to obtain the getaway car.

Two dark mornings later, on March 14, 1941, at the newly appointed time Max Manus cast his line again—and felt an answering tug. Soon he reeled in the heavy rope, and with the help of nurse Astrid Olsen, made it fast to the hospital bed. Nurse Olsen then helped her patient onto the window sill, from where he leaned down, kissed her in gratitude, then struck her soundly on the jaw—as planned—for she must not be connected to the escape.

With his useless right arm hanging free, Manus squeezed through the hatch, wrapped his feet about the rope, and slid to the ground. The snow against his bare feet, and the cold wind whipping through his flimsy hospital gown and his bare back felt good—for they meant freedom. The rope, which Astrid Olsen had untied was gathered up, and once again she concealed the fishing rod beneath her skirts.

Max Manus was given a pistol by his rescuers. Together they ran across the hospital garden, through a hole already cut in the fence, and into the safety of the waiting car. The day nurse was seated in the back and prepared with an injection of stimulants. As the fugitive car drove along Kirkeveien toward Røa some twenty miles away, they heard the sirens of police cars on the way to investigate the escape.

From the outskirts of Røa, Max Manus and a companion skied through the forest. Physically, Manus was hardly prepared for the strenuous journey, but with a stop for brandy, and the drug the nurse had supplied, the two reached the cabin deep among the snow-covered woods.

When the convalescing Manus was left on his own in the forest hut the accumulated tension kept him awake, despite the greatest fatigue he had ever known. He became terrified by the silence within, and felt the Gestapo must be quietly closing in. Max could stand it no longer, and—still not strong enough to walk after the exhausting journey—crawled into the forest, where he spent the day dozing while burrowed in the brush. When darkness fell he crawled back to the hut, muscles aching with every movement, and prepared dinner. Max Manus regained his strength over the ten or twelve days he remained in the hut—the silence broken only by visits of his comrades, and the masseuse brought to help him recondition his muscles.

Back in Røa, on the first leg of his flight to Sweden, Max Manus was startled to see his face on a poster, with a warning underneath beginning: "He will be shot who . . ." The escape through Oslo, then to Hamar, Elverum, Flisa, and through the forest to Sweden was essentially uneventful—although Manus and his guide Andreas Aubert came face to face with Germans all along the way to Flisa.

Max Manus traveled a tortuous route to reach the Norwegian Forces in Great Britain—plane to Helsinki, across Russia to Odessa by train, then by ship to Istanbul, Port Said, and finally England. Manus was then commissioned a first lieutenant in the Norwegian infantry. Greater tasks on behalf of his native land lay ahead.

NORWEGIANS IN NAZI CONCENTRATION CAMPS

23. Leo Eitinger in Auschwitz and Buchenwald

One hundred and fifty-eight Norwegian Jews—men, women, and children—had been herded aboard the *Gotenland* on February 24, 1943.[1] With this second transport Vidkun Quisling had surpassed his master. Except for the scattered few hidden by beneficent protectors and those "lost" among hospital patients, the Norse Nazi had made his country *Judenfrei*. As Leo Eitinger trudged up the gangplank of the murder vessel he nurtured a single, distant hope for survival—the end of the war.[2]

On arrival in Stettin, the human cargo was sent rolling to Berlin— tightly packed in closed freight cars. The Norwegians were gathered in a large synagogue in the German capital where—with two thousand other Jewish captives—they were forced to deed their worldly goods to the Nazi state. In return, they were promised, all their needs would be provided for—until death.

From Berlin the prisoners were loaded aboard another train in groups of fifty packed in cars built to hold eight horses. A single piece of bread supplied to each captive and a single bucket of water for the entire car had to suffice for twenty-four anxious and oppressive hours until the locked cars were opened outside the Buna-Monowitz section of the Auschwitz concentration camp. Women and children were rudely separated from the men and—except for a few young girls—were hustled aboard trucks that were dispatched directly to the gas chambers. Another selection later, all males between twenty and forty, and a few husky eighteen- and nineteen-year-olds, were set to the side to become slave laborers. Among those "privileged" to survive were Leo Eitinger, Robert Weinstein, and Fritz Lustig. The last despairing group of younger boys and older men followed the women's path to extermination.

The Germans made little use of the many prisoner-physicians in their traditional role of relieving human suffering. Shua Eitinger's assignment to the *Revier* (dispensary) of the main camp bore no relation to his medical

211

qualifications. The Nazis had called for a prisoner combining two particular skills—typing and knowledge of the conquerors' tongue. Eitinger's years in German language schools coupled with typing proficiency won him the job that he regarded as his "life's darkest work." In characteristic teutonic orderliness, the camp warders kept index card records of how any prisoner died, whether in the hospital or after an "escape attempt." Eitinger typed those cards.

The description of prisoners said to be fleeing was standard. Each was reported to have been examined and found to be well nourished and, aside from the fatal injury, in good condition. The bullet wounds were always to be found in the back of the head or the shoulder, signifying flight. Notation of any sign of external violence was forbidden. Leo Eitinger's writing table overflowed with new cards daily. The designation "shot while attempting to escape" exceeded all others.

Occasionally Polish prisoners risked flight, for once outside the camp they could expect shelter from patriotic countrymen. Jews, however, were denied refuge beyond the barbed wire. Some attempted to flee as a final means of ending their misery. Others were goaded into flight by camp guards murdering for profit. SS troopers received fifty marks and three days leave for each prisoner shot to death in an actual or feigned escape. Signs of maltreatment or frontal wounds notwithstanding, Shua Eitinger was permitted no deviation in the cards he completed. Every hospital patient was reported to have received extraordinary care—despite which, death was unavoidable.

Auschwitz was efficiently organized for slave labor as well as extermination. All physically able male prisoners worked either in the I. G. Farben factory at Buna or in heavy duty about the camp. The gas chamber or the protection of the hospital were the only alternatives. Each day the sick and the wounded formed a line to be inspected by an SS physician. Those whose ailments would allow return to work within fourteen days were admitted to the *Revier*. All others were quickly dispatched by *Spritz*, an intracardiac injection of carbolic acid.

Hardened Polish prisoners and German criminals, long accustomed to Nazi callousness, laughed at Eitinger's expressions of horror. Protest was impossible for it brought only punishment. One new friend, a Slovakian Jew Eitinger called "the good Mittleman" offered this advice:

> If you wish to live, you must never show what you feel or think. Informers are everywhere. One word to the SS is enough that you will receive an injection as well. I have written death notices for my father and my three brothers as well. I have noted how a Polish prisoner, wishing to become an

informer, had spied on me and tried coax me into saying something. That pleasure I will never give. I *will* survive. That you must also will. Be hard! Show nothing that is within. We must close our minds until we are free men again."[3]

A short distance from the *Revier* lay the infamous Block 10—site of heinous human experiments performed by Nazi doctors, led by the despicable Joseph Mengele. Block 10 was carefully shielded from prying eyes. Windows were covered by whitewash, and entry denied to all without official duties. Eitinger learned of the inhuman experiments— implantation of cancer into the living womb, castration, radiation, and other acts of pseudo-research by depraved physicians—through a fellow Czech, an elderly painter.

A few words of advice to a nephew who had been conscripted by the Germans had led to the painter's imprisonment in Auschwitz. "Do not forget the measures of which your mother has spoken," wrote the painter in a letter—and that was enough.[4]

The Czech was first summoned to the *Revier* by the camp doctors to paint three small gypsy patients with "noma," a rare and striking affliction limited almost entirely to the undernourished. The Nazis wished to depict the massive gangrenous and spreading destruction about the mouth. Pleased with the results, the amoral physicians engaged the Czech painter to sketch changes twice weekly in "experimental subjects" in Block 10. Disclosure of happenings in Block 10 were, of course, punishable by death, but Eitinger had provided better clothing and leather shoes for which the painter felt indebted. In his native Czech tongue, Eitinger learned of the horrors within the forbidden barracks.

Robert Weinstein appeared at the hospital in May with severe diarrhea. Since Shua had last seen his friend, Weinstein had become a "musselmann"—so emaciated that his skin stretched tight and glistening over his bones. Without Dr. Eitinger's help, Bob would have been doomed to an *Einspritzung*, or journey, to the gas chamber. Shua ministered gently to his friend—sheltered him in the *Revier* and secured extra rations. Soon Weinstein recovered and Eitinger managed to place him in the hospital office.

Weinstein's good fortune was brief—for he fell victim to the irrational rage of SS Dr. Entress. The Nazi physician came across typographical errors in Weinstein's work—Oneumonia instead of Pneumonia—and two other mistakes. The misfortune was enough to banish the unlucky Norwegian Jew from the *Revier* to the most dreadful of barracks in the main camp.

Eitinger was not spared the Nazi's fury. Never, Entress had shouted, did prisoners die of inanition—but always of some illness. He threatened that Eitinger should soon write a history of himself, including a cause of death.

Shua Eitinger could scarcely tolerate the agonies he was forced to submerge within. He asked the personnel officer for transfer and in June was assigned to a small "hospital" in a newly constructed sub-camp at Auschwitz, the *Eintrachthutte* (Harmony Hut). Even though slave laborers still worked twelve-hour shifts—day or night—in the anti-aircraft cannon factory, conditions were far better for all. The goal was hardly humanitarian, but merely to keep prisoners fit for work. The factory overseers were civilians and the hospital commander was not a hardened Nazi.

Dr. Eitinger's clinical quarters in the *Eintrachthutte* hardly resembled a hospital. In two rooms, he and his colleague, Czech surgeon, Sperber, handled illnesses and injuries of as many as two hundred prisoners each day. Two tables occupied the room that served as first-aid station and office. One was covered with bandages and a few poor instruments that were inadequate even for first aid alone. The second table was occupied by a typewriter that served Dr. Eitinger's internal medicine service.

The clinic boasted not even a stethoscope, and medication was virtu-ally nonexistent for concentration camp inmates. A few aspirin tablets, cough lozenges, and a little charcoal constituted the entire pharmaceutical armamentarium of the internal medicine service. Patient care was of little import to the Nazis; records and reports were paramount. The captors insisted on a daily flow of information and accounts. For the Nazis the typewriter was the most important of instruments.

Dr. Sperber became a dear friend as well as a colleague with whom Shua Eitinger could discuss medicine and science. The Czech doctor had been educated in Prague, then took a position as ship surgeon to a British tourist vessel. When war erupted Sperber served aboard a merchant ship that was torpedoed by a German U-boat. Initially Sperber was treated as a prisoner of war. The Nazis soon discovered his Jewish origin, however, and sent him to Auschwitz.

German physicians did not bother themselves with the *Eintrachthutte Revier*, but gave full authority to lowly non-coms. The first, Corporal Glowinski, considered himself a doctor, having passed through a three-week course in Berlin. After Glowinski was transferred, his replacement, Wloka, a mason from Dresden, was more realistic. He told his prisoner-physicians, "You are doctors and understand disease better than I. You know the rules and what should be done. If everything goes well I will not mix in. But God help you if I get into a mess with the Camp Physician because of you."[5]

Eitinger and Sperber did take chances whenever they could help fellow prisoners in their *Revier*. Too many patients required more than fourteen days hospitalization. German industry at Auschwitz paid the Nazis three marks a day for each slave laborer—and was reluctant to continue the pittance beyond the two-week period. For the skilled worker, however, factory managers were more than willing to make exceptions. The two doctors would bypass the rule merely through signing the prisoner out, then readmitting him for another fourteen days, often repeating the process. Now and again data cards were falsified and at times hidden away. Too few, however, could be helped through these subterfuges.

Shua used a different approach to save one of his favorite patients. Two discharges and readmissions brought a teen-aged Polish Jew, Mendel Barberer, to the end of six weeks in the *Revier* and the brink of catastrophe. Barberer had become too familiar a face. Dr. Eitinger had been unwilling to surrender his young patient. When he found the German *Oberscharführer* in good humor Eitinger approached him with a "humanitarian case" to consider. He had a boy who had lain in the *Revier* for fourteen days with pleurisy. According to the rules he should be discharged, but he had improved to such a degree that within the space of a week—at the most two weeks—he would be fit to work again. The patient was a particularly clever worker. Perhaps the *Oberscharführer* would allow the youth to remain until truly capable of work again. The German agreed and Barberer remained a patient until his pleurisy had cleared.

Another time, a sixteen-year-old youth from Sighet in Transylvania was admitted to the hospital because of a massive infection on the sole of his foot early in Jauary 1945. Life or death depended on the success of treatment. Were the young Jew unable to walk and to work, survival was impossible. Dr. Eitinger examined the infected foot. There was only one possible recourse—surgery. Shua himself did not operate, but promised the lad he would be present at the procedure. More than a dozen years later the patient described his life-saving treatment.

> The doctor, a great Jewish doctor, a prisoner like ourselves, was quite definite: I must have an operation! If we waited, the toes—and perhaps the whole leg would have to be amputated. . . .
>
> The doctor came to tell me that the operation would be the next day. "Don't be afraid," he added. "Everything will be all right."

At ten o'clock in the morning, they took me into the operating room. "My" doctor was there. I took comfort from this. I felt that nothing serious could happen while he was there. There was balm in every word he spoke, and every glance he gave me held a message of hope.

"It will hurt you a bit," he said, "but that will pass. Grit your teeth."

The operation lasted an hour. They had not put me to sleep. I kept my eyes fixed upon my doctor. Then I felt myself go under. . . . When I came round, opening my eyes, I could see nothing at first but a great whiteness, my sheets; then I noticed the face of my doctor bending over me:

"Everything went off well. You're brave, my boy. Now you're going to stay here two weeks, rest comfortably, and it will be over. You'll eat well and relax your body and your nerves."

I could only follow the movement of his lips. I scarcely understood what he was saying, but the murmur of his voice did me good.

Suddenly a cold sweat broke out on my forehead. I could not feel my leg! Had they amputated it?

"Doctor," I stammered. "Doctor . . . ?"

"What's the matter, son?"

I lacked the courage to ask him the question.

"Doctor, I'm thirsty. . . ."

He had water brought to me. He was smiling. He was getting ready to go and visit the other patients.

"Doctor?"

"What?"

"Shall I be able to use my leg?"

He was no longer smiling. I was very frightened. He said:

"Do you trust me, my boy?"

"I trust you absolutely, Doctor."

"Well then listen to me. You'll be completely recovered in a fortnight. You'll be able to walk like anyone else. The sole of your foot was all full of pus. We had to open the swelling. You haven't had your leg amputated. You'll see. In a fortnight's time you'll be walking about like everyone else."

I had only a fortnight to wait.[6]

The young author-to-be was Elie Wiesel.

It was never a surprise to see a prisoner beaten senseless by the SS. It was unusual, however, for *any* German to exhibit significant concern. An elderly Pole who had been discovered smoking in the factory—as did many workers—had aroused the ire of an SS officer. The prisoner had been thrashed and stomped into unconsciousness and brought moribund into the *Eintrachthutte Revier*. Treatment, such as was possible, was to no avail. Three days later the patient was dead without ever recovering consciousness. On each of those three days, Herr Frenzl, a civilian functionary in the factory, visited the motionless Pole, initially accompanied by the camp commandant, and then alone. The two doctors were questioned pointedly, but caution prevented them from telling Frenzl little other than that death had followed brain injury.

Wloka was amused by the attention. "If that had happened on an ordinary work-command, out in the forest, in the quarry, or another place where civilians were not to be found, no one would have spoken of the matter," he noted. "I have seen thousands of such cases, and I do not bother myself with it. But to beat a man to death in the middle of civilians, or for that matter just to beat, that is so stupid that he shall pay just for that."[7]

In the course of his visits Frenzl became friendly with Sperber and Eitinger. For the most part the German did the talking when the three were together, for he spoke of dangerous things. He wished victory for Germany, of course, but not for the Nazis. Frenzl continued to visit the *Revier* after the Pole's death, for he had injured his foot and was treated daily. Frenzl also brought the two captive physicians to the factory first-aid station, where he supplied medication and some surgical instruments.

Herr Frenzl questioned the two doctors about personal matters and discussed prisoner psychology with them. Sperber and Eitinger soon became convinced the German took their problems seriously and spoke more freely. Frenzl was aghast when informed of the gas chambers and the ever-growing mounds of personal belongings taken from the doomed. He tried to reach higher authorities in the *Wehrmacht*, hoping an end could be put to the atrocities. It was, of course, useless. Finally Frenzl was denied entry to the camp. Shua had given his German friend the names and numbers of Norwegian prisoners in Buna-Monowitz, with the hope Frenzl could be of some help.

The hope was not in vain. Frenzl managed to have two young comrades from Eitinger's Nesjestranda days, the Lustig twins, transferred from Monowitz to the *Eintrachthutte*. He had convinced the Nazis that Hans and Fritz Lustig had particular skills of value to the German war effort. The news the Lustigs brought was shattering. Most of their fellow Jews on the *Gotenland* transport had perished. Some succumbed to typhus, diphtheria, or pneumonia; others froze or were beaten to death, "shot in flight," executed, or merely disappeared. One day they were there—the next gone.

June 1944 brought a flash of hope to the prisoners—the Allies had landed at Normandy, and Russian troops had already crossed into Poland. Allied forces moved slowly, however, and the flash receded to a glimmer.

The relative safety of the *Eintrachthutte* was threatened by the appearance of Prisoner Number 1, Bruno Brodniwiecz. At about fifty

Brodniwiecz, a hardened criminal, had already been imprisoned for half his life and was indeed the first to be confined to the concentration camp at Auschwitz. Brodniwiecz was head of camp *kapos*, prisoners who had been placed in charge of their fellows in the barracks. He functioned with no less authority than an SS trooper, and was not to be outdone in bedevilment of his charges. He dressed entirely in black—black boots, black riding breeches, black jacket and a black hat—and his vicious behavior earned him his title—The Black Devil. He had presided over prisoners in the larger camp, but drunkenness had brought a string of demotions until he was reduced to being chief prisoner in the smallest of camps, the *Eintrachthutte*.

Soon after The Black Devil's installation twelve Russian prisoners had escaped. From their barracks they had tunneled beneath the barbed wire encircling the compound, and disappeared. Brodniwiecz and his like shared the Nazi's rage. Prisoner Number 1 furiously forbade any reading of the Nazi newspapers that lay about in his quarters. Prisoners might be tempted into an action forbidden under pain of death—discussion of politics.

Bruno's ban had little effect in quenching the thirst for news to confirm the rumors of impending Nazi defeat that continually raced through the camp. The two doctors used every possible ruse to visit SS quarters where they could gaze surreptitiously at the three- or four-day-old newspapers lying about and memorize the daily communiques.

Unable to detect violators of his rules, Brodniwiecz set about to entrap. He recruited *provocateurs* who seduced prisoners into tunneling beneath the barbed wire fence while all others slept. In the middle of the night the SS rounded up twenty the *provocateurs* had ensnared. The unfortunates were confined between the two lines of electrified barbed-wire—a space but fifteen inches wide—to await their "trial." The very next night, after the charade of a hearing, the twenty were driven away in trucks to punishing labor in a coal mining camp.

Only two young lads in their twenties were seen again. They were returned to mount the gallows in full view of all the prisoners.

With the fate of the tunnelers in mind, Leo Eitinger had good reason for fear when he found himself between the lines of electrified barbed wire together with the entirety of *Revier* personnel. Wloka, their protector, was away on leave. The thunderous threats of the commandant brought even greater distress. This was to be their last night. They were a band of murderers and criminals. They were to be tried and hung in the morning. With such as they, the process would be short. The case against them had already been proven.

The hearing followed shortly—with charges so incredible that even the Gestapo found belief difficult. The accused were supposed to have placed dynamite to blow the SS barracks to pieces. *Revier* personnel had hidden the explosives in trunks on their premises. Shua Eitinger was purported to have provided poison for injection into Martin Schmitz, one of the cruelest camp *kapos*.

The ludicrousness of the charges gave even the Gestapo pause. Wloka, who had just returned, demanded, "Either you are convinced that my people are guilty of what they are accused of, or they should immediately return to work! I must have doctors for the patients, and if this can not be dropped I must telephone the Chief Physician and explain the matter and have new doctors sent."[8]

The freedom that followed Wloka's efforts was still tenuous, for Bruno had followed with a long and rambling complaint filed against *Revier* personnel. Both Eitinger and Sperber, however, had noted Brodniwiecz's small pupils that failed to react to light—a hallmark of central nervous system syphilis. Wloka agreed to have Prisoner Number 1 tested. The blood serology was positive, and the tormenter was transferred.

At this point the two doctors had become too dominant in *Ein-trachthutte*. The camp commandant returned them to Monowitz-Buna in October 1944. With foresight, Shua had prepared a letter that Wloka had endorsed. The two physicians, the missive stated, had been sent by order of the SS chief physician for service in the hospital. That letter protected Eitinger and Sperber for the duration of their internment in Auschwitz.

Life took on a new tone for Shua Eitinger in the Monowitz *Revier*. The hospital functioned independently of the remainder of the camp. Polyglot physicians—from France, Hungary, Poland, Czechoslovakia, and other lands—ministered to the ill and injured with humanitarianism as a principal intent. All strove to overcome "selection" of patients who had passed the fourteen-day limit. Six times a comrade who had shared imprisonment at Falstad with Leo Eitinger had been saved after having been ordered to the gas chamber. His prison number was simply and conveniently lost.

Rumors thundered into reality as Russian cannon boomed in the distance. Prisoners oscillated between jubilation at thoughts of freedom and fears concerning the Nazis who still held the power of life and death. Finally the uncertainty ended. The camp was to be evacuated. The ten thousand prisoners who had filled Buna-Monowitz were to set out on foot through the snow-covered winter countryside. A contingent from the hospital, bearing whatever medication and supplies they could manage, was to follow in the wake of each thousand. A few doctors, along with patients too ill or too elderly to be moved, were to be left behind. To what fate? Eitinger did not believe witnesses could survive when the Nazis had already dismantled the gas-chambers and crematoria.

Eleven days after the prisoners had marched away toward Germany a liquidation force of SS troops appeared at the camp hospital. Patients were routed from their beds and, with the *Revier* personnel, were hounded into the deserted camp where the SS had set up banks of machine guns. A Soviet air attack put a halt to the murderous attempt. Prisoners were hounded back into the buildings and the SS fled. Two days later Russian forces entered the camp.

Shua Eitinger's group was the last to follow the marching prisoners out of Monowitz-Buna on January 15, 1945. Behind him were only the women from the bordello, the *kapos*, and criminals who had served as guards.

The trek began not too badly, but after the first night's stop, weakened prisoners began to fall in their tracks in the deep snow. Those unable to rise, despite kicks and blows, were shot by the Nazi guards and left to the side of the road. Doctors and hospital personnel helped where they could, but too often assistance was futile.

Fatigued, overworked, and weakened with a high fever, Shua Eitinger came close to falling victim. Only the support of his former patients and his friends and colleagues kept him from receiving the fatal shot.

The nightmare march—broken only by short pauses and filled with shouts, blows, and shots—covered the snowy and windswept forty-five miles to Gleiwitz. A concentration camp that had been built to accommodate eight hundred overflowed with twenty thousand prisoners. Nearly more dead than alive, hospital personnel fell into the small infirmary.

The prisoners received no better treatment in Gleiwitz than they had along the route. A group of common criminals from Krakow who already filled the camp set upon the exhausted and helpless arrivals, stripping them of everything useful—particularly shoes and clothing. Those who resisted were beaten to death.

Febrile as he was, Dr. Eitinger still managed to join his colleagues in pitifully inadequate attempts to treat the cuts, bruises, and frostbite that had afflicted virtually all the marchers. Time was short, medication even shorter, and dressings non-existent—but each man soothed and did whatever he could.

Surviving prisoners were divided into two groups and sent off by train in open cars—one to Mathausen, and the second to Buchenwald. Shua and four Norwegian comrades—Assor and Asriel Hirsch, Julius Paltiel, and Sammy Steinmann—managed to cling together for six days until they reached Buchenwald.

In panic over the approaching Russians, the SS beat prisoners unmercifully as they hounded them into open cars, up to eighty in each. Hospital personnel were more fortunate. Eighty had two cars to themselves, in each of which was some medication.

The train passed through Poland and Czechoslovakia before entering Germany. Only the Czechs offered relief. In Bohemia and Moravia sympathetic villagers threw food aboard the cars as the train stood in the stations. In Pardubice children from a passing school train flung their lunches to the starving prisoners. Hunger, thirst, and the cold were more than malnourished prisoners could tolerate. Thousands died en route. Only half those leaving Monowitz-Buna reached their destination alive.

From the relative safety of the hospital in Monowitz-Buna, Eitinger had been plunged into the despair that was Buchenwald. When he heard a Norwegian tongue call out the question, *"Er det noen fra Norge her?"*[9] (Are there any from Norway here?) the despair evaporated into the foul air of the dingy barracks. The voice belonged to a student—one of those rounded up and sent off to Germany when the Nazis closed down the University of Oslo. He had arrived to see how students could help their countrymen.

About five hundred Norwegian students had survived Buchenwald through the "privileged" existence the Nazis provided to their fellow "Aryans." The students lived together in their own barracks, did no work as slave-labor, wore their own clothes, and received packages of food from the Danish and Swedish Red Cross to supplement the miserable camp diet.

That evening the students sent warm clothes, underwear, and food—along with hope for the future—to their Jewish countrymen.

Eitinger and his four young Norwegian friends were moved into the all-Jewish Block 22 and were instantly accepted as comrades by the long-time Buchenwald inmates. The spirit and discipline in the Jewish barracks was uplifting to the new arrivals, and the nearness of the Norwegian student quarters made visiting simple.

Shua Eitinger felt restored with each evening visit to his newfound countrymen. The students were kept firmly apart from the rest of the camp—with an SS overseer in their barracks from morning until evening, when the quarters were locked. Students had a key, however; so Eitinger and his friends could enter freely by night. For the first time since he had left Nesjestranda Shua entered a friendly and humane atmosphere—in which everyone spoke Norwegian.

When slave labor factories at Buchenwald became frequent targets for Allied strikes late in the war a bomb struck the camp, wounding scores of prisoners. Quickly the hospital became filled to overflowing. Norwegian students reacted with compassion, voluntarily converting a floor of their barracks to a temporary hospital, even though they were forced into crowded quarters where two slept in the same bunk. They readily took over the care and nursing of the patients to whom they had relinquished their quarters.

Once again, good fortune was fleeting. Representatives of the Danes and Norwegians in the camp were ordered to list their countrymen. The five Jews were included by the Norwegian students but struck from the list by the Nazis. The listing was but the prodrome to departure of their friends and protectors. Once again, Eitinger and the four youths were defenseless.

Day by day transports of prisoners arrived in Buchenwald from concentration camps in the ever-shrinking German Reich, for the Nazis wanted none to "fall into the enemy's hands." Day by day the prisoners' concern for their future increased. The rapidly growing underground in Buchenwald looked to that future.

Political prisoners in Buchenwald—particularly Communists and Social Democrats who shared little but their anti-Fascist beliefs—took the lead in Buchenwald's Underground Movement, with Stefan at its head. Stefan was experienced in concentration camp existence, for he had known no other life for a dozen years. His most important function at Buchenwald was screening prisoners for transport. Buchenwald was overflowing with prisoners. The gas chambers no longer functioned and the Nazis wished to move out those most able to travel. The remaining prisoners were to be liquidated. Cunningly, the camp underground worked to frustrate that plan. Time and again Stefan sent prisoners who were unfit to travel to the transport, and they were returned to camp. He aimed to preserve, as much as possible, those who could contribute to the future. "Concentration camps are to kill ten thousands of human beings every year," Stefan told Eitinger. "The only thing we can try to do is to keep those alive who can do something positive in the world we live in."[10] Meanwhile, members of the underground attempted to smuggle in weapons, should final defense be required.

As American forces steadily neared Buchenwald, forty-eight of the camps most noted prisoners were ordered to appear at the SS political section. Few questioned the intent. Among those summoned were prisoner-chiefs of the hospital and the typhus block, and prisoners who had seen human experimentation. All could testify at a War Crimes Trial to the atrocities committed against the prisoners. The forty-eight disappeared into the camp—changing their clothes, names, and numbers. They were not to be found.

On that very day, April 4, 1945, Himmler ordered death for every Jew. On April 5, Eitinger, his comrades, and all his co-religionists all became the quarry.

Repeated calls over the loudspeaker summoned all Jews, but none responded. The sound of an air-raid siren ended the calls. For the day, at least, the danger had passed. The responsibility was shifted to the barracks chiefs the following day—each should identify all the Jews. The underground leadership countered. Every barracks chief was to burn his card files—none should reveal who was a Jew or who was not. The Norwegian youths who lived in the Jewish barracks were transferred to quarters of the German political prisoners, and hidden in the loft.

Shua Eitinger forged a death certificate, declaring his own death, then took the name and number of a Czech prisoner who had died the previous night. He would live with a dead man's identity. Eitinger then sewed a Czech prisoner-stripe on his jacket and went out into the camp. The announcement of the fictitious death ultimately reached the Red Cross. The political prisoner, Leo Eitinger, was listed as having died the night of 6/7 April.

At the evening line-up all Jews were commanded to step three paces forward. Among the few who did so was a Norwegian Jew. "I am too old to live illegally," he said. "Now that God has protected me until this day, I continue to place myself in his hands."[11]

The SS swept through the camp, dragging out Jews wherever they could be found. The young Jews in the attic armed themselves with an iron bar and resolved to sell their lives dearly, but they remained undetected.

About four thousand Jews were transported, never to be heard from again. Still, some two thousand remained in the camp—among them Shua Eitinger and his four young friends.

The passive resistance continued. Those unfit to travel were sent time and again to the gates, and sent back again. All others refused to heed the call to assemble. Little by little, however, the Nazis managed to send transports from Buchenwald. One included Dr. Sperber. Somewhere along the march, however, Sperber managed to slip away and hide until he was saved by an advancing British column. The Russians suddenly volunteered for transport, were collected, and left. With smuggled arms they fled after overpowering their guards en route.

Finally five hundred heavily armed SS troops marched through the camp routing out resisting prisoners from the barracks. The going was

slow, for none went willingly. Blows, threats, and kicks were uniform, and
some were shot. By evening twenty thousand prisoners still remained in
Buchenwald. No sounds were heard in the camp until ten o'clock the
next morning. The shriek of the siren announced the enemy was near,
and shouts over the loudspeaker proclaimed, *"Alle SS-Angehorige verlassen
sofort das Lager!"* (All belonging to the SS leave the camp immediately).[12]

From his rooftop observation post Leo Eitinger could see the SS
scurrying away in disarray—riderless horses, soldiers fleeing in virtually
a forced march, and automobiles speeding recklessly.

Two American tanks swung off the highway and turned toward the
camp. Prisoners scrambled from the camp in welcome. The Americans
paused only long enough for a few words before they headed to Berlin.

Free men then, the ex-prisoners raided SS supplies to add weapons to
the few they had already smuggled in, and took charge of the camp. A
Resistance group searched the surrounding woods for SS stragglers and
flushed out more than a hundred. The tables turned, former prisoners
guarded the SS. None of the newly captured Germans were beaten or
murdered. The former prisoners behaved responsibly.

The danger was yet to pass. The ex-prisoners maintained an uneasy
watch, for the Gestapo headquarters at Weimar was but five miles away.
Some hours after liberation of Buchenwald the telephone rang in the
camp office. The chief of Gestapo at Weimar was on the line, asking for
the camp commandant. "Heil Hitler," responded a prisoner, who then
reported the commandant to be out, and asked if there were a message.
It was nothing special the caller replied, just that some shots had been
heard. That was just as usual, the chief was reassured, but the commandant
would return the call.

The Gestapo called again at midnight, and again was put off. The
ex-prisoners held the camp alone, and were in no position to fend off the
Germans, if curiosity should bring them to Buchenwald. The following
day the Americans overran Weimar. Two days later they took responsibility for Buchenwald. Death still plagued the camp when the liberators
arrived, weakened as the occupants were by disease and malnutrition.
Thanks to the concern and kindness of Norway's students, Shua Eitinger
and his four Norwegian friends had had the food and clothing needed to
survive.

Eitinger's work in Buchenwald was not over. It was a month after
liberation before he finally managed to leave. In the meantime survivors
were no longer prisoners, but had become displaced persons. Shua was
well occupied and finally able provide adequate medical care to his fellows.
All patients had been transferred to the former SS hospital and to the

SS barracks. The Americans flooded the facilities with equipment and medication—all with the war still in progress hardly thirty miles away. Leo Eitinger once again became a physician with the means to practice when he was given the responsibility for a medical service.

24. Odd Nansen
in Sachsenhausen:
A Daybook of Despair

How fine! thought Odd Nansen cynically as he passed through the gate to the Sachsenhausen Concentration Camp beneath the shining white sign, "ARBEIT MACHT FREI" (Work makes free).[1] Were it not for the placards posted along the electric fence warning potential fugitives they would be shot on sight, the carefully tended entrance and garden paths would have suggested peace and tranquility. Before the day was out Nansen had discovered how wrong that suggestion was to be.

The new arrivals from Grini stood for hours. All belongings were taken—money, watches, suitcases, and even the clothes from their backs. A bundle of forms were thrust forward to be completed and signed. The prisoners were then led naked into another room to be roughly shorn of hair, first pubic and then from the head. The crude debasement was followed by soapless showers in icy water, smearing of bodies with anti-vermin ointment, and the distribution of ill-fitting rags to replace the clothes they had so recently surrendered.

Dr. Sven Oftedal appeared, "as calm, as balanced, and as sedate as ever,"[2] to provide solace and support to his downcast countrymen. Norwegians were far better off than all other prisoners, Oftedal told Odd. They had escaped, more or less, the major indignities and punishments heaped on other prisoners—especially the Ukrainians and Jews. Scandinavians were permitted packages in unlimited numbers—not only from home, but those generously supplied by the Swedish and Danish Red Cross. "Beyond doubt, what keeps the Norwegians alive and in relatively good condition is the food parcels from home and from Sweden and Denmark,"[3] Nansen wrote.

Dr. Oftedal himself was often as crucial in keeping Norwegians alive as he was in maintaining their morale. Seriously ill prisoners characteristically were placed aboard the *Todestransport* to be hauled away for "disposal." Oftedal had "a big job saving Norwegians from this transport. And he has in fact saved them all—even our friend Henry Hansen, on the pretext that he's on the eve of a new operation that will cure him," wrote Nansen. "Oftedal is doing magnificent work here altogether."[4]

In Auschwitz Shua Eitinger suffered the nightmares of the victim. At Sachsenhausen Odd Nansen endured the despair of the compassionate. The diary that he meticulously maintained for the year and a half of his imprisonment in Germany overflows with empathy and despondence. Very quickly he learned that many of his fellow Norwegians had already perished. In the parlance of the dreaded concentration camp, they had "gone up the chimney."[5] All about he observed "*mussulmen*," emaciated and expressionless, shuffling about in skimpy and filthy rags, and he saw the frenzy with which the starving fell upon even the most revolting of nourishment. After a meal of pickled herring supplied by the Norwegian Red Cross, refuse lay heaped on the rough table before the more fortunate Norsemen—scales, skin, bones, and offal. An emaciated Ukrainian was seen reaching between Norwegians, seizing the refuse and stuffing his pockets with the remains.

Prisoners were tallied daily at morning roll call and again in the evening. The figures *had* to be right. Those who had perished during the night were carried to the parade ground to be counted with the living. The SS made certain that none were missing. "The dead and dying," Nansen wrote in his diary, "often lay on the ground in great heaps of twenty, thirty or forty men alongside the column."[6] In October 1943 the count showed two men extra at morning roll call. Two prisoners were selected and kept standing by the gate the entire day. When the evening count gave the same number, Odd heard two pistol shots from the gate house, adjusting the figures. After speaking with a young Soviet flyer Nansen noted:

This is a hell for Russian prisoners. About fifteen thousand of them have marched through the gate from time to time, and there are only eight or nine hundred left in the camp. The rest have been starved to death, beaten to death, or otherwise done away with. Seven of the young Russian airman's comrades were hanged here. . . . These hangings take place on the parade grounds and everyone has to look on. Our Norwegian comrades have seen any number of them. Nor are these executions lacking in their "heroic episodes." A German was hanged for attempting to escape. He talked of

freedom on the scaffold, freedom for the German people which would
soon come. He turned to the Commandant, who attends the executions,
and calmly said, Well it was his turn now, before long it would be the
Commandant's. When the rope was put around his neck he raised his
hand and waved and smiled to his comrades for the last time.[7]

Odd Nansen wrote as bitterly about those of his own countrymen who
had become completely insensitive to the degradation of others as he did
about his captors.

> Everyone is thinking about himself. Everyone is grabbing for himself,
> few share with others. The average Norwegian, even treats a Ukranian
> worse than he would a dog at home. He knows the Ukrainian is starving,
> everyone does for they get no parcels "from home." He just doesn't think
> about it, simply drives him away as he would flies or vermin. I suppose the
> Ukrainians and Russians are the worst beggars, as is natural. Their lives
> are at stake. The Norwegians did the same when their lives were at stake
> before they started getting parcels.[8]

Odd Nansen befriended two small groups of Jews in the camp brought
for their special skills: watchmakers to repair the hundreds of thousands
of watches stolen from Nazi victims, and printers to forge documents
and counterfeit the money of Germany's enemies. From the watchmaker,
Keil, who had spent 1936 in Norway as a refugee in Hønefoss, he learned
of the death of so many his Norwegian Jewish friends in Auschwitz.

Amidst all the degradation and inhumanity, it was paradoxical that
Hauptsturmführer Steger called for Nansen just before the end of December 1943. The young German officer had read much about Fridtjof
Nansen and discovered that the great man's son was a prisoner of the
Nazis in that very camp. The *Hauptsturmführer* told Nansen he knew of
his father's efforts in science and on behalf of humanity, and apologized
that the son of such a distinguished person should be treated as he was.
The officer regretted that he had no choice but to treat Odd as a prisoner,
but he could be transferred to a separate room where he could read, write,
draw, and be more comfortable.

Odd thanked the German, but said that he was all right where he was
and preferred to go on living with his friends. For the time being, Steger
responded, he would let that be. In the meantime, should Odd wish to
see him again he would be admitted at any time.

Despite his desire to remain close to his friends, the fame of the Nansen
name brought Odd notice and transfer to another work squad. Norwegian
Scott Isaksen overheard two non-commissioned officers arguing whether

Fridtjof Nansen had or had not reached the North Pole. Isaksen told them it was easy enough to find out since the explorer's son, an architect, was a prisoner in the camp. The two Germans "invented" the need for an architect—Odd was ordered shifted over. The actual transfer was averted when a supervisor interceded on Nansen's behalf. He was already working on architectural plans for enlargement of the camp, it was claimed, on work just as vital to the war effort as that on the intended assignment. In March, however, the work squad was broken up. Odd Nansen was assigned to calculate the cubic content of all the wood used in the camp workshop.

By May 1944 deaths in the camp grew more and more frequent. In addition to the executed, and the ill who were transported, two to three hundred died each month, particularly of pneumonia. Norwegians fared better than the other prisoners, sustained as they were by the continual flow of packages, but several still succumbed to illness.

In June a nineteen-year-old Ukrainian was first given fifty blows with a rubber hose then hanged during the evening roll call. He had taken two leather bags from the shoe factory where he worked and had cut soles from them. Nansen could not bear to see the hose thudding again and again into the young man's flesh, and tried to turn away. Only a single protest arose from among seventeen thousand witnesses. A Dutchman shouted, "It's shameful! It's vile!"[9] He was one of a group of "Bible-searchers" who had been imprisoned for rigidly held beliefs matching Johan Scharffenberg's. Hitler was a false prophet, and as such, a disaster to Germany. The Hollander was taken away for his own punishment, and the execution continued.

On December 14, 1944, well into his second year in Sachsenhausen, Odd Nansen filled his diary with pages of despair for his fellow prisoners, and repeated his bitterness against those of his well-off countrymen who had become insensitive to the suffering of others:

> Yesterday I had a letter from Kari! and one came on my birthday itself. Every one of these letters is a gleam of light in the darkness. I can't help thinking of all the thousands who have no such gleam. How profoundly thankful we should be, we who are well off, who are not in want, and who have good news from our dear ones at home. But these ideas which arise whenever one looks into the faces of the starving, shattered human beings who surround one everywhere in the camp, makes one sad and heavy hearted. It isn't well to be "well off" among many who are badly off. The only possible relief is to share the material goods which are divided amongst us so unequally and unjustly. To see a starving, broken-down Ukrainian eat his fill is a far richer and deeper satisfaction than most this life can offer.

But his dog's eyes while he's eating and afterward are unbearable. And its so infinitely little one can do to help.

To tell the truth, of the senseless abundance in the Norwegian blocks only a distressingly small amount is given away without a demand for something in return. . . .

This unfairness has a very bad effect, not only on the relation between the Norwegians and the others, but on the Norwegians themselves. . . . We howl with the Germans and with others: *Verdammte Juden*! A Norwegian of my acquaintance, a decent chap on the whole, gave himself away the other day when we got to talking of all that these unhappy Jews suffer.

"Well it serves them right!" said he. "I know them; I live in the same block with them. . . . Never sharing with anyone, always cheating and swindling each other! No, I've had enough of Jews. Thank goodness we had only one at home in Ålesund. He was bad enough."

"Well you can certainly count on being rid of him now," said I. "No doubt he was disposed of in Auschwitz along with a thousand more Norwegian Jews, so you may rejoice, if you can!" And then I said a lot more, for I get so easily worked up. . . .

A Norwegian of the highest social class hoarded in his bed, boxes, and cupboard to such a point that action was taken. It was monstrous the amount he had! Then he was said to be ill. For he was a "Norweger"—and not a Jew, not a Ukrainian, Russian, or Pole. If a good Norwegian steals, he's a "kleptomaniac" . . . But the disgrace of a single Jew—whether "good" or "bad"—is divided equally among all Jews. And it's the same today with Poles, Ukrainians, and to some extent, Russians in this camp. They are "grundsatzlich" (fundamentally) scum.[10]

On February 12, just five weeks before leaving Sachsenhausen on a voyage to freedom, Nansen wrote, "The language is exhausted. I've exhausted it myself. There are no words left to describe the horrors I've seen with my own eyes."[11]

As the Allied forces pressed into Germany from the east, the west, and the south, Norway's government-in-exile and its Legation in Stockholm moved to protect and salvage their countrymen held captive in Germany. Each month the government added five thousand packages of food to those provided by the Danish and Swedish Red Cross, and by families and friends at home. On November 10, 1944, Norwegian authorities appropriated 8.3 million kroner toward the expense of returning their citizens home. Rector Didrik Seip, who had already been released by the Nazis, and other Norwegians in Germany, including lawyer, J. B. Hjort and the Norse Seamen's Pastor in Hamburg, journeyed from camp to camp, preparing a list of their countrymen still held captive. The seventy-five hundred names collected were transmitted to Stockholm through the Swedish Legation in Berlin.

Concern over the fate of Norwegian prisoners had mounted as reports from Germany suggested that concentration camp commandants had been ordered to liquidate all prisoners as Allied forces approached. On their part, the Allied military had concluded that no rescue missions would be carried out before the involved region in Germany had been conquered.

Norway's minister to Sweden, Niels Christian Ditleff, who had labored mightily in Czechoslovakia and Poland in the refugees' cause, became the driving force in the move to save his countrymen prisoners. Count Folke Bernadotte, vice president of the Swedish Red Cross, readily agreed to lead Ditleff's rescue effort.

With the support of both the Swedish king and government, Bernadotte first contacted Ernst Kaltenbrunner, second in command to Gestapo Chief Heinrich Himmler, then Foreign Minister Joachim von Ribbentropp. Finally, on February 19, 1945, the Swedish humanitarian met with Himmler himself. Nazi self-interest was served by promoting better relationships with Sweden, but the Gestapo leader did not wish to risk that the freed prisoners would join the Reserve Police he knew had been training on Swedish soil.

Folke Bernadotte then proposed that only the ill, the elderly, and mothers would be taken to Sweden. The Swedes would transport all others to a common camp still within Germany, and the Swedish Red Cross would assume responsibility for their care. Himmler claimed the entire operation could not be great, for the camps held only two thousand Norwegian prisoners. Bernadotte knew better. More than seven thousand had already been tallied by Seip, Hjort, and their group, and Bernadotte reckoned that number to be little more than half the actual.

Norwegians survivors dwindled sharply in number during the disastrous winter of 1944–1945, as the Nazis transported their victims in open railroad cars from camps threatened by Allied advance. In the transport from Gross Rosen scarcely a thousand Norsemen survived of the nearly twenty-four hundred who had begun the journey.

In accord with the agreement forged by Count Bernadotte, Norwegian prisoners were to be sequestered under Swedish care in the camp at Neuengamme in the vicinity of Hamburg. In the meantime Norse prisoners began arriving at Sachsenhausen from the outlying camps. Many, especially the women from Ravensbruck, were in a debilitated condition.

A column of thirty-six buses—each painted white and emblazoned with a Red Cross and a Swedish flag—crossed the Danish border in Jutland and entered Germany. Trucks, mobile kitchens and workshops, and automobiles, a total of ninety-five vehicles with personnel of three hundred, headed toward the concentration camps on their errand of mercy. Sachsenhausen was to be the first stop.

The order for Norwegians to travel reached Sachsenhausen on March 15, 1945. It was not until March 18, however, that Odd Nansen saw the outer gate to the camp open and a Swedish Officer, whom he described as nearly seven feet tall, stride through. Thirteen white buses were soon filled with the first contingent to leave—thirty men to a bus. Each man received a package with food and cigarettes before the buses departed.

Later in the day, before all Norwegians had left the camp, a huge air raid struck nearby factories. Three bombs landed on the camp itself, one striking a shelter and killing all the occupants. Seven trips were required before the camp was emptied of twenty-two hundred Norwegians and Danes. With the list supplied by Rector Seip and his group, the buses fanned out into Germany, visiting one forgotten camp after the other until thirty-two hundred Norwegians had been safely transported to Neuengamme.

In the dark of early morning of March 20, it was Odd Nansen's turn to board a white bus. The desolation of impending defeat gave the roads "the impression of disintegration and confusion, hopelessness, misery, and disaster."[12] Swedes and their buses were forbidden entry to the camp itself at Neuengamme. As the Norwegians struggled on foot over the kilometer from the gate to their barracks, the sense of liberty they had so recently treasured evaporated. The familiar stench of garbage and sewage that had permeated Sachsenhausen returned to reinforce a sense of helplessness that had barely begun to drop away. Nansen recorded in his diary:

> The Swedish Red Cross has obviously been taken in. There is already typhus in the camp. The dungheaps lie open, sewage and filth are afloat everywhere. Lousy, sick, and dying mussulmen drag themselves around and hang by barbed wire fences around the yard. . . . Every day a hundred or a hundred and fifty men are dying in the camp. . . . Shooting and hanging, too go on continually.[13]

Thousands of mussulmen were "transported" to their deaths to make room for the arriving Scandinavians. Where four to five emaciated prisoners had piled together in a bunk, a single Norwegian or Dane occupied the same space. They were, however, not anxious to take over the vermininfested quarters.

> The SS had miscalculated if they thought they could get Norwegians and Danes in their right senses to move in and go to bed in this hell of filth.

Our block doctor unhesitatingly took the responsibility of going against orders, and gave directions for a general spring cleaning of the whole house from floor to roof. And then began a cleanup the like of which this camp and its rulers, at any rate, had never seen. Norwegians and Danes went at it—literally—in contempt of death all night through, and are still at it far in the afternoon.[14]

Characteristically, Nansen was unable to accept his own good fortune without concern about the effect on those still suffering.

Now every Norwegian and every Dane is to have his bunk; one man in each bunk! Of course it causes bad feeling and the other prisoners can't see—or understand—why it is, let alone why it should be so. . . . but the bitter thing is that now in the gallery of their mortal enemies we now have a place. It was we who took their bunks and huts from them, we who drove them out of "house and home," out on a transport. And what a transport means to them, they all know too well.[15]

On Good Friday of 1945, March 30, Count Folke Bernadotte and the Swedish Commission paid a visit to their fellow Scandinavians in Neuengamme—to be shown about by the infamous Nazi Commandant Pauli. Sverre Løvberg, speaking for the prisoners, described the conditions clearly and without hesitation, while the SS stood about. There was no fear of consequences, for the conversation was entirely in "bewildering" Scandinavian tongues.

Bernadotte discussed possible evacuation of the camp with Pauli. Until that moment, the Swedes had no permission to move Scandinavian prisoners. The Allies had advanced so swiftly, however, that even Neuengamme lay close ahead in their path. Count Bernadotte convinced the commandant to send Danes and Norwegians north to Schleswig or Denmark if the camp was evacuated.

On Easter Sunday Professor Lundberg and two other members of the Swedish Commission returned to the camp with eight *lottas* (military nurses) who took up regular duties in the *Revier*. The Swedish visitors responded to the requests of prisoners with plans to provide recreation materials, including musical instruments. They also indicated that Bernadotte was negotiating liberation of Scandinavians even before the end of the war. "It's incredible what Bernadotte has achieved so far," stated one of the Swedes. "Why shouldn't he achieve that too?"[16]

The confidence was justified. On April 5, Bernadotte reported that all women, a number of students, Rector Seip and his wife, and all patients with chronic illnesses were to be dispatched to Sweden at once.

When Dr. Leif Poulsson appeared in the camp at Neuengamme on April 7, Nansen barely recognized him. Paulsson had been the leading head doctor in Natzweiler at a camp so neglected and hidden that it would have been unknown to the Swedish Commission if not for the endless efforts of the Norwegian Seamen's Pastor in Hamburg. Starvation was everywhere among the Natzweiler prisoners. Thirteen of the Norwegians who had arrived three months earlier were already dead—and the rest nearly so from typhus, pneumonia, or pure exhaustion and malnutrition. Initially Dr. Poulsson made rounds daily. When that became more than he could manage, he had remained in bed a day each week to regain his strength. As he weakened Poulsson spent more of each week in bed. When the rescuing commission arrived he could manage only a single day a week caring for his patients.

Odd Nansen and Poulsson's other friends nursed him gently and carefully fed him in small amounts. Two days later he was evacuated to Sweden with the first transport of the ailing. Frode Rinnan, Nansen's colleague and companion from Grini, was sent by another such transport to Sweden five days later.

As the war moved closer to Neuengamme Odd Nansen could hear cannon and bursts of machine gun fire, and see planes overhead. No vehicle moved without peril. Even Red Cross buses had been targets of gunfire, and a driver had been wounded. On April 19, when Hamburg fell, Bernadotte's unceasing efforts reached fruition—Scandinavians in Neuengamme could move off to Denmark.

Half of the Swedish Red Cross personnel had already returned to their home country, but the Danes had prepared well for the liberation of Scandinavians in the Nazi camp. With the underground movement, the Danish administration had prepared a "Jutland Corps" for the task of transport. In the course of a single night 120 buses, with 290 drivers, doctors, and nurses were assembled to cross the border into Germany and speed south to Neuengamme. For their part, the prisoners had managed effectively, and the entire operation went quickly and smoothly. Between April 20 and May 3, 4,225 Scandinavian ex-prisoners celebrated their freedom in the small Danish border town of Padborg. From Padborg the Norwegians were separated then joyfully received and lodged in a number of different locations in Denmark.

Odd Nansen made the last entry from foreign soil into his diary on April 28, 1945. From a country house called Møgelkaer, just outside Horsens—with Denmark still under German control—the notation contained a message to Kari: "I'll soon be home."[17] In the first days of May, Odd Nansen began to telephone his wife from Ramlosa to share with her the joy of safety in neutral Sweden. He had forgotten his telephone number, and needed assistance to complete the call.

At home in Lysaker in the house Fridtjof Nansen had built, Odd appended a postscript to his diary.

> One thing is certain, hate, revenge, and retribution are not the way. They lead us back to the abyss. . . . If we nourish the rising generation on them it is tantamount to spiritual murder and to signing the death notice of our culture. . . .
>
> . . . . Whatever one might feel about the Germans and others who were fighting against our country during the war, surely in the course of time, even though it might require an effort, one can think and feel differently about the growing generation. . . . It does not square with justice that they should suffer for the sins of their fathers. Let them have a fair chance. Don't forget it is they who must rebuild Europe, along with you and me. We are in the same boat. If they sink, we sink as well. Don't let us be like the wise man of Gotham, who sawed off the bough on which he was sitting. . . .
>
> . . . . The worst crime you can commit today, against yourself and society, is to forget what has happened and sink back into indifference. What happened was worse than you have any idea of. And it was the indifference of mankind that let it take place.[18]

THE MARCH TO FREEDOM

25. The Occupation's End

In June, 1940, after deciding not to accompany King Haakon and the Norwegian government to Great Britain, Levi Kreyberg spoke with Foreign Minister, Halvdan Koht about serving in Norway's legation in Finland. Koht supplied the following letter of support:

> To the Legation in Helsingfors.
>
> Professor dr. Kreyberg, who has been in active service since the first day of the war, and must now depart the country following orders from the commanding general, since his continued presence in Norway is no longer possible, is recommended to the legation's assistance, and possible usefulness.
>
> Halvdan Koht[1]

No offer of a position followed and Kreyberg was embittered by the turn of events. Aside from General Ruge, who had offered an invitation with a specific assignment, no one seemed to have a use for him. He sought out Minister of Health Karl Evang, who was himself preparing to flee to England. "Pull yourself together, man. Your life is not yet over," Evang responded to Leiv's obvious depression. Evang then added, "Why not journey to America? With your qualifications and position, you can be of use to them over there."[2]

Evang's proposal struck a receptive chord. On June 8, 1940, Leiv Kreyberg and Hans Jacob Arnold, set sail for the New World aboard the fishing smack *Grimsøy*.

The *Grimsøy* reached New York on July 17, 1940. The reception in the United States left Leiv in shock and dismay. Leland Stowe's report in the *Chicago Daily News* has been dismissive of Norwegian resistance. The headlines read "Oslo Natives Fraternizing With Nazis,"[3] although in the end, the two months of Norwegian combat exceeded that of any other nation subjugated by the Nazis. France itself had survived the German onslaught for only seven weeks. Belgium and Holland were overrun in nine days. Dr. Kreyberg felt Norwegians were viewed in the United States as a nation of traitors.

As a first assignment in exile Kreyberg was ordered to organize the medical service in Toronto in an army camp preparing to train upward of a thousand Norwegians. He continued his responsibilities in the New World for two years. Kreyberg was then was transferred to Norwegian headquarters in London where he was assigned the responsibility for the sanitary unit. He devoted his efforts to development of delousing equipment, preparation of concentrated rations for the anticipated invasion of his homeland, and investigations on the treatment of frostbite. Kreyberg's impatience and intolerance of ineptitude often led to friction with his superiors, enhancing his reputation as a "stormy petrel."

In March 1945 Kreyberg accepted an invitation from the *Hospital Beaujon* in Paris, arranged by Lieutenant Colonel Bernard Pisani, chief of the American School Center. The hospital, which had been taken over by the U.S. Forces as the 108th General Hospital, was staffed by physicians from Loyola University Medical School in Chicago, under the command of Colonel L. M. Rousselet. Frostbite, an area of Kreyberg's expertise, had become a major problem for American troops in Europe.

During the two month sojourn in Paris General Paul Hawley invited Leiv Kreyberg, as acknowledgement of his work, to a tour of the Front where the Allies steadily pushed toward victory. Together with the American neurosurgeon, Colonel Roy Spurling, Leiv left Paris aboard an Air Force Dakota. At Darmstadt each transferred, to a single-engined Piper "Cub." Buffetted by strong April winds, the two planes landed on a small strip at Hersfeld and were led to the 121st Evacuation Hospital. At the hospital Kreyberg heard of the liberation of the nearby concentration camp at Buchenwald. Since he knew Norwegians had been among those held, Leiv asked to be taken to the camp.

Freedom had come to Buchenwald so recently that bodies still lay piled in heaps about the camp. Kreyberg, then a major, demanded the Nazi camp commandant collect all Norwegians who hed been held prisoner. The German managed to assemble only the five Norwegian Jews who had survived the extermination camps and the death march from Auchwitz—among then Dr. Leo Eitinger. The Norwegian students had long-since departed. Appalled as always by injustice and official ineptitude—that Norway's Social Department's organization for "displaced persons" had yet to aid norwegian Jews as long as ten days after liberation—Kreyberg dispatched telegrams to Norwegian Legations in Stockholm and Paris, and to the Embassy in London recommending notifying friends and surviving relatives.

Early in April, having returned to London, Major Kreyberg received orders that would bring him back to Norway.

The German thrust into Norway signaled a halt in Dr. Gunnar Johnson's medical career. As a reserve officer he had fled north in 1940 with still resisting Norwegian forces, then crossed over to England. For the five bitter years of Occupation he functioned purely as an intelligence officer. As the war entered its final phase Johnson turned to relief of human suffering in the Nazi-ravaged Norwegian North.

Soviet troops, accompanied by a small Norwegian contingent, crossed the Arctic border into Norway in October of 1944, driving the Occupation forces westward. The retreating Germans torched every structure in Finnmark, set fire to forests, and destroyed all means of communication. Johnson personally viewed the devastation when he returned to his country in November 1944 as an intelligence officer with the "Crofter" expedition. Surveying the destruction he felt compelled devote himself to the care of the sick and to the relief of an entire population rendered homeless by Nazi savagery. Mustering every possible transport—fishing smacks, launches, and all small craft that had escaped German destruction—he brought the sick and the homeless to safety. During the Christmas season alone he rescued more than nine hundred of his countrymen—usually in foul weather and often under fierce Nazi pursuit.

In January, 1945 Dr. Johnson discovered yet another thousand Norwegians who had been driven from their homes and were hiding in mountain caves on Sarøya. He set off immediately for London to organize the rescue mission. On the 6th of February he was en route back to Sarøya aboard a Norwegian Catalina Flying Boat. Nine days later British destroyers carried the fugitives to safety in Murmansk, and Johnson returned to England.

Perils mounted in the north as the Nazis continued to scorch the Norwegian earth. The following telegram to the government-in-exile in London described but a small part of the danger facing Norwegians attempting to escape the threatened region.

> The Germans still continue their hunt for people who have hidden themselves in West Finnmark and in the Troms-district. Boats still come to Tromsø with the forcibly evacuated, some weeks more than 500. But they are treated as prisoners, and are taken to concentration camps at Krokebaersletta.[4]

Gunnar Johnson's first proposal for additional relief of his beleaguered people received no official support, since all available resources were directed toward Germany's final defeat. He then came up with a more wide-ranging but acceptable plan that would bring him back to Norway. Two officers and two enlisted men were to be sent to the German occupied area as an "anti-sabotage" unit. The four men were to travel about the north, instructing the populace to hide food and fuel in caves and among the rocks, to sink boats in shallow water, and to remove planks from the docks. In general they were to secure reserve supplies and make destruction of existing facilities more difficult for the Nazis. Leiv Kreyberg was selected as the second officer and departure was scheduled for May 9, 1945.[5]

The pace of military action accelerated rapidly throughout all battle areas leading the two physicians to fear their Catalina aircraft would be requisitioned for other use. Allied contingents were scheduled to land almost simultaneously in Oslo, Bergen, Trondheim, Stavanger, and Tromsø. Two days before their scheduled departure Johnson proposed yet another ingenious plan. He pointed out to the commander of the Norwegian armed forces that huge areas of Northern Norway with large numbers of German troops and significant local populations were to be left without any Allied military presence. He proposed that the tasks of his anti-sabotage group be altered. Within minutes the unit metamorphosed to an "advance administration party" that would disembark in Vesterålen, make contact with surrendering German forces, then serve as Norway's first military presence in the north.

Gunnar Johnson had correctly anticipated the confusion that would arise up on the liberation of his country. Five years of occupation with a government still functioning from abroad in the face of a local German *Nasjonal Samling* administration made the transition to civilian rule an obstacle course. For example, the Nazi-infiltrated police force had to separate officers who were traitors from those who were still loyal to their king and country—often functioning as valued double agents.

Between three and four hundred thousand fresh, battle-ready, and superbly equipped German troops remained in *Festung Norwegen* (Norwegian Fortress). Realistic fears arose that Nazi commanders would follow Hitler's directive to drag all Europe down with him should he fall. Against these well-disciplined forces the Norwegians could muster the fourteen thousand "Reserve Police" trained in Sweden, some forty thousand lightly armed irregulars scattered throughout the country in *Milorg* units, and the fourteen thousand troops being held in English bases in readiness for return to Norway.

Then too, Quisling was surrounded by his fanatical, and armed *Hird* and fears arose that the unstable traitor would plunge the country into civil war. At the very least, the bitterness loyal Norwegians felt against all quislings had flourished during the long Occupation. If vented in its fullest, this could lead to retribution in a night of "long knives."

The long and impatiently awaited announcement of Germany's capitulation was heard on the radio in Oslo on the afternoon of May 7, 1945. During that night both the Home Front leadership and *Milorg* defense units began to surface. The following afternoon the Allied Armstice Commission arrived in Oslo. Quisling and his band of traitors remained to be addressed. The would-be dictator had entrenched himself together with some of his ministers at Gimle, the rightful residence of the Norwegian Crown Prince on the island of Bygdøy, just outside Oslo. Surrounded by his *Hird* and Norwegian Nazis who had volunteered to fight side-by-side with the Germans on the Russian Front, Quisling demanded to be treated as a defeated head of state.

Concerned about the possibility of a violent confrontation with the volatile Quisling, the Home Front leadership decided to dispatch an envoy to Gimle on May 8, to negotiate surrender with the turncoat. The task was delicate, for Quisling, more rigid and unstable than ever, had always marched in Hitler's footsteps. A dependable, diplomatic, and resourceful envoy whom both the Norwegians and Quisling could trust was essential. In the mind of the lawyer, Lorentz Brinch, chief of the Home Front leadership, Dr. Bjørn Foss was the choice.[6]

Brinch considered Foss's medical background to be a critical factor in his selection—not only because of the societal trust it implied, but because it could be important in dealing with Quisling's mental instability. As chief of *Sanorg*, Foss had completed the tasks—initiated by Carl Semb and Kristian Kristiansen—of building up medical stores sufficient to support an Allied invasion, thus obtaining the confidence and respect of Resistance leaders. Through dealings with both Germans and local Nazis in his official role as chief of the medical service of civil anti-aircraft defense, he had achieved acceptance by both groups as well as experience in dealing with the enemy. In the meantime he had succeeded in keeping his underground activities well hidden.

Still unaware of his selection Dr. Foss moved at a hectic pace. He had mobilized the twelve hundred physicians and nurses of his *Sanorg* medical corps and prepared the four aid stations in Oslo for action even before word of German capitulation came over his concealed radio receiver. He wasted little time rejoicing at the Nazi defeat, but went immediately to headquarters of the civil anti-aircraft defense, then to the prison at *Møllergata 19*.

A mass of impatient Norwegians had assembled outside the structure that had witnessed the torture of so many political prisoners and now held their friends and relatives. Many armed Nazi guards were present and Foss feared they might fire into the crowd should it push forward. With Police Inspector Andreas Bjørbaek, Foss made his way through the human mass and entered the prison. They found no guards at the doorways, and inside the hallway policemen stood about, aimless and perplexed.

Two *Nasjonal Samling* police lieutenants within the office informed them that neither the chief of police nor his adjutant were in the building. "You ought to go home now boys," said Foss. "You have lost the war, and we must not have confusion here."[7] The two officers moved menacingly and drew their pistols. Foss and Bjorbaek avoided further provocation by withdrawing into the hallway. There Foss spoke with the gathered policemen. He asked all non-Nazis to remove the hated insignia from their caps. When every Fascist emblem had been torn off Foss ordered the police officers to arrest the two quisling lieutenants. Just after the arrest was completed, Harry Söderman, the Swedish police chief, and godfather of the Norwegian troops in Sweden, appeared.[8]

Söderman addressed the excited crowd outside *Møllergata 19*. In soothing tones he explained why the political prisoners could not be released immediately. Thieves, informers, quislings, common criminals, and drunkards were intermixed with the victims of Nazi persecution. They must all be transported to Grini and sorted out before release would begin. Bjørn Foss prepared to go to Grini to prepare for the prisoners' arrival.

One more task remained before Dr. Foss could complete his night's work. Söderman wished to meet with the leadership of the Home Front police in order to set the release apparatus into motion. Foss made the necessary contacts then returned to his home in the late hours of the night. He was awakened at 7:00 A.M. on the morning of May 8 by the call from Lorentz Brinch with a mandate for a meeting with Quisling. The Home Front wanted no more bloodshed, and it was up to Foss to dissuade the traitor from ordering his forces to make a final, desperate stand.

Bjørn Foss contacted Quisling through a captain in the state police, setting the meeting for 8:00 A.M.[9] Quisling demurred saying the time was not suitable, proposing 11:00 A.M. instead. Foss replied that the victor should set the time, which he then did, for 1:00 P.M.

Diplomats could be distinguished by their clothes, and this was a diplomatic mission, Foss reasoned. He selected an impeccable, dark blue suit. For his drive to Gimle he secured the best vehicle he knew to have been hidden away during the war, a seven-passenger limousine.

Dr. Foss passed several hundred armed *Hird* on his way into the elegant villa at Gimle. Returning Quisling's bow, in proper Norwegian fashion he presented himself by name. Quisling did not reciprocate. The traitor then led his guest to the fireplace where two of his *Nasjonal Samling* Ministers rose to introduce themselves. The joyous celebration from the city of Oslo could be heard clearly through the window as the four men sat without speaking. Bjørn Foss broke the silence. "You know why I am here" he said after he had refused Quisling's offer of a cigarette. What I wish is that it will not develop into a battle action. I have the mandate to offer you and your wife the protection of the Home Front Forces in a villa on Holmenkollen until your trial comes up. You can take whatever is necessary for you and your wife!"[10]

Quisling responded with a question: "Why is it exactly *you* who comes?" Dr. Foss, however did not feel compelled to reply, for in truth, he himself did not know why it *was* he who was selected as envoy.

Quisling appeared unwell, but once the silence was broken he spoke without interruption for an hour and a half, in a voice that was often tearful. He began with a bitter complaint that the Germans had tricked him, and that his battles had always been fought for, and not against, Norway. He had thirty thousand men in the vicinity of Oslo, while *Milorg* could muster but four thousand, he said. On that day he could win, but he knew his defeat was inevitable. The Allies were certain send aid to his enemies, and against their might he could not prevail. He did not wish Norway to become a battleground anew.

Bjørn Foss sat silently through the entire soliloquy, but he had difficulty maintaining his composure as Quisling concluded:

> I am disappointed in the Norwegian people. In ten years they will see that I am right. Then they will see the danger from the East. I know that I am condemned to death by the Norwegian people, and I know that the simplest thing for me is to take my own life, but after mature consideration I wish to see history's judgement on that,—and I believe that in ten years I will be a new St. Olaf.[11]

Quisling made it clear that he would not allow his followers to plunge the country into civil war, but he also refused the protection of the Home Front. He would not accept the refuge at Holmenkollen unless the offer applied to his ministers as well. That, the Home Front was not prepared to offer.

As Foss rose to leave Vidkun Quisling followed him to the doorway, placed a hand on Foss's shoulder and said, "I give you my assurance there will be no battle."

"Thank you for that," Foss replied. "If you have the need to speak with me, you can ring me at Møllergata 19."

"Thanks," responded Quisling. "That might possibly come to pass."[12]

A telephone call from Gimle, indeed reached no. 19 that very night inquiring for Bjørn Foss, but through some misunderstanding the caller was told the doctor was not in.

Dr. Foss's open manner had convinced Quisling a trial would be fair. Without protest, the Norwegian traitor responded to an ultimatum that same evening, and with some of his ministers reported to *Møllergata 19* early on the morning of May 9. He was, however, indignant at being placed in an ordinary cell, now demanding the Home Front offer of protective isolation in a villa on Holmenkollen, and completely disregarding his earlier refusal.

26. Leiv Kreyberg: Caring for Norway's Allies

On May 9, Norwegian, British, and American troops entered Oslo. On that same day Dr. Gunnar Johnson set out directly for the British air base at Woodhaven. Leiv Kreyberg, meanwhile, gathered a bundle of cigarettes, a sack of coffee, a British flag, and a Norwegian pennant, then traveled by taxi to the airfield. Late that afternoon the two physicians took off for Norway and, aboard the plane, studied their orders. It was soon clear they were to have command of virtually the entire northern region.

Heavy winds battered the aircraft as it passed through snow-laden clouds over the North Sea, but the skies cleared as they reached the Trøndelag Coast. A crewman felt the need for a cup of coffee and, lacking a kerosene stove, decided to ignite a small container of gasoline with a match. After the makeshift apparatus had set fire to the flooring and the flames had been extinguished by a blanket of foam, the crewman repeated his act with the same result. As the airman began yet a third attempt Kreyberg envisioned a plaque at his university "Gave His Life for His Country,"[1] in truth for a cup of coffee. Kreyberg's explicit threats put an end to any further effort.

It was still daylight in the far north as the two doctors landed at Langøya at 1:00 A.M. on May 10. Gunnar Johnson had been in Norway less than three months earlier, but for Leiv Kreyberg it was an emotional return to his home country after a five-year absence. An extended wedding celebration was in progress, and the newcomers were welcomed as unexpected guests. They reciprocated, serving coffee from their stores—a beverage that had long since disappeared from Norwegian homes.

Kreyberg then telephoned Dr. Nils Brodersen at Stokmarknes Hospital, saying simply, "It is Gunnar and Leiv."[2] Brodersen needed nothing else. The two returnees arranged transport by motorboat and by 6:00 A.M.

met Brodersen at the hospital dock. Even before breakfast the three physicians drank a *skål* from a bottle that, as in every loyal household, had stood for five years awaiting this moment.

Quickly, the three men contacted local Home Front leaders to prepare for confrontation with the commander of the occupying German Forces. Contact with the Home Front in Oslo had yet to be made, so Johnson, Kreyberg and the local patriots drafted a dozen rigid demands for presentation to Norway's former enemies. They had no idea what agreements might have been reached in Oslo or how they could enforce their will on the hundred thousand or more heavily armed, Nazi troops. The demands were outlined as follows:

1. German troops were to be interned at Haug and Flatset.

2. All enlisted men were to be disarmed. Officers were to be allowed to keep their handguns.

3. All telephone communications with their German superiors were to take place only after permission of the Section Commander at Hadsel.

4. All radios were to be delivered with the exception of two for each camp—one for enlisted men and one for officers.

5. All confiscated Norwegian goods were to be gathered together for redistribution.

6. All minefields were to be exploded.

7. All vessels were to be abandoned, with all materiel remaining aboard.

8. The vessel commanders and section commanders were to be personally responsible to see that no sabotage is carried out.

9. All alcohol was to be delivered immediately to the Chief of Police at Hadsel.

10. Automobiles and bicycles were to be delivered.

11. All German camps were to be supervised by the Section Commander at Hadsel.

12. All communication with the civilian population were to cease immediately.

In return, Norwegian military authorities—at that time consisting of only two physicians and two enlisted men—committed themselves to the following conditions:

1. Safety of German troops would be guaranteed.

2. The German forces were to keep their existing rations of food.

3. A Norwegian guard would be placed in protective positions around the German camps so the troops would not be molested.

4. The repatriation of German troops would begin as soon as possible.[3]

Dr. Brodersen then telephoned the German commandant, announcing the arrival of an "Allied Commission" that required the German officer's presence at Dr. Brodersen's abode precisely at 3:00 P.M.

A table was then set up in center of the Brodersen dining room. Norwegian and British flags were fixed to the wall behind. Just before the appointed hour two enlisted men, Sten guns in hand, were placed on the outside stairway. Their instructions were strict. Look at the Germans only from a distance. When the Nazi officers passed on the stairway, the sentinels were to stare steadfastly ahead.

Minutes before 3:00 five officers appeared, clothed in foot-length green capes, and resembling "five bottles of Mosel Wine."[4] They were forced to wait outside until the third chime of the living room clock had faded—the enlisted men playing their part to perfection. As the Germans entered they found Johnson and Kreyberg seated at the table and backed by the Norwegian and British flags. Ludvig Brandtzaeg represented the Home Front and Dagny Brodersen, who happened to be a second cousin to Leiv Kreyberg, was also present. Mrs. Brodersen was given the role of secretary as compensation for events of the previous day, when she had raised the Norwegian flag, only to have it hauled down by the Nazis, accompanied by insulting remarks.

Two days later Major Kreyberg sailed from Stockmarkenes and arrived in Narvik at 11:00 P.M. In the Grand Hotel he met with the commanding officer for Norwegian forces in north Norway, Colonel Munthe-Kaas, who detailed Kreyberg's new and vital assignment. During the war the Nazis had imported thousands of prisoners of war into northern Norway as slave laborers in both the fish filet factories and on the Nordland Railroad. Conditions in the POW camps were abysmal, particularly in the last years of the war, and countless prisoners had perished. Munthe-Kaas appointed Dr. Kreyberg as chief of all camps for allied prisoners of war in Nordland County. He was to be entrusted with the rehabilitation and repatriation of the forty thousand Soviets, eight hundred Yugoslavs, and twelve hundred Poles who still existed in misery in the northern camps—all malnourished and many seriously ill. The report from but one such camp indicated the dimension of the task:

> About 800 Russian prisoners arrived in camp in Trofors, 15 April, 1945 after being held captive in Dolstad Church about four months. The camp consists of four barracks. Half a barrack serves as a dispensary. Each barrack is made up of two rooms measuring about 11 x 2.75 meters with a height of 1.75 meters. On the day of our inspection 63 sick men occupied

the dispensary. On 18 May, 74 men were lodged in the same room. One Russian doctor and three *feldschers* were available for medical assistance. The doctor only had 1 knife and 1 pair of forceps at his disposal, together with some gauze. . . .

Most of the patients suffered from general weakness, inanition, edema, some with tuberculosis, and many with acute gastroenteritis with bloody stools. The rest of the soldiers were distributed in the remaining seven rooms, (i.e., 355 men in 200 square meters with walls 1.75 meters high).

The buildings appeared hastily slapped together from poor materials. . . . The Russians lay in bunks of two levels with up to 5 centimeters separation between the boards of the bunks. No straw was to be found in the camp. Each man had only a single wool blanket for cover. No washrooms were to be seen. The latrines were built with walls only along the length, but none across and lay about three meter south of the dispensary. Excrement lay uncovered, and produced a dreadful stench.[5]

Dr. Kreyberg's responsibilities stretched far beyond caring for the health of the prisoners of war. He was charged with organizing self-government in the camps in order to free the small Norwegian forces from administration and guard duty as much as possible—and then arrange, together with the state police, for those guards still needed. He was to organize the "welfare" of the POWs, arrange for provisions (including the use of German sources), and transmit reports at least every fifteen days on conditions in the camps.

During the war local Norwegians could not help but recognize the misery, disease, and death that prevailed in the prison camps. They did all they could for the wretched prisoners—but always at risk, and always in secret. They passed food to them whenever possible, and encouraged them at every opportunity, but it was not enough. Thousands died and thousands still faced death in the camps. When it became obvious that Germany's collapse was inevitable Norwegians gathered fish, cod liver oil, and potatoes. Under the leadership of Dr. Anton Johnson, contact was sought with the German command to allow shipment of the nourishing foods to the prisoners. At times the attempts were successful, and at other times they were rebuffed. The overwhelming majority of foodstuff and clothing clearly remained in Nazi hands. The surrender agreement required German cooperation, which was given grudgingly. If prisoners were to survive, the Nazis had to give up some of their own food. Kreyberg organized forays through the defeated enemy's camps to search out potatoes they had secreted away for their own use.

Leiv Kreyberg turned immediately to Anton Johnson, who was Gunnar's brother. As district chief of *Milorg*, he also was nominally Kreyberg's superior. They drafted policies that would bring the prisoners as quickly as possible to health and freedom. They could not, of course, manage the enormous tasks independently, so other members of *Milorg* were recruited. The area was divided into five subsections—each under the responsibility of a local physician.

The Germans at times refused to take orders from civilians, or did so grudgingly. Accordingly, Kreyberg collected a bag of "stars," and Mrs. Frostad sewed three on her husband's windbreaker and another three on her son's scout cap. The next morning the German officer in Saltdal clicked his heels together with a *"Jawohl, Herr Hauptmann"* as the Home Front's Dr. Frostad was transformed into Captain Frostad. Other regional chiefs were made "officers" by the same device.

The Germans expressed concern about growing unrest among the prisoners, and feared they could no longer control the Russians without gunfire. It was clear to the two doctors, however, that Norwegians lacked the power and desire to master the prisoners. Rather, the doctors believed the liberated soldiers should be treated as the free men they indeed were. Kreyberg planned to make it clear that Norwegians were friends who would provide all possible help and appeal to the prisoners' own sense of discipline and responsibility.

Throughout the late spring and early summer of 1945 Leiv Kreyberg moved from camp to camp, seeing to the care of the harshly treated and malnourished ex-prisoners. His travels required an automobile, which could only be obtained through German sources. Vehicles were grudgingly given and commonly sabotaged. Three times the engine caught fire—and each time Kreyberg found an electric cable had been short-circuited close to the fuel supply. The third experience occurred in Mosjøen, where he had received a new car that had been recently "adjusted" by a German mechanic. As he drove away, Kreyberg placed a German officer in the seat beside him, until that vehicle too began to blaze. Dr. Kreyberg then returned to the German garage, commandeered General Alfred Jodl's own *Horch*, and drove off without further adjustment. On another occasion the exhaust pipe that was sawed through and held together with string collapsed during an inspection tour.

Day and night were virtually indistinguishable, for the dark disappears from the Arctic Circle at that time of year. In 1945 the weather neared perfection. Major Kreyberg kept a sleeping bag, radio, and typewriter in the car and for the most part, spent sunlit nights in his sleeping bag at the side of the road. Only rarely did he turn in to a camp or hospital to sleep.

Within the first ten days of receiving his assignment Major Kreyberg had visited a large number of Soviet camps throughout the entire area, always following the same ceremony. All prisoners able to stand assembled, and were greeted in a friendly manner. No longer were they prisoners, Kreyberg told them, but were free soldiers of the famous Russian Army. They were soon to return home and were requested to show discipline worthy of Generalissimo Stalin. The soldiers were responsible for their own organization. Food, clothes, and medicine would be sent as soon as possible.

At the outset Kreyberg used a Ukrainian-born Norwegian to convey his messages in Russian. Dr. Kreyberg soon realized the interpreter was adding statements of his own. Leiv then substituted Gunnvor Haavik, a nurse from Bodø Hospital, who had studied Russian as a hobby. Before long she knew the contents of Kreyberg's talk, and spoke independently after the doctor had greeted the prisoners.

By the time of his second official report (May 21) Kreyberg had visited or had received reports from all camps. Aside from the thousands of prisoners with signs of gross malnutrition he calculated that three to four thousand were severely ill, requiring hospitalization. Deaths were daily occurrences. Hundreds were found to have open tuberculosis. The need for hospital beds was critical.

At first barracks within the camp, as well as those requisitioned from the Germans, were equipped and staffed with both Norwegian and Soviet personnel. Not only were there some doctors among the Russians, but *feldschers* were also employed. *Feldschers* stood somewhere nurses and physicians. They performed minor surgery, assisted at operations, and carried out other tasks usually performed in the West by only the medically qualified. Because of the shortage of physicians in the Soviet Union *feldschers* were common in both civilian and military life.

German hospitals, along with their physicians and other personnel, were also employed, but unsatisfactorily so. German doctors were frequently careless, and the Russians had little or no confidence in them.

Dr. Kreyberg then sent out an urgent plea for aid to Oslo and to the Swedes who, in turn, appealed to their Red Cross. The Norwegian authorities sent a field hospital of one hundred and twenty beds under the direction of Dr. Hjalmar Wergeland. Dr. Sven Oftedal set up a program in Drevja that cared for five hundred patients, many seriously ill with tuberculosis. In all about two thousand beds were improvised in the course of a few weeks. The hospital was staffed by Norwegian physicians who, like Oftedal, had been held prisoner by the Nazis in German concentration camps.

In the early days food was as critical as medical care. The Allied high command ordered the Germans to transfer a thirty-day supply of provisions immediately to the prison camps. The Germans complied, but not without contemptuous suggestions that everything would be consumed long before the thirty days had passed. The Russians proved them wrong, for the rations were weighed with meticulous accuracy and distributed evenly throughout. The Swedes sent white flour, barley, and powdered milk to Bodø on aircraft of Colonel Bernt Balchen's group, and the British flew in smaller quantities of food. Rapid overeating caused some of the most starved of prisoners to become ill. In general, however, the return to health was remarkably rapid.

Clothing represented a far more difficult problem. On June 14, more than a month after he had taken command Kreyberg reported that only one hundred and fifty shirts were available for six hundreds patients in Drevja. The next day he found patients in Fauske in a wretched condition with ragged shirts and no sheets for their bunks. He telephoned the German commander, Colonel Buchweiser, and in the name of humanity, "demanded the shirts off his and his soldiers' bodies and sheets from his and his soldiers' beds until the Russian needs were filled."[6]

On June 17 he sent the following telegram to General Richter in Mo i Rana:

There are still to be found many hundreds of Allied ex-prisoners of war in my district who need immediate hospital treatment because of German mistreatment. We do not have enough places in our hospital because those places are occupied by those who have become healthy but cannot travel because they have no clothes. From both humanitarian and logical sides that is such a shocking condition that I will repeat directly to you what I have said to the Colonel: This condition cannot continue and I will not be silent to its continuing existence. Militarily I cannot give you this command, but in humanity's name, and possibly in your own interest arrange immediately to collect sufficient clothing so that we can extend all possible help to the mistreated, even if it costs the shirts off your own and your soldier's bodies. I speak now as a physician and a human being.

Kreyberg[7]

The following day Kreyberg received a message that six hundred complete outfits had been dispatched to the facility in Mo i Rana, and similar shipments sent to hospitals in Mosjøen, Drevja, and Fauske. The Swedes sent a supply of antiquated, "almost prehistoric" army uniforms with coats and peaked hats that had lain in storehouses since the eighteenth century.

Prisoners returned rapidly to health if starvation was the only problem. When tuberculosis accompanied the malnutrition the outcome was too often rapidly fatal. Once full vigor returned the prisoners became impatient. The Germans, in particular, but Norwegian and Allied authorities as well, became concerned about the Russians' behavior now they were no longer controlled. The Germans had continually maintained between 2,000–3,000 guards, backed up by the occupying force of 50,000 well-armed troops. The Norwegians could only muster 150 men from the Home Front and another 110 from the State Police and the Reserve Police. From the time of his original discussion with Anton Johnson, Kreyberg had steadfastly maintained that the prisoners must be their own masters and be responsible for their own discipline. The Norwegians simply did not have the needed manpower, and use of German troops was unthinkable. Assignment of guards to the camps would be degrading.

After Dr. Kreyberg convinced Major MacDonald, Lieutenant Colonel Laidlaw, and Colonel Wilson, representing the Allies, that his solution was the only practical way to manage the dilemma, prisoners took charge of the camps. Permits were issued that allowed a percentage of the freed prisoners to leave the camps each day.

The remarkable discipline exhibited by the Russian soldiers justified Kreyberg's confidence. Small incidents were more humorous than damaging. For the most part the incidents were directed against the Germans, whose officers still rode fine horses, drove about in elegant automobiles, and consumed real coffee and French liqueurs and wines. Now and then prisoners would stop German cars, throw the passengers into the river, and commandeer whatever property they could find. On one occasion a German colonel complained to the amazed Major Kreyberg that the Russian prisoners had helped themselves to 150 bicycles. The doctor could only ask if the colonel had lost all sense of propriety. Many of the bicycles and much of the other German "property" had been taken by force from the Norwegians.

Although they had nothing but disdain for their former wardens, the prisoners behaved most properly and graciously to their benefactors. The day the Swedish hospital began operation, bicycles belonging to the nurses disappeared and the chief surgeon, Dr. Nordwall, discovered his radio missing from his room. The Swedes, though distressed, did not complain. Leiv Kreyberg, however, alerted the Soviet commander. The Russian officer immediately expressed his regrets to the Swedes, for his men had assumed the hospital was German. In a gay procession the stolen property was returned. The bicycles were festooned with wild flowers and covered with messages of apology.

During the long Occupation the Russian slave laborers in the fish filet factory had fed a number of pigs with the seafood refuse. Despite the sentimental bonds the prisoners had developed with the animals, they decided to butcher the pigs as they prepared for a memorial banquet to their companions who had perished in the camps. When news of the anticipated slaughter reached Norwegian headquarters in Bodø, local agricultural authorities objected. They had intended to breed the pigs to replenish the depleted Nordland stock. The Russians threatened forcible resistance, and a messenger was dispatched to Bodø requesting armed troops to protect legitimate Norwegian interests.

Dr. Anton Johnson drove to the fish filet factory himself and prevented the confrontation. He found most pigs to be castrated and useless for breeding. There was, however, a single pregnant sow. In Solomonic judgement he turned the fertile animal over to the Norwegian authorities and gave all the sterile pigs to the Russians. The Soviet commander, Captain Paul, climbed upon a chest and, praising Johnson offered a pig as reward for his wisdom. The doctor, in the long tradition of independence of Norwegian judges, declined the gift. That midnight, however, a ham was surreptitiously placed on Johnson's doorstep.

Kreyberg's fearless, almost belligerent, advocacy of any measure that could contribute to the health and welfare of the prisoners often brought him into conflict with the Germans. Although he was inclined toward reason and diplomacy wherever former prisoners or the Allies were concerned, he exhibited no such tolerance toward his former enemies. Complaints about his behavior poured into Allied and Norwegian head-quarters from German sources throughout Nordland County.

On June 16, the day following Leiv Kreyberg's reproach to Colonel Buchweiser regarding the prisoners' lack of clothing the Norwegian received a call from Colonel Munthe-Kass, who inquired if he was happy in his position and wished to continue. The peculiarity of the wording suggested something amiss. Kreyberg immediately dispatched a letter to his superior, ending with: "I place myself at the disposal of the Zone-Commander completely, and will be more than happy to continue in that zone with high authority. I think I have prevented many episodes by taking a strong stand against our enemies and for our Allies."[8]

That very day the British zone commander, Brigadier Sandars arrived by plane from Tromsø and summoned Kreyberg to a conference. "What are you doing Kreyberg?," asked the British brigadier. Kreyberg quickly realized that the Germans had complained. He replied that he had attempted to carry out his assignment in the best possible manner. Sandars continued, "Be careful that you do not overstep your authority. What would you do if five Russian Divisions were sent to Norway because the Germans revolted? We do not have enough people to handle such a situation." The doctor answered that he had operated with an open mandate the entire time, and had no difficulty with the Germans until, behind his back, and without advising him, some person or another, had reduced the mandate to that of an "Inspection Officer", a position he would never have taken, as he was unwilling to *inspect* peoples' deaths. In his opinion the Allies had not done enough for the prisoners. "May I be permitted to return your question in a slightly different form?" Kreyberg asked. "What would you say, Brigadier if five Russian Divisions were sent here because we do not do enough for the Russians? You neglect the Russians out of fear of the Germans. I look after the Russians without fearing the Germans."[9]

The two men then drove to a camp outside Bodø, that was indeed one of the better, then on to the camp in Fauske. There Dr. Sadownikov, the Russian physician fell about Kreyberg's neck and wept in gratitude. The camp had received a large supply of linens during the night. Sandars' visit served only to strengthen Kreyberg's position.

The eight hundred Yugoslavians in their camp near the Arctic Circle were better nourished and better clothed than the Russians since they had received aid from America and from the Red Cross. The prisoners were largely intellectuals—teachers, artists, and university faculty. For the most part they were committed supporters of General Tito. Those considered to be traitors had been eliminated in the first days after the liberation. The relationship between that camp and the neighboring Russian compound was excellent.

Leiv Kreyberg described the twelve hundred Poles as the area's "spoiled children."[10] Many were arrogant and without particular inhibitions. The Polish soldiers were healthy on liberation and well clothed in their national uniforms, again through aid from America and the Red Cross. Some prisoners were said to be pro-Russian, while others were so anti-Soviet as to express open preference for the Germans as the lesser of two evils. The tensions between the two groups often ran high, especially during political discussions. Tactless expressions of anti-Russian sentiments led to a complaint from Russian officers.

During their long imprisonment the Soviet officers had "lost themselves" among their enlisted men. They had removed all insignia of grade and disguised themselves as common soldiers since Germans were expected to execute officers. Once liberated, the officers reemerged and took command. Discipline was superb among the Soviet soldiers, and even after the former prisoners were allowed to move about freely there were no crimes of violence. Camps that had been slovenly under German control now became models of cleanliness. Kitchens were swept and washed, and the cooking vessels cleaned and polished.

The Russians had little trust of their former captors and considered every treatment ordered by German physicians a manifestation of deviltry. On the other hand they obeyed orders from Norwegians and their own physicians without hesitation. During their imprisonment, surgical instruments available to the Soviet doctors were scandalously scarce. Nevertheless they performed abdominal surgery in crude barracks illuminated by oil lamps using equipment hardly adequate for even minor procedures.

As quickly as possible the Russians assumed the responsibility for their own hospitals. In Mo i Rana, for example, a Russian major announced late one afternoon that the Soviets wished to take over two German hospitals that had treated ailing prisoners. After concluding that an administrative officer, two physicians, a couple of *feldschers*, a chief cook, and kitchen personnel of eight to ten, as well as a nursing staff would be needed for each hospital the major decided to begin the takeover at 9:00 A.M. the following morning. Within days the miserable German hospital filled with lice-infested, dirty-footed patients was clean and provided good medical and nursing care. The Swedish Hospital functioned exactly four weeks before the Soviets took over the management.

On the surface the relationship between the newly emerged officers and their men appeared good. The joy of liberation seemed incomplete, however. A number of Russian prisoners refused to conform to the party line and others were even followers of the anti-communist Russian General Vlasov, who had fought with the Germans against his countrymen. Tribunals were established to mete out punishment with sentences ranging even to death. The secrecy of the executions prevented the Norwegians from ending the practice until some time had passed.

Leiv Kreyberg worked well with the Russian officers and moved to increase their cooperation and confidence with a series of small dinners in their honor wherever he traveled. At the Mosjøen dinner a Russian officer rose for a toast: "We know your great artists, Grieg and Hamsun. We heard that the latter became a fascist in his old days. We will forget the old man's erring in gratitude for what he had given."[11]

Norwegians, however were not so forgiving of their Nobel Laureate embracing both Nazism and the German presence. At that very time, Kreyberg noted, many Norsemen burned Knut Hamsun's books in anger and protest at his wartime behavior.

Only one really unpleasant incident soured Kreyberg's memory of Soviet officers—the visit of General Ratov. He wrote:

> I parked at the side of the road outside of Mo [i Rana] from 1900 hours in order to show the utmost courtesy and meet him [General Ratov] at the

"border." At 2300 hours [July 14] I was informed that the general had left Rognan and would arrive before 0230 [July 15].

At midnight the ship "Nordkyn" arrived, and since I had work connected with that ship I went to bed at 0100. I was awakened at 0230 by a British (Canadian) interpreter, who informed me that the general had arrived. I asked if I were wanted, and the answer was "Yes, right away." Ten minutes later I was greeted by the general in the hotel with a couple of insignificant questions, who then declared himself too tired to work. He asked me to return at 0900 in the morning.

At 0800 I was on my feet to see that all was in order. I came to the hotel at 0900, as agreed, and found the general in a deep sleep. I waited until 1030, without a sign of life. I then proceeded to the Brigade Headquarters for pressing telegrams and telephone calls. With the kind help of Major Rongstad, arrangements were made for lunch for the Russian guests. . . .

. . . Major Rongstad bade the guests welcome, and a general conversation developed. Ratov very soon expressed displeasure over our failure to control anti-Russian propaganda in the camps, and turned to Major Rongstad. The major passed the ball to me, for good reason—and then the general directed his displeasure toward me. We then began an argument through his interpreter. In a short time the hall became hushed as a result of the attack, so I found it appropriate that I give some facts, and rose for a short speech:

"Our honored guest, General Ratov, has chosen the lunch table to criticize our efforts, so I presume it necessary to remind our honored guest of some facts. With the collapse of German resistance in Norway we had over 26,000 Allied ex-prisoners and a great number of armed German troops in the North of Norway—in a part of our country without Norwegian resources and with very few men. I myself was one of the very few Allied soldiers in that region for several weeks. Even before the German collapse, the Home Front had planned to help our unfortunate Allies, and my mission was to coordinate that help from the Home Front with our Allies' policies. The picture was one of many thousand sick and mistreated prisoners, badly clothed and spiritually depressed. I saw my principal task thus: To bring food, clothing and medical assistance, at the same time re-establishing discipline and faith.

In the first few days the only food we could supply was fish, potatoes, cod liver oil, and bread. That streamed in. Later we obtained food from the German camps as well—an effort that was sabotaged to some extent by the Nazis.

In the course of three weeks we had more than 2000 ex-prisoners hospitalized under treatment of good physicians, in a district that normally had means to hospitalize but 500. The British and Swedes also aided in the form of trained personnel.

The question of clothing was very difficult, and I pressed the Germans
—even to demanding the shirts off their backs until the Russian needs
were filled. Later British and Swedish supplies poured in.

The prisoners' morale has been raised to the highest, and I wish to say
that Generalissimo Stalin has never had better ambassadors in our country
than those well-behaved, good-natured, and fine soldiers. And may I add a
personal remark. Never in the course of five and one half years of war have
I done any work that has personally given me greater satisfaction. What
can be more inspiring than to see broken, mistreated, sick, and degraded
human beings restored to mental and physical normality.

I had never expected to be thanked for that work, because the most
essential aspects were performed by others, but I have the right to demand
respect for that which was done. The only thing I have heard today
is criticism that I have not occupied myself with combatting political
propaganda in the camps. To that criticism I will reply: You have, General,
had four majors and one Lieutenant-Colonel traveling up and down
this sub-sector for four weeks—visiting the camp and making contacts
almost every day, and not a single one has mentioned that propaganda a
single time.

Allow me to use a picture: If I am standing on a quay and see some
children in danger of drowning, I will certainly jump into the water to try
to save them—even if there is a political meeting on the quay. These eight
weeks my principal work has been to save Russian lives, and to help them to
get food and clothing and to be sent home. That has been a humanitarian
effort.

Ratov raised yet another point: Men in the camps had disappeared, and
I was supposed to have allowed them to escape. My reply was an invitation
to the general that he visit a Norwegian hospital where a Russian lay who
had escaped death by stoning by his comrades. "The general drops the
matter," said the interpreter.

I ended by proposing a toast for friendship between our two great
peoples and continued cultural and humanitarian cooperation. Skaal for
King Haakon VII. Skaal for Generalissimo Stalin. After some grumbling,
Ratov departed, offering me his hand with a sort of a smile.

The British interpreter came toward me: "That devil, he has behaved
like this everywhere." The pleasant Russian interpreter in her captains'
uniform, even expressed regrets that she had been obliged to transmit such
unpleasant remarks.[12]

As the time of repatriation to their homeland neared, a smoldering
fear surfaced among the Soviet ex-prisoners. Their apprehension was
well founded, for Stalin considered capture by the enemy to be a crime.
A good Soviet soldier fought to the death. The Yalta agreement had
raised similar apprehensions among the Poles with its stipulation that

all soldiers of Russian origin would be repatriated to the USSR. Polish soldiers who were born in Polish territory usurped by the Soviets were included by being considered Russians as well.

The Soviet officers inspecting the camps were extremely reserved toward their newly liberated countrymen. The ex-prisoners, on the other hand, became almost hysterical in attempting to demonstrate their loyalty. They decorated Stalin's portraits with leaves and flowers, and composed verbose messages of gratitude. Camp Commandant Ulanov dispatched the following message from Bodø on behalf of his command.

To Comrade Stalin.
Moscow, The Kremlin

We, prisoners of war in the special, hard-labor camp in the city of Bodø (Norway) extend a hearty thanks to our great victorious Red Army, and to you personally, Comrade Stalin, Leader and Commander, the brilliant organizer of victory in the war against fascism, against the menace of eternal slavery and medieval barbarism in the battle that has no parallel in history. We are grateful to have been saved from fascism's beastly yoke, from annihilation, from inhuman drudgery, from insult and degradation, and from starvation unto death.

During the entire imprisonment, and in spite of all the terror—killing on the spot, torture and hunger, illness, slave-labor, threats and insults— we did not lose faith in our great people, our courageous Red Army, and in you our leader—faith in our righteous cause and in an eventual victory. We did not lose hope to return to our socialist fatherland, and to once again work for the welfare and future of our peoples, for our fatherland, and for our mothers', fathers' and childrens' freedom.

We have suffered irreparable losses, we have been witness to how many thousands of our comrades perished, we felt the consequences of hunger and disease, but were, and are not bowed, exactly the opposite, we are strengthened. We have ourselves experienced the feeling of what fascism means, and our hatred will live as a legacy to our children and grandchildren.

We, who found ourselves in a foreign land, in the harsh nature of the Polar Circle, we rejoice in the victory, together with our great victorious people, together with all the freedom-loving nations of the world. We take the opportunity to thank the Norwegian people for all their help in spite of the prohibition and persecution by the German occupiers. Many of us have only the Norwegian people to thank that we came through with our lives intact.

We are proud today, during the universal celebration and cheering, to lift our red banner over the region where the melancholy camps previously lay.

Long live our beautiful socialist fatherland and our people!

Long live our courageous, victorious Red Army that has liberated the fatherland from the fascist villains!

We wish you—our leader—commander of the Army and organizer of the historic victory—still many years of work for our peoples' welfare, and for the flourishing of our socialist fatherland.

Signed, having been given the mission by the camp,

Bodø, 14 May, 1945
Camp Commandant Ulanov[13]

The repatriation of the Soviet former captives began near the end of June and was virtually complete by mid-July. For the most part the ex-prisoners marched quietly to the quay to begin their fateful journey to Russia. Some few managed to escape, including "the well-educated young man who sang so transportedly at the departure celebration in Mo i Rana when Ratov and his followers were present."[14] By the next morning he had disappeared without a trace.

27. A Tragedy in the North

Even in a nation of hikers and skiers Dr. Hjalmar Wergeland's special skills in ski-jumping and gymnastics stood out. The young physician combined the daring of the athlete with the ingenuity of the scholar in his acts of Resistance.

Wergeland's father, as director of a teachers college, had felt the brunt of *Nasjonal Samling* pressure early in the Occupation.[1] The native Fascists, having failed to force Nazi propaganda into the school room, shifted their tactics to the education of the teachers. The senior Wergeland was discharged from his position in the first step of a Quisling move to infiltrate the faculty with fellow travelers and foist the Nazi line on the future teachers. Student applicants were then screened, and those selected consisted principally of candidates whose records indicated Nazi leanings.

Borrowing his father's key, young Wergeland entered the college office under cover of night to conduct a screening of his own. His list complete, Dr. Wergeland then wrote all non-Nazi students applying for admission to the school, advising them of the circumstances and urging all loyal Norwegians to withdraw their applications. The advice was followed uniformly—the college could not open the term because so few students enrolled.

The imprisonment of teachers and thousands of other loyal Norwegians placed a heavy burden on family members, and the Home Front worked mightily to provide food and financial support to the distressed families. Dr. Johannes Heimbeck's financial wizardry, together with money smuggled in from the government-in-exile, supplied funds distributed through a network of couriers, among them Hjalmar Wergeland and his wife, Helga. On one occasion when Helga struggled to board a train bearing a case stuffed with half a million kroner she appealed to a nearby Nazi officer for aid. Anxious as the Germans were in the earliest year of the Occupation to cultivate Norwegian friendships and obligations, the officer willingly bore the contraband aboard.

Unlike Denmark, a self-sufficient and even an exporting agricultural nation throughout the war, Norway was hard-pressed to supply its own needs. Only 4 percent of its rocky land was arable, and even in the best of years Norway used much of its precious foreign exchange in the import of food.

German demand for much of the native foodstuff added deprivation to the other stresses of the war years. Yet Norwegians stretched every means to care for those stripped of their livelihood by the Nazis. Farmers who had habitually milked twice daily were forced to yield much of the product to the forces of the Third Reich. Secretly the dairymen added a third milking, much of which was passed on for Home Front use. Norway's physicians were critical to the third milking distribution network, for they had easy and frequent contact with both producer and recipient.

Wergeland was in charge of the Telemark network. Just as the Nazis in Oslo descended upon the University and interned students, the Gestapo became aware of his role. Warned by *Milorg*, Hjalmar concealed himself in Telemark's forests for two weeks, then made his way across the border to Sweden, a crossing that had become crowded with fleeing students.

In Stockholm, Hjalmar Wergeland was assigned to assist Carl Semb and Kristian Kristiansen in administration of the Health Camps, organizing the deployment of refugee physicians and medical personnel. He was still in Stockholm shortly after the German capitulation in May 1945, when a catastrophe in Finnmark dampened Norse jubilation. As Norwegian and Soviet troops had pursued the fleeing German army in the far north, the Nazis had strewn the area in their rear with land mines. Following German surrender, Norwegian explosive experts began to clear the area—heaping mines in a huge mound as the search for others continued. While demonstrating sounding, an officer accidently set off the mine underfoot. The detonation spread to the perilous heap, and within seconds twenty-two Norwegians were dead and many others injured.

The call for emergency medical aid went to Carl Semb, who found all but one surgeon under his command attached to field hospitals they were unable to leave. The single surgeon available was so heavy that parachuting into the area would certainly make him a casualty himself. Semb's only alternate, the relatively untrained Hjalmar Wergeland, was eager to help. He had had only three years of surgical experience on the wards of a small hospital, but time and urgency left no choice. Wergeland prepared to travel.

Without a moment's instruction in jumping, Wergeland and a surgical nurse volunteer donned parachutes and set out for Finnmark in a small

Bernt Balchen plane. Dense fog covering the drop area made the jump too perilous, especially for the inexperienced duo, and the rescue mission was forced to return to a Swedish air base. Carl Semb, chafing all the time his surgical team was in the air, succumbed to his inner urgings and joined in the effort. While waiting for the fog to lift the trio had some hours to practice for the jump under the guidance of Norwegian experts.

Harry Söderman, acting as intermediary in the preparations, anxiously awaited word of a safe arrival. A bell rang as he fretted. He opened the door to two Jehovah's Witnesses, who explained in halting Swedish they had come to speak about God's solutions to problems on earth. All this, Söderman wrote later, "while I have Carl Semb in the Arctic air . . . 500 meters above Karasjok."[2]

As they traveled toward their goal the two doctors laid plans. Hjalmar Wergeland, young, fit, and with the skills and confidence of athletic training felt secure. The landing could be no more difficult than flying through the air, landing with a shock, and balancing on two thin skis while still speeding downhill. For Semb it was different—he was fifty years old and without jumping experience. Wergeland was to jump first, survey the situation, then radio to Semb still circling above. Only if his surgical skills were needed would he jump.

Hjalmar Wergeland easily completed the task of jumping, but once below he was unsure. Another physician on the scene took responsibility and radioed Dr. Semb for help.

As he prepared to leave the plane, Semb was reluctant to allow the nurse to make the drop as well. She had been air-sick through the entire flight. Still she resisted Semb's order to remain aboard the plane—and threatened to leave the plane without a parachute if Semb denied her permission to leave with one.

The fears were for naught. All traces of air-sickness disappeared after the pair's safe landing. The nurse assisted Semb and Wergeland as they operated for twenty-four hours without stop. Several of the injured were saved, then transported to the hospital in Bodø for further treatment.

Dr. Wergeland's next mission was to join Leiv Kreyberg in caring for the maltreated Russian ex-prisoners of war in the north of Norway.

THE AFTERMATH OF WAR

28. Leo Eitinger's Long Journey Home

For the second time a welcome voice called for Norwegians over the Buchenwald loudspeaker—not in their native tongue but in English. The caller was Severt Stackland,[1] a U.S. Army corporal, born of Norse parents from Westland and raised in Iowa. Severt took pride in the little Norwegian he spoke and understood, but he wrote laboriously and phonetically. Severt wished to bypass military censors and reasoned— correctly—that letters in Norwegian could convey everything he desired, yet remain mysterious to censoring eyes.

The Norwegian Jews helped their new American friend as, together, they wrote Severt's parents in their native language. In a few short weeks Stackland and the "displaced" Norwegians became virtually inseparable. Severt was a warm and caring human being and particularly well placed to help others. His special task was a daily drive—Sundays excluded—into Jena for the rations that fed the camp.

When Stackland first arrived in Buchenwald bodies remained heaped in the camp, to be collected by German soldiers who had exchanged prisoner status with their former captives. One day as Severt passed two Germans tossing corpses into a wagon, he noticed slight movement in a body. "*Halten!*" he shouted, then sent a passing G.I. for a jeep. The Americans wrapped the woman carefully, and sent her off to the hospital in Kassel.

On a trip to Jena he found a young woman blocking the center of the road. As Stackland maneuvered his truck to the left, the girl moved as well. Climbing down from the vehicle, he discovered the young woman was Czech—held prisoner in enforced servitude to a German farming family. She had prepared for a homeward journey, but had no way to carry her luggage. Severt completed his duties, then picked up the young Czech and her bags. Behind the picket fence the German matron cried out, "I have treated her like a mother." Two youths, standing along the

267

fence either "smiling or crying" had used their Czech prisoner as a sex partner at will, said the woman. Stackland drove the former captive to Weimar, then found her a room for the night. By the next morning she had boarded a bus for her homeland.

Severt Stackland worked mightily to start his Norwegian friends on their way home. He approached his superiors, seeking ways to send them to England while the war was still in progress—to no avail. Once news of German capitulation in Norway was announced over the radio he tried every means to send them northward—again without success until he met British chaplain Captain H. J. Woodall.[2] The chaplain's driver, a young Austrian Jew, had fled to England and enlisted in the British Army. He had volunteered for service in Germany in hope of finding his father, who had been imprisoned as a Social Democrat. The British soldier discovered most Austrian Social Democrats had been held in Buchenwald, then prevailed upon the chaplain to journey the hundred miles from their station in Hamburg to the concentration camp.

Woodall's journey to Buchenwald was truly a golden deed. Father and son were reunited, for the older man had managed to conceal his Jewish identity throughout the ordeal. Initially the chaplain was hesitant to start the five "displaced persons" on the way to Norway. Woodall was moved, however, by the joy of the reunion and the miseries the prisoners had experienced in Buchenwald.

Leo Eitinger added another young Norwegian to Woodall's passenger list. Alf Knudsen had barely reached the state of conscious recognition when the group set out. He had suffered both typhoid fever and an encephalitis that had wiped out all knowledge of the period—even an awareness of the end of the war. The patient was placed on a mattress on the floor of the small lorry that began the trip to Hamburg on May, 15, 1945. Stackland loaded his friends with preserves, sausages, and other provisions, and supplied them with U.S.-issued documents of identity. For Shua, Stackland had one more parting gift. Some time earlier the young corporal had been beckoned by a youthful Jew, insistently stammering, "Kommen sie mit" (come with me). The former prisoner refused to be denied, and finally persuaded Stackland to accompany him to the camp quarry. There he tugged at a great boulder. Stackland summoned three G.I. friends, and together they nudged the rock to disclose a cavity below. Inside were four suitcases: the first packed with eyeglasses and jewelry, the second with Russian paper money, the third with old style, oversized U.S. currency, and the fourth with watches. Severt accepted five watches. One he gave to a little boy, one he kept for himself, and three were presented to Shua and two other departing Norwegians.

As darkness fell the happy group reached Celle, not far from Hamburg, where Reverend Woodall sought lodging for the night. The chaplain was turned away from a number of military units before his passengers recognized themselves as the obstacle—only the captain and his driver would be lodged. The Norwegians told their benefactor they had slept in all sorts of places, and could well sleep in the small lorry. Woodall would have none of that, and finally found quarters for the lot.

The following day they reached the shattered remains that had been Hamburg, then started off toward Kiel where Chaplain Woodall thought the chances of finding further transport to the Danish border were better.

Before reaching Kiel, however, the group encountered Kristina Söder-baum, driving a car flying a small Swedish flag. Kristina, who was then looking after Sweden's interests in Germany, readily offered assistance to her fellow Scandinavians. After well over a hundred miles aboard the small British lorry, the Norwegians said grateful goodbyes to the captain and his driver. Kristina then drove the group to Kiel, where she canvassed every British Military Office seeking permits for her charges to cross the Kiel Canal. Everywhere she came up empty-handed. Still lacking the necessary papers they started out for the canal, but were stopped and turned back. In Kiel they sought overnight lodging in a variety of places including a collecting station for voluntary civil workers. The collecting station manager, a Canadian descendant of Norse parents from Trøndelag, made room for the former prisoners in the crowded quarters.

On May 17, 1945, the day Norwegians celebrated their national holiday in their homeland as free citizens for the first time in five years, the small band searched for transportation to Denmark. By chance they found a former Russian prisoner who had managed to steal a German car. They exchanged a share in Stackland's largesse for a ride to Flensburg on the Danish frontier. Still lacking proper papers, the travelers painted a Norwegian flag on the auto, and stuck Eitinger's Red Cross armband on the window. The decorations served their purpose. The travelers crossed the Kiel Canal unmolested, and arrived at the border unchallenged.

The Danish consul in Flensburg treated his fellow Scandinavians as if they were his own children. "It would be my principal task and greatest pleasure to help you over the border today, the 17th of May," he told them.[3] Some hours after the consul had driven into Denmark he returned with a Red Cross worker. "You need worry no longer," she told the waiting Norwegians. "You are now in the hands of the Danish Red Cross."[4]

Passports were unnecessary as the freed men crossed over to the Danish side. They were met with a shower of chocolates and cigarettes, and apologies there was not more to give. The first evening on free Scandinavian soil was celebrated with a festive dinner as guests of the townspeople of Padborg.

On the following day the six Norwegians were taken by bus to be examined at a Copenhagen hospital. By then Knudsen was much improved. After a week they boarded a ship for Oslo together. The joy of return was blunted by the bitterness of a second group of passengers—Norwegian military officers who had been interned in Germany during the war. The Nazis had issued a call early in the Occupation to which the officers had responded voluntarily. Their countrymen were critical and unforgiving—the officers should have fled to Sweden rather than passively surrender to the Germans. No Norwegians met the disgraced officers as the ship slid into her pier in Oslo.

Assor and Asriel Hirsch recognized their brother waiting on the quay. He had survived the entire war in Norway, hidden away as a "patient" in Gaustad Mental Hospital. Augusta Helliesen, sister to Sigrid Helliesen Lund, had been notified by the Danish Red Cross and welcomed Shua Eitinger on the pier. She brought the five returning Jews to a temporary Red Cross hospital in the Norwegian Broadcasting System Building near Ullevål Hospital. The new arrivals were examined, found fit, and released to resume their lives in Norway.

Within days Leo Eitinger traveled to Nesjestranda—a solitary returnee. Nora Lustig and the Taglichts had perished in the gas chambers, and Robert Weinstein had disappeared after being sent to clear the ruins of the Warsaw Ghetto. Hans and Fritz Lustig had been rescued from Mathausen in deplorable condition, but had survived. For the time being, they had returned to Czechoslovakia.

Nesjestranda sorrowed over the fate of their Czech friends whose ashes were covered by neither grave nor marker. In Sølsnes Churchyard, villagers raised a stone, carved with the names Nora Lustig, Robert Weinstein, and Vera and Tibor Taglicht.

At the unveiling of the memorial stone, Pastor Aksel Kragset spoke these words:

> This memorial stone is not only carved from the rock, but has also sprung out from our hearts.
>
> Was there ever a time in Norwegian homes or in the country of Norway when it was the custom to hand over to the hangman those who had sought protection in our homes? Had it not always been the custom in Norway to help and protect the defenseless who lived in our homes?
>
> We are deeply ashamed of the atrocities that took place in Norway, when hundreds of peaceful people who had come for protection in our homeland

were handed over to suffering and death. This is without comparison the worse disgrace that ever took place in Norway and the worse stain on our history.

I then unveil this memorial stone with the wish that in times to come it will remind the community of Veløy about this: Each man, no matter of what race he may be, is your brother, and with the wish that he always brings about the cherished memories of four dear brothers and sisters from another country. Peace be with you[5]

Nesjestranda had been like a home to the Czech Jews, Eitinger then told his friends in return. He thought of the small village as a bright spot held before him as a precious memory in dark and troubled times.

Shua Eitinger could not linger long in Nesjestranda regardless of his bonds with Aksel Kragset and the warm-hearted villagers, for he was committed to continue humanitarian work. Dr. Sven Oftedal, who had ministered to his countrymen so caringly in Grini and Sachsenhausen, had collected volunteers to treat Russian ex-prisoners of war under Leiv Kreyberg's jurisdiction in Northern Norway. Eitinger had much to do for few full-fledged physicians were among the many volunteers. Most were medical students whose training had been interrupted. Eitinger was appointed superintendent of the hospital in Mosjøen.

When Leiv Kreyberg arrived in Mosjøen he had no words for Shua Eitinger, who followed him around dutifully on the inspection tour then on to the hotel. It was as if the older doctor had no recollection of their meeting in Buchenwald. At the hotel Kreyberg suddenly turned, and asked a favor. "Could you come and visit us when we are in Oslo?,"[6] Leiv requested. Eitinger, of course, readily agreed.

In Mosjøen, Dr. Eitinger received a telephone call from his former superintendent in Bodø, wondering what in the world had happened to him. "Why aren't you here?," Shua was asked. "You have your position here."[7] That Eitinger's work permit was revoked was of no import. The time had come for him to move on with his life's work.

29. Judgment Day: The Trial of Vidkun Quisling

Five years of preparation for liberation began to pay dividends on May 7, 1945. In anticipation of that day The Norwegian government-in-exile had authorized the Home Front to accept the German surrender, maintain order, and assume temporary responsibility for Norway's civil administration. At the same time the Reserve Police of fourteen thousand men were to cross the border from Sweden and cooperate with the Home Front in the effort. Over the next twenty-four hours *Milorg* units—about forty thousand strong—emerged to take over their assigned tasks.[1]

Identified only by armbands and makeshift uniforms of knee-pants and a jacket, *Milorg* leaders accepted the surrender of battle-ready Nazi forces, then moved against their country's traitors. The jail at *Møllergata 19* and the prison camp in Grini were emptied of victims of Nazi tyranny and filled with collaborators and both Germans and Norwegians accused of war crimes.

Milorg units began a search for the greatest of the criminals, while the Nazis attempted to frustrate that search. The German High Command issued secret orders to hide and protect members of the *Nasjonal Samling* Security Police who sought their aid. Many were issued enlisted men's uniforms and concealed among the masses of ordinary German soldiers. Siegfried Fehmer, the infamous chief of the Gestapo in Oslo, who had usurped the home that later became Ole Jacob Malm's abode, resorted to the subterfuge of a private's uniform only to be betrayed by his love of a dog. After donning the *Wehrmacht* uniform he slipped in among the German troops interned at Solørkanten. *Milorg*, well aware of the fondness of the cruel "Gestapist" for his pet shepherd dog, monitored telephone conversations between German camps. When Fehmer called to inquire about his dog, he was discovered and arrested.

The *Milorg* unit that hurried toward Skaugum, the residence of Crown Prince Olaf that *Reichskommissar* Joseph Terboven had requisitioned for his own quarters, was turned back by heavily armed Nazi troops. In the meantime Terboven and SS General Wilhelm Redeiss barricaded themselves in a bunker the occupying forces had constructed. Their chief of security then touched off an explosion that saved Norway the trial of the two who topped the list of war criminals.

Heinrich Fehlis, head of the Gestapo in Norway, took refuge with seventy of his men in a German military base near Porsgrunn. When *Milorg* units demanded he be turned over, Fehlis first swallowed poison, then shot himself.

Two members of Quisling's cabinet, Minister of Justice Sverre Riisnaes, and Minister of Police Jonas Lie, sought cover at a Skallum farm, together with the Quisling Chief of Police Henrik Rogstad. When Riisnaes emerged to surrender to *Milorg* forces surrounding the farm, he reported that Lie and Rogstad had taken their own lives.

Led by a flotilla of minesweepers, and accompanied by the British cruiser *Apollo*, the cruiser *Devonshire* that had borne him away almost five years before returned Crown Prince Olaf to his homeland on Sunday, May 13.[2] The crown prince, who doubled as commander in chief of Norway's Armed Forces, was greeted at the dock by Chief Justice of the Supreme Court Paal Berg, Mayor of Oslo Einar Gerhardsen, a number of other functionaries, and a tumultuous crowd of welcoming countrymen. In an open car with Max Manus, he was driven to the Royal Palace at the end of Karl Johansgate. Disregarding the deplorable state of the palace, despite the vigorous efforts of the royal staff, Crown Prince Olaf decided to spend his first days back in Norway in the palace—at home.

The greater celebration was reserved for the return of King Haakon and Crown Princess Marthe on June 7, 1945.[3] Thousands of small boats escorted the vessels bearing the king and his party in a welcome unseen since Fridtjof Nansen sailed the *Fram* up Oslofjord. Flags and banners draping the buildings and strung across the wide avenue virtually obliterated the sky above Karl Johansgate as the king was driven past the jubilant crowds to face the hundreds of thousands clogging the streets and *Slottsparken* surrounding the palace grounds.

There could be but a single choice to greet the king who had become the nation's hero in exile—the man who had set the Resistance in motion and had provided counsel and moral support throughout the Occupation—Johan Scharffenberg. The decision, that had been made by the Home Front leadership as he sat in his cell at *Møllergata 19* in 1940, reached fruition on the joyous day in June 1945. Dr. Scharffenberg, having become a confirmed *ex-republican*, thanked the king warmly for his defense of Norway, for maintaining the principle of sovereignty of his people, for his *no* to the German demand for a Quisling government on April 10, 1940, for the second *no* on July 3 to the Nazi demand he abdicate, and for serving as the standard bearer for his peoples' freedom and independence. Scharffenberg then turned to the masses and directed them to repeat his simple words to King Haakon and the Royal Household: "Welcome home to Norway!"[4]

Human costs of the war had been enormous for Norway's tiny population of about three million. From the time their government had departed and organized military action had ceased, about nine thousand Norwegians had lost their lives—almost half in the Resistance movement or in German concentration camps. More than eighty had died as a result of torture during interrogation or had committed suicide. Forty thousand loyal Norwegian men and women had been imprisoned for political crimes, almost nine thousand of whom were sent on to concentration camps in Germany.

The bitterness that had been building throughout the five years of Nazi and *Nasjonal Samling* brutality was expressed in the intensity with which the oppressors were searched out to be placed on trial—not in the ferocity of revenge. The nineteen-year-old *Milorg* youth who ordered the seventy-four *Gestapists* assembled in the square in front of *Viktoria Terrasse* to "*Hinlegen*" (lie down) and "*Auf*" (up) over and over again was hardly repaying the infamous tormentors in kind.

Members of the *Nasjonal Samling* whose only crime was belonging to the party and those whose activities were minimal were spared. More active traitors, collaborators, and *provocateurs* were arrested—all under written warrant—and tried. In all, forty-six thousand guilty verdicts were handed down. Eighteen thousand received fines alone, and twenty-eight thousand were sentenced to prison. For the most part sentences were brief. By the end of 1945, barely eight months after the proceedings had begun, ten thousand had been released.

Norway had long since abolished the death penalty in the Penal Code of 1902. The Military Penal Code, however, maintained that punishment. The Norwegian government-in-exile had also decreed on October 3, 1941, that the death sentence could be enforced after the war had ended. Thirty Norwegian traitors and German war criminals were sentenced to death. Twenty-five of those sentences were carried out. Among the executed were Siegfried Fehmer, Henry Oliver Rinnan, and eight of the "Rinnan Gang." The despised *provocateurs* were not only themselves murderers, but had exposed more than a thousand Norwegian Resistance operatives. Several hundred of those had been arrested and tortured, and over a hundred had perished as a result. Rinnan himself had made a last desperate but unsuccessful effort at escape on May 7, 1945, when he had taken two hostages in Trondheim and attempted to barter their lives for freedom and safe passage to Sweden.

Almost uniformly Norwegians adhered to the rigid regulations forbidding illegal reprisal against either Germans or local traitors. On the few occasions when emotions overruled instructions against unauthorized punishment, Norwegian perpetrators were charged with criminal offenses. Some collaborators who had offended Norse morality more than the national welfare suffered the greatest indignities. "German tarts" who had welcomed Nazi soldiers as companions or lovers were set upon— their hair shaved, and at times they were beaten. As protection the government took into custody a thousand—a number of whom were common prostitutes—until fury against them had abated.

Once again, Johan Scharffenberg swam against the stream of his countrymen's opinions. Even during the Occupation he had considered the code covering traitorous behavior to penalize excessively, particularly in regard to those who were merely passive members of the *Nasjonal Samling*. Speaking during the memorable celebration of the first May 17 celebration since liberation, he stressed that concepts of justice should take precedence over those of politics. Too little regard was afforded to subjective guilt, and too much to revenge and reprisal. He hoped, therefore that amnesty would be given to those whose only crime was membership in the *Nasjonal Samling*.[5]

Of all the trials, none was more meaningful and thorough, and none attracted more world-wide attention, than that of Vidkun Quisling. Despite the sentiments of many that the traitor should be summarily executed, the Norwegian government was determined to try him fairly. The would-be dictator remained confined to *Møllergata 19* for more than three months—with none of the amenities he demanded as a chief of state—until the trial began in Oslo's Freemason Lodge on August 20, 1945.[6]

Vidkun Quisling was tried by a court of three judges, chief of whom was Erik Solem, and four assessors. Two of Norway's most distinguished lawyers were appointed: Annaeus Schjødt to manage the prosecution and Henrik Bergh for the defense.

The defendant was accused principally of the following crimes:

1. Proclaiming himself head of the Norwegian government on April 9, 1940
2. Revoking orders for military mobilization on April 9, 1940
3. Calling for voluntary war efforts on behalf of Germany
4. Formation of an illegal government on February 1, 1942
5. Complicity in the deportation of Jews, that cost almost all their lives
6. Responsibility for execution of death sentences passed on Norwegians by Nazi military courts
7. Assisting the Germans in planning the attack on Norway, and receiving financial aid from the Nazis

Despite the rancor of the Norwegian people, the trial was a model of fairness. An observer of the proceedings, Swedish attorney A. Hemming-Sjoberg, published an account of the trial in which he wrote: "The principal parts in the great drama has thus been placed in the most qualified hands, and accordingly the proceedings were distinguished by objectivity, simplicity, concentration, and dignity."[7]

Four physicians were involved with Vidkun Quisling during his imprisonment and trial: Leo Eitinger, Georg Monrad-Krohn, Sigvald Refsum, and Johan Scharffenberg.

Asriel Hirsch and Leo Eitinger[8] were called as witnesses on behalf of the Jews who had been persecuted by the quislings and those who had perished in Auschwitz and Buchenwald. Vidkun Quisling denied personal responsibility or even knowledge that deportation was tantamount to execution. Dr. Eitinger's testimony in response to Schjødt's questioning gave clear evidence of the defendant's foreknowledge.[9]

"Was this thing, that which went on in Germany, commonly known among Jews here in 1942"?
"No, they did not know."
"But they presumably knew of the Nuremberg laws and the act of tyranny that occurred?"
"Yes."
"But they did not know of the gas chambers?"
"No."
"They presumably knew of the concentration camps?"
"Yes. May I be permitted to state a second thing? I read in the newspapers that Quisling had expressed that he knew nothing of the persecution of the Jews before they were sent under guard on the 'Donau' and that he would have liked to have helped them. The 'Donau' departed at the end of November, and from the day the 'Donau' left, completely until the end of

February we were located at Bredtvedt, and during that time Quisling gave a talk in Trondheim where he defended that which had happened. The Nazi Minister of Justice was at Bredtvedt and looked at us, and Skancke was there and spoke with an old man from Trondheim who had been terribly beaten at Falstad. But there was nothing done that we should not be sent to Germany."

Justice Solem asked Eitinger when Quisling's talk was held.
"It was in December, 1942 that the talk was held."
The judge then turned to Quisling, asking,

"Can you remember that you held that talk in Trondheim where you defended persecution and transport of the Jews?"
"I gave a talk there in any case."
"How did you defend that?"
"I cannot remember, it was an ordinary talk."

Asriel Hirsch added to Eitinger's information, responding to the following questions by the prosecutor:

"How were you treated by the Norwegian State Police who took you to Bredtvedt?"
"We were beaten, both old and young. When we came we were beaten and chased into the cars. They showed little consideration, they placed revolvers in our backs and led us into the cars."
"Were old people beaten by the Norwegian State Police?"
"Yes, both women and men were beaten, there was no difference in that."

Until the two Jews' testimony Norwegians knew little of the extermination camps—and they reacted with shock when the details appeared in the newspapers. The *Aftenposten* legal correspondent wrote, "None of the Jews' earlier tragedies can measure up to this horror. It was deathly still in the courtroom when the two Jews spoke. . . . It was like a solemn memorial in a church, when in thoughts of sympathy encompassing millions of the desperate, it was as if the ashes bore witness to one of the world's greatest outrages."[10]

Vidkun Quisling had been an enigma to those aware of his involvement in Fridtjof Nansen's humanitarian achievements in Russia, Armenia, and the Balkans. Among them, Professor Georg Monrad-Krohn wondered how the those activities could be rationalized with his subsequent inhuman behavior.[11] Were it possible, the neurologist wondered, that

Quisling's turn to the anti-social embracing of fascism might have been a reflection of some organic neurologic disease.

Professor Monrad-Krohn prevailed upon the President of the Court, Erik Solem, to halt the proceedings to allow a complete examination to determine whether indeed, Quisling might suffer a disease capable of impairing his judgement and altering his behavior.

When the trial was recessed, Vidkun Quisling entered *Rikshospitalet* for an examination by Dr. Sigvald Refsum, Monrad-Krohn's next-in-command. As Dr. Refsum entered the examination room, Quisling, in characteristic Norwegian fashion, extended his hand. Sigvald Refsum, ordinarily the very soul of propriety, thrust his own hand behind his back, refusing the offer. In a gesture of anger and frustration, Quisling flung the rejected hand quickly behind his own back. To the end of his own fatal illness, the ever-proper Refsum wondered if he had behaved appropriately. Vidkun Quisling was, after all, a patient, and every patient deserves to be treated by his physician with dignity.

Quisling's study was complete—with an extensive clinical neurologic examination, an electroencephalogram, and the most rigorous and traumatic procedure available at that date, the pneumoencephalogram. All were normal. With Monrad-Krohn's question answered, Quisling was returned to trial.[12]

Vidkun Quisling spoke finally in his own defense—holding forth for hours—rambling and rationalizing in self-justification. He began with the story of his childhood, and ended with his "unselfish" efforts to protect Norway's interests during the Nazi occupation, concluding,

> To me, politics is not a matter of party interests, professional job seeking, or personal ambition and lust for power. It is a matter of self-sacrifice and practical action in the service of the historical development for the benefit of one's own country and to promote the realization of God's Kingdom on earth which Christ came to establish. If my activities have been treasonable—as they have been said to be—then I would pray to God that for the sake of Norway a large number of Norway's sons will become traitors such as I, but that they will not be thrown into jail.[13]

The self-serving harangue came to naught, of course. The crimes were too blatant and too heinous. On September 10, 1945, the Criminal Court in Oslo sentenced the most notorious traitor in Norwegian history to death. The verdict was upheld by the Supreme Court of Norway on October 13, and the request for reprieve filed by the Russian-born Maria Quisling was denied.[14]

Johan Scharffenberg had repeatedly characterized Adolf Hitler as insane and not responsible for his actions. Initially he held the same opinion of Vidkun Quisling. In September 1942, Dr. Gabriel Langfeldt, professor of psychiatry at the University of Oslo, had been approached by an agitated Johan Scharffenberg who proclaimed Quisling completely mad. The "Fører" had warned that university students would be arrested and certain faculty "heads would roll" if *Nasjonal Samling* students were not given preferential admission to medical school. Scharffenberg proposed, without success, that he and Langfeldt declare Quisling insane and have him committed.[15]

In the final analysis, Dr. Scharffenberg formed a different opinion. The psychiatrist's forgiving nature had led Vidkun Quisling's wife to write Scharffenberg, requesting him to visit her husband in jail. Characteristically, Johan Scharffenberg acceded to the request and met with the condemned tyrant three times. The visits were long and searching. The psychiatrist concluded that indeed Quisling was sane—but lacking both a sense of reality and common sense. Scharffenberg recognized that objective guilt was enormous, but looked at the traitor's subjective guilt with greater compassion than most. Still, once the death sentence was passed, Johan Scharffenberg refused to support Quisling's request for a reprieve. "Were I in his place," Scharffenberg had declared, "I would have found it unworthy to either seek or accept reprieve."[16] Nevertheless he still had tears in his eyes as he departed the cell. Shortly before the execution the doomed man wrote he had always had a premonition that he would come to suffer "Christ's and St. Olaf's fate."[17]

Georg Monrad-Krohn, still uneasy and not yet completely convinced, requested that the condemned man's head be spared from the fatal fusillade. The neurologist wished to examine the tyrant's brain and leave no uncertainty. The request was denied.[18]

Vidkun Quisling died before the firing squad early on the morning of October 24, 1945. He was cremated, and his ashes interred in his native village. He had not become, as his few followers had hoped, a martyr around whose memory future fascists would rally. For a time the definition of a quisling as any traitor ruling his country as the vassal of foreign power remained throughout the world. To America's youth his name is largely unknown, some fifty years later. In Norway, however, the word *Quisling* is as infamous as *Hitler*. It left a scar that shall forever endure in the nation's history.

Epilogue

Norway steadfastly continued her march along the road toward a true humanitarianism throughout the Nazi Occupation. Buoyed-up and strengthened by the Home Front, the people maintained allegiance to king and country against the insidious penetrations of invaders and the machinations of rogues among their own countrymen. Yet, as Odd Nansen bitterly reported, even in the hell that was Sachsenhausen, anti-Semitic, anti-Ukrainian, and anti-Russian prejudices still stained the souls of a few of his Norse fellow prisoners.[1]

Koordinasjon Kommitteen paroles had bound the captive nation together, firming the national resolve to resist the occupiers. No *parole* had been issued, however, to warn and assist Norway's Jews facing arrest and deportation to extermination camps in Poland. Only the state church, under the enlightened leadership of Bishop Eivind Bergrav, spoke out firmly and openly against Nazi and *Nasjonal Samling* persecution of Norway's tiny Jewish community. Private citizens of conscience needed no directive, however. Placing their own lives at stake, they aided and gave comfort to their Jewish countrymen and refugees who sought haven from Nazi terror. Unguided by *paroles* the Underground still provided the massive assistance that salvaged half of Norway's Jews and guided them to safety in Sweden.[2]

Once reestablished in Oslo in 1945, the government moved quickly to counter the prejudice that had scarred the *Nasjonal Samling* and had contaminated small numbers of loyalists. Norway's authorities offered refuge to over seven hundred Jews recently freed from Nazi terror—compensating in number for their Norwegian co-religionists who had perished in German concentration camps. Norway was unique among nations in welcoming the ill and the infirm. The blind, the deaf, and the tubercular who were denied entry elsewhere were admitted to the country and treated.[3] Some three thousand refugees were welcomed into a land of just over three million.[4]

Despite desperate economic conditions consequent to the ravaging of the north, loss of half her merchant fleet, and the cost of carrying out war from a foreign base, Norway reached out beyond her borders to aid refugees and displaced persons. The Norwegian Red Cross and the

Norwegian People's Aid joined forces, forming Norwegian Aid to Europe. Six hundred local committees raised funds and provided assistance to refugees. More than 2.5 million dollars in aid was distributed to twelve countries. One hundred and twenty-five tons of clothing were dispatched to South Korea during the war with communist forces in the north. Elderly Armenians refugees in Greece who first received aid through Fridtjof Nansen in 1922 received assistance from the Norwegians. Further refugee relief was provided in Hong Kong, the Middle East and North Africa.

Norwegian efforts to implement peace throughout the world have had a particular impact on the Middle East. Ralph Bunche, Menachim Begin, and Anwar Sadat have each become Nobel Laureates following their efforts to bring peace to a region that had known only strife for well over half a century.

Norway's Foreign Minister Johan Jorgen Holst; his wife, Marianne Heiberg, who is head of the Norwegian Institute for Applied Science; Terje Roed Larsen; and Larsen's wife, Mona Juul, of the Norwegian Foreign Ministry, played important roles in expediting the peace negotiations between Palestinians and Israelis. In 1993 the Committee again brought to world attention that those who appear to be the most implacable of enemies can indeed negotiate peacefully as it awarded the Peace Prize to Nelson Mandella and Frederik W. De Klerk, then in 1994 to Yitzhak Rabin, Shimon Peres, and Yasir Arafat.

In 1965, the community of Baerum chose Jo Benkow, one of its handful of Jewish residents, as representative to the Norwegian *Storting*—the first of his faith to be elected to national office. In the ensuing years Benkow rose to occupy his country's highest elected position. He was chosen by his peers in Parliament as their President; his rank in diplomatic protocol exceeded only by that of King Olav.[5]

In the post-war years President Benkow has witnessed the completion of Norway's transformation from a country officially espousing bigotry in the nineteenth century to one that has served at times as the conscience of the civilized world in awarding the Nobel Peace Prize to those who aid the underprivileged and fight for human rights. The Office of the United Nations High Commissioner for Refugees, sucessor to the League of Nations Office first headed by Fridtjof Nansen and later bearing his name received this award twice. Three other organizations aiding refugees were also honored with a Nobel Peace Award. The defense of civil and human rights by organizations like Amnesty International and individuals like Andrei Zacharov, Adolfo Perez Esquivel, Bishop Desmond Tutu, Martin Luther King, and Albert Luthuli were brought to world attention, lauded and rewarded by the action of Norway's Nobel Committee.

No better example of reversal of anti-semitic bias can be found than the Norwegian Nobel Committee's selection of a Jewish author—a spokesman for victims of the Holocaust—as the 1986 recipient of the Peace Prize. Leading Elie Wiesel's nominators was the President of Norway's Parliament, Jo Benkow. The celebration and presentation of the award in Oslo reunited Elie Wiesel with Leo Eitinger, the "great Jewish doctor" of Wiesel's last days in Auschwitz.

Numerous Norwegians—physicians and others—who appear in the preceding account had already distinguished themselves before the Nazi Occupation, including Carl Semb, Hans Jacob Ustvedt, Leiv Kreyberg, Johan Scharffenberg, Jan Jansen, and Gunnar Johnson. They continued their concerns for humanity and proceeded unhesitatingly toward the summit of achievements—professionally and as humanitarians—joined in the ensuing years by many who were mentioned above. An astonishing number achieved the uncommon distinction of election to the Norwegian Academy of Sciences and Letters on the basis of scientific achievements. Following are brief summaries of their many accomplishments.

Robert Andersen returned to his life of music. He arrived in Minneapolis in 1948 to teach at the music school of the University of Minnesota. Shortly after beginning his duties at the university he found himself in difficulty with the immigration authorities—his visa allowed no employment. Like wartime refugees in his homeland he was reduced to whatever secret work could be obtained. The problem was finally resolved when he reentered the United States through Canada. Andersen resumed teaching and became a member of the first violin section of the Minneapolis Symphony Orchestra. He continued with the orchestra until his death in 1961.[6]

Konrad Birkhaug had continued his responsibilities to the Red Cross throughout the Occupation—but not without running afoul of the Nazis. At Christmas in 1944, as the Germans neared defeat, he was denounced by a Norwegian Nazi, Jacob Johannesen, for "malicious defamation of *Die Wehrmacht* and Quisling's government at a public Red Cross meeting."[7] The investigating SS officer ordered a year's imprisonment in Sachsenhausen where he could keep his "damned Telavåg friends company." Birkhaug managed an appeal to Gestapo Commander Herman Muller, with whom he had negotiated relief of Televåg prisoners. Muller was satisfied with a harsh reprimand, interdiction of any public talks or showing of film, and a fine of five thousand kroner.

With the Occupation ended, Birkhaug felt hunger in his heart for the "green valleys" of his youth in the United States. American authorities were unwilling to quickly renew his passport, however, until they had "obtained positive information about . . . national deportment during the German occupation of Norway."[8] The positive information was slow in coming, and it was not until April 14, 1946, that Birkhaug was able to sail from Gothenburg aboard the Swedish freighter *Vretaholm*.

Konrad Birkhaug, long a champion and developer of the anti-tuberculosis Bacillus Calmette-Guerin (BCG) vaccine, spoke frequently and wrote of its benefits after his return to the United States. The vaccine, conceived and developed in Paris by Albert Calmette and Camille Guerin, had achieved widespread use in Europe and Asia, but had not been employed significantly in the United States. Birkhaug was engaged by Dr. Herman Hilleboe, New York State commissioner of health, to develop the vaccine for use in the state. The vaccine was controversial in the United States, however. Many felt it had relatively little use because of the sharp decline in incidence of tuberculosis. As a result, the BCG project was discontinued in New York state in October 1953, thus ending Birkhaug's scientific career.[9]

Leo Eitinger remained in Bodø for three years. At the outset he was isolated from his past life. His identity had been destroyed in Buchenwald; the issuance of a false death certificate led friends, the remains of his family, and close contacts from his earlier years in Czechoslovakia to believe he was dead. His "loss" was particularly painful to Lisl Kohn, a woman for whom he had developed a special fondness while they were comrades in Jewish youth movements. As a Sudeten Jew, she had managed escape to England even before Hitler's invasion of her homeland. During a visit to her sister, then a refugee in Stockholm, she chanced to learn the miracle of Eitinger's survival. Lisl wrote Shua and the correspondence led to marriage in Stockholm in 1946.

Dr. Eitinger took a position at the University Psychiatric Clinic in 1950, and was appointed professor and head of the department in 1966. His investigation of mental disorders in refugees in Norway—displaced persons from Germany, and the Russian, Polish, and Yugoslavian prisoners of war from the north who had managed to remain in the country— served as Eitinger's doctoral thesis. He subsequently extended that work with a seminal study of the variations in psychological problems between Norwegian Christian concentration camp survivors and Jewish counterparts in Israel. The publication of these studies finally convinced

West German authorities that psychosis and personality disorder did indeed arise from the concentration camp experience. Victims were then eligible for German government compensation.

Throughout the years Leo Eitinger has remained active in the cause of human rights—particularly in Amnesty International and in the establishment of a Center for the Study of Torture in Copenhagen. He was elected to the Norwegian Academy of Sciences and Letters and was named a Commander of the Order of St. Olav. The Lisl and Leo Eitinger Prize—established in 1986 in their honor—is awarded annually in Oslo for accomplishments either in humanitarian endeavors or in psychiatric interests.[10] The initial award went to Elie Wiesel. The 1991 prize was presented to Eigil Nansen for continuing the caring tradition of his father Odd and his grandfather Fridtjof.

Reidar Eker served as director of the Radium Hospital in Oslo from 1947 to 1975, and as head of the department of pathology until 1974. He was a key participant in developing the Norwegian Radium Hospital and the Norsk Hydro Institute for Cancer Research into a university hospital and an internationally recognized cancer center. He was a recipient of an honorary plaque from the Nordic Cancer Union and was made a Knight of the Royal Order of St. Olav in 1977.[11]

Tove Filseth continued her humanitarian activities after arriving in Sweden in 1942. Swedish authorities immediately recognized her accomplishments and asked her to oversee the care of refugee Norwegian and stateless Jews. In 1943, she was given the same responsibility for the recently rescued entire population of Danish Jews. Tove was particularly diligent on behalf of the Jewish children—making every effort to find placement in Swedish homes rather than resort to orphanages. While in Sweden she met the publisher Max Tau, himself a refugee from Norway, and they subsequently married.

Tove was particularly taken by a group of fifteen- and sixteen-year-old boys who had survived the gas chambers through being "mistreated" by the Nazis. The wish to emigrate to Israel burned fiercely among most of the boys, and their wish was finally fulfilled. Years later Tove Tau, through Youth Aliyah in Jerusalem, received an invitation to be the guest of these now young men at a *kibbutz* near Haifa, on the Mediterranean coast. She spoke of her reaction to the visit:

> They had arranged a reception in such a wonderful way. They had long *tisches* [tables] where they had Swedish flags, and Israeli of course. . . . They had married and they had kids of their own, on their knees, and

they had made the most marvelous place . . . this was in the evening when
the dark begins. It was a wonderful atmosphere . . . singing Swedish songs
and [telling] tales, and they were speaking so nicely to me and they were
giving speeches. It was so marvelous I never experienced anything like this
evening. The finest thing is when I think of these boys coming to Sweden,
undernourished, unhappy, and you know everything was so sad and looked
hopeless. And now they were so fine and happy, and self—what do you
call it—confident and happy, and they knew exactly what they wanted and
who they were.[12]

Tove Filseth Tau was awarded the Danish Liberty Cross by King
Christian X for her work in Sweden with wartime refugees from Denmark. On return to Norway after the war she established several childrens'
homes for orphans from Eastern Europe. She then received a degree in
social work and worked in the University of Oslo Psychiatric Clinic until
1975. Her husband, Max Tau, died in 1976. After the death of her close
friend, the wife of Haakon Natvig, she and Dr. Natvig were married
in 1985.
Tove Filseth Natvig died on August 4, 1994.[13]

Bjørn Foss continued in the practice of ophthalmology in Oslo. In
1949 he was awarded his doctorate (Dr. Med—the equivalent of a Ph.D.
in medicine), with his thesis, *Experimental Anaphylactic Iridocyclitis*. He
served as chief medical officer in the Norwegian Home Guard from 1945
to 1949. Following his work for the Home Front, he became involved in
an international organization of World War II Resistance activists.[14]

Viktor Gaustad became Norway's first geriatrician and was appointed
head-physician of the newly established geriatric department at Ullevål
Hospital in 1952. In 1963 he was appointed chief epidemiologist of the
Oslo City Board of Health. On his official retirement in 1977 he remained
active supervising nursing homes and leading the effort in rehabilitation
of the city's psychiatric hospitals until 1986.[15]

At the time of this writing Per Giertson continued his practice of
medicine in his office on the ground floor of his dwelling. The room
beneath the rug-covered trap door remains as it was in the days of the
Resistance.[16]

Berthold Gründfeld termed his life in Sweden "a haven or a paradise.
Everything was calm, peaceful, ordered. You bought everything you
needed. All sweets you could get—chocolate and nuts—so it was fantastic. . . . the Swedish school system was a well-ordered, disciplined system

with traditions long back in Swedish history, putting heavy emphasis on scholastic knowledge, which suited me very well."

The Jewish community in Gothenburg took charge of the fourteen orphans who had been rescued by "Nic" Waal, Sigrid Helliesen Lund, and their circle of women. The Oslo orphanage was reconstituted just outside Gothenburg with the addition of more than a half dozen other refugee children from Austria, Germany, and Hungary. For virtually the first time Gründfeldt felt both security and excitement. Earlier life had been, as he said,

> a series of separations—abandonment in a way. . . . [Those were] my most important years of life, when you awake and get a consciousness of being a human being—discovering that there is a world outside you, that there are newspapers, that there are books, that there is knowledge. You awaken as an intellectual person, and its a very dramatic feeling, and particularly during those years when the world was burning. It was very dramatic, because in a way we crystallized—we were the very symbol of what happened. It was a type of life and death. We didn't know at that time it was a fight where almost the total Jewish population in Europe were systematically exterminated. But we knew it was a fight against Nazism, which meant it was a fight against our enemies—and that made us very early mature—and very conscious about history and destiny . . . and it gave us a push forward, which made us mature in a way or precocious intellectually. . . . We were clever pupils, not necessarily because we were intellectually superior, but because we were earlier mature.

Once the Nazis were driven from the country, the young refugees—except the few who had found relatives in England, Canada, or the United States—took up residence again in the Jewish orphanage in Oslo.

In the early 1950s the refugee orphans were no longer children and the Orphan's Home was officially closed, although the young people continued to live in the same quarters for a time. Berthold Gründfeld continued to excel in his studies, and astounded all Norway. As a youth who had spent more than half his life on foreign soil, he finished first in the country in Norwegian in the *Artium*, the national examination on completion of *gymnasium* and the basis for entry to the university.

Gründfeld moved into a room in the same building that housed the orphanage. Supported by the American Joint Distribution Committee, he entered the University of Oslo as a student in the faculty of medicine. On completion of his training he was appointed to the department of social medicine of the University of Oslo at *Rikshospitalet*, and became Norway's first specialist in the management of sexual dysfunction.[17]

Gunvor Haavik, who had served as translator for Leiv Kreyberg while he addressed the Soviet ex-prisoners of war, found good use for her linguistic skills, first in the Norwegian embassy in Moscow, then in the Foreign ministry in Oslo. While in the Soviet Union she became enamored with, then entrapped by, a young Russian who was a KGB agent. Fear of revelation held Gunnar Haavik hostage. She became a pawn of the Soviets, passing the KGB information, first from the embassy, then from the foreign ministry. Gunvor's spying remained undiscovered for nearly thirty years. On January 27, 1977, she was arrested by Norwegian police after having handed Foreign Office classified documents to a Soviet Embassy official. Gunvor Haavik was imprisoned until August 5, 1977 when she was found dead in her cell of heart failure. She had never been brought to trial.[18]

Wilhelm Harkmark returned to complete his medical education at the University of Oslo. He then entered graduate studies and achieved his doctoral degree by defending his thesis in the *Aula* of the University of Oslo. He was appointed *Prosektor* in the Anatomical Institute of the University of Oslo. In 1952 he assumed directorship of the recently established neuropathology laboratories of Ullevål Hospital. The following year he traveled to the United States where he spent two years obtaining additional training in neuropathology at the University of Minnesota and a year in his research specialty, neuroembryology, with Victor Hamberger at Washington University.

On return to Norway he was appointed professor and head of the department of anatomy at the University of Bergen where he spent the remainder of his career.[19] He died in 1988.

Johannes Heimbeck devoted his medical career to the study and treatment of tuberculosis after the war ended. He was a proponent of the use of BCG and served as president of the First International Congress on BCG in Paris in 1948.

Jan Jansen resumed his full-time duties as *Prosektor* in the Institute of Anatomy at the University of Oslo. His outstanding work on the anatomy of the cerebellum coupled with his extraordinary abilities as teacher and administrator won him the appointment as professor of anatomy and director of the Institute of Anatomy. Both Jansen and the institute became particularly renowned for imaginative and exacting research on the anatomy of the nervous system. For his original and influential research, Jan Jansen was elected to the Norwegian Academy of Sciences and Letters in 1934. He was the recipient of honorary degrees in Kiel, Leiden, and Aarhus; was an honorary member of the American Neurological Association; and was named a Commander of the Order of St. Olav. Jan Jansen died on November 4, 1984.[20]

As important as was his own work, Jansen was committed to the development and advancement of members of his institute. Many, including Jan Jansen, Jr., followed the elder Jansen's induction into the Academy of Sciences and Letters.

Dr. Marianne Jaroschy, a physician like her Jewish husband, Wilhelm Israel Jaroschy, escaped the fate of Norway's Jews, since she fulfilled the Nazi definition of an aryan. She was imprisoned first in Oslo, then transferred to Grini Penitentiary for the remainder of the Occupation. After release on May 8, 1945 (at the age of 48), she remained in Norway, resuming her professional life at the Orthopedic Hospital at Stavern.

Leiv Kreyberg had already been elected to the Norwegian Academy of Sciences and Letters when he left his post as pathologist of the Norwegian Radium Hospital to become professor and head of the Institute of Pathology at the University of Oslo. His expertise in both cancer research and frostbite investigation brought him honors and prizes including the UICC (International Cancer Union) Award of Merit in 1960, and the Fridtjof Nansen Award in 1963. He became a Commander of the Order of St. Olav in 1966, and received honorary degrees from the University of Perugia in Italy and the University of Brno in Czechoslovakia.

For his relief work in North Norway he received the Medal of King Haakon VII. There was no word from governments of prisoners of war Kreyberg had aided until 1964 during Nikita Kruschev's visit to Norway. The Soviet leader arrived in Oslo bearing a huge ceramic vase that he dispatched, along with his calling card, to Leiv Kreyberg. The Yugoslavs waited still longer, awarding a decoration in 1973. From the Poles Kreyberg heard nothing. Leiv Kreyberg died on September 6, 1984.[21]

Kristian Kristiansen returned to *Rikshospitalet* as senior resident in neurology under Georg Monrad-Krohn. He then completed three years of training in neurosurgery at the Montreal Neurological Institute under the direction of the most outstanding neurosurgeon of the time, Wilder Penfield. In Montreal Kristiansen worked together with Penfield on experimental surgical procedures for the management of intractable epilepsy. The influential book authored by Penfield and Kristiansen, *Cortical Seizure Patterns*, described the physiological and anatomical basis for the procedures, and served as the foundation for the further development of the surgical treatment of convulsive disorders.

Kristiansen returned to Oslo to establish the neurosurgical service in Carl Semb's third surgical department at Ullevål Hospital. He was named professor at the University of Oslo, was elected to the Norwegian Academy of Sciences and Letters, and became a Commander of the Order of St. Olav. Kristian Kristiansen died in Oslo on April 19, 1993.[22]

Ole Jacob Malm returned to Sweden from London in 1944 with administrative responsibility from his government-in-exile. He felt compelled to remain in Stockholm for a week after his country's liberation, arriving in Oslo on May 15, 1945. Three weeks later, at a chance meeting on Karl Johansgate Carl Semb discovered Ole Jacob was still jobless after his four-year absence. Semb immediately offered Malm a post as assistant surgeon.

Later Dr. Malm spent two years in the United States at the Rockefeller Foundation. He became an American citizen during an eight-year stay beginning in 1953, but relinquished that citizenship to return to Norway as a consultant. He was awarded a Professorship in surgical pathophysiology at the University of Oslo, with a base at Ullevål Hospital where he had developed the renal transplantation program. The Ullevål Hospital unit performed the first kidney transplant in Scandinavia in 1963.

In recognition of the importance of the Resistance Movement a number of geographic landmarks in Norway's territorial claim of Queen Maud's Land were identified with the names of key Underground operatives. Ole Jacob Malm Ridge now appears on detailed maps of Antarctica.[23]

When *Yom Hashoah* (Day of the Holocaust) was commemorated in Oslo in 1995 Erling Malm was declared "a righteous gentile" by *Vad Yashem* (The Israel Holocaust Memorial) for sheltering Dr. Jaroschy and his wife during the Nazi round-up of Jews in November 1942—an act of compassion that led to Malm's death. Ole Jacob Malm was presented with a medal and a certificate on his father's behalf. Forty members of Ole Jacob's family observed him as he lit one of the six ceremonial candles memorializing the six million Jews who perished. In particular, Malm dedicated the lighting of his candle to Dr. Jaroschy. Leo Eitinger was among those lighting the remaining five memorial candles.[24]

Georg Monrad-Krohn completed his term as dean of the medical school of the University of Oslo and returned to direct his Department of Neurology at *Rikshospital*. He retired from the university in 1957 and died September 9, 1964.[25]

Odd Nansen re-entered architecture on his return from Sachsen-hausen. Nansen Relief, having fulfilled its mission of rescue, was disbanded. Nansen, however, maintained his fathers legacy through continuous devotion to humanitarian causes. As Fridtjof had served the League of Nations, Odd worked on behalf of the United Nations. His observations of 1947 and 1948 served the UN, as he traveled throughout Europe, recording the desolation in the aftermath of the war. He became President of *Nasjonalhjelp*, an organization providing aid to Norwegians in need, and of the *En Verden* (One World) movement in Norway. Odd Nansen took up the cause of the defeated as well, working on behalf of German prisoners of war, and with UNESCO in providing aid in educating German youth.[26] He became chairman of the Nansen Committee Against Anti-Semitism (now known simply as The Nansen Committee). He was succeeded in that office by his son Eigil.

Haakon Natvig was director of the department of food control for the City of Oslo through 1951. In 1952 he was named professor and head of the department of public health at the University of Oslo and subsequently became dean of the faculty of medicine. He was appointed Knight, 1st class, and then Commander of the Royal Order of St. Olav. He is an honorary member of Helsinki University and received the Danebrog Order from Denmark.[27]

During the Occupation Sigvald Refsum had uncovered a peculiar familial disease involving both the visual and nervous systems. He searched the medical literature at the University library assiduously, sitting throughout the winter in gloves and overcoat in the unheated reading rooms and found no mention of the condition whatsoever. He delayed reporting his finding, because publication was considered unpatriotic as long as the *Nasjonal Samling* remained in control.

Once the war ended the findings were published in both Norwegian and German medical journals. The unwieldy designation of *Heredopathia Atactica Polyneuritiformis* made it certain that the condition would forever be known as Refsum's Disease even after the cause became recognized as intolerance to the commonly occurring natural substance, phytanic acid.

Refsum first traveled to the United States to study the burgeoning field of electroencephalography in Chicago under one of its pioneers, Frederick Gibbs. He returned to the United States in 1949 and remained for three and a half years as visiting professor in medical schools at the University of Illinois, University of Minnesota, and University of California. On return to Norway he first assumed the chair in neurology at the University of Bergen, then in 1957 succeeded his mentor, Monrad-Krohn, at the University of Oslo.

For more than three decades, beginning in 1957 as member of a state-appointed commission, Refsum worked actively on behalf of Norway's disabled veterans and concentration camp survivors. From the time of his retirement in 1977, at age 70 in accord with Norwegian law, he served as consultant to the Disabled War Veterans Association, traveling over the oceans to find and examine those still entitled to Norwegian government benefits.

Sigvald Refsum's international contributions were formidable, particularly in relation to the World Federation of Neurology, of which he was president from 1973 to 1981. More than twenty foreign neurological and medical societies saw fit to invite him to honorary membership. He received honorary degrees in Sweden and France as well as in his own country. Refsum's honors abroad were matched by recognition at home. He was elected to and became president of the Norwegian Academy of Sciences and Letters, and was awarded numerous honors, including his country's highest—the medal of St. Olav.

Sigvald Refsum died in Oslo on July 8, 1991.[28]

Johan Scharffenberg had reached the Norwegian retirement age of seventy more than four months before the Nazi invasion of his country. He had continued to work, at Bot Penitentiary, the Oslo Asylum, and in journalism until he was forbidden to publish and removed from his Oslo Asylum position by the Nazis. He functioned as a physician and psychiatrist for only a few months after the liberation for he was in his seventy-sixth year. He continued to be in demand as speaker and writer. Together with Lorentz Brinch, Oslo District Home Front commander; Didrik Seip, rector of the University of Oslo; and Einar Gerhardsen, mayor of Oslo, he addressed the massive gathering in the square before Oslo's City Hall on May 17, 1945—the first National Holiday Celebration since liberation. On September 2, 1945, he spoke to the first Student Association meeting of the year, where "he was greeted with a hurricane of enthusiasm from several thousand members when he spoke of the 'Academic Spirit'."[29]

Scharffenberg continued to speak and write articles until just a few months before his death. His final contribution appeared in *Morgenbladet* in September 1964. One month later he was admitted to Ullevaal Hospital with a broken hip. On February 1, 1965, at the age of ninety-five Scharffenberg's career and life ended. On his deathbed he had fretted that he had lost his clarity of thought.[30]

Carl Semb served as chief medical officer of the Norwegian Forces after the war ended. He then returned to Ullevål Hospital were he resumed responsibility for the third surgical department. He continued to add to his scientific accomplishments in the field of thoracic surgery. Semb was a principal in the formation of the Norwegian MASH Unit during the Korean War, and of the Scandinavian Teaching Hospital in the National Medical Center in Seoul.[31]

Severt Stackland was transferred to France, where he had an opportunity to use his skills in plumbing and sheet metal work. Before completing his service abroad Stackland was assigned to the Wharton School in England, which provided technical refresher courses for U.S. military service personnel. He brought his English bride back to Eagle Grove, where they remained briefly. The two moved first to Clarion, then to Estherville, Iowa, where they established a permanent home and raised three children. Now a widower, Stackland remained in Estherville and is semi-retired. Although he had returned to Norway to visit his mother's relatives he had lost contact with Leo Eitinger. Only through interviews for this book did the rescued and the rescuer learned of each others lives and activities in the intervening years.[32]

Dr. Caroline "Nic" Waal returned to her position on the staff of Gaustad Hospital for a time. She then journeyed to Topeka, Kansas, for a period of study in adult and child psychiatry at the famed Meninger Clinic. On return to Oslo in 1948 Dr. Waal became among the earliest Norwegian specialists in child psychiatry. When she was unsuccessful in establishing a children's psychiatry unit at *Rikshospitalet*, "Nic" Waal formed her own institute in Oslo. Beginning with modest quarters in a cellar, the institute soon moved into a more spacious clinic in a converted apartment building. The institute, once firmly established as a cornerstone of child mental health, finally came to occupy a structure designed to meet its needs.

Dr. Waal attracted a group of active collaborators, with whom she developed a team approach to therapy. They contributed importantly to the educational system in child psychiatry. Caroline "Nic" Waal died in Oslo in 1960.[33]

Hjalmar Wergeland became director of psychiatry at the Children's Medical Center of the University of Oslo and consultant in psychiatry to a number of institutions providing medical care to children.[34]

Notes

Chapter 1

1. S. Abrahamsen, "Wergeland and Article 2 of the Norwegian Constitution." *Scandinavian Studies*, 38 (1966): 102–123.
2. J. Andenaes, O. Riste, and M. Skodvin, *Norway and the Second World War*. Oslo: Johan Grundt Tanum Forlag, 1974, p. 18.
3. R. Petrow, *The Bitter Years*. New York: William Morrow and Co., 1974, pp. 93–96.
4. O. Riste, and B. Nøkleby, *Norway 1940–1945: The Resistance Movement*. Oslo: Johan Grundt Tanum Forlag, 1973, pp. 59–61.

Chapter 2

1. K. Larsen, *A History of Norway*. Princeton, N.J.: Princeton University Press, 1950, p. 387.
2. The acquired name of Jean Baptiste Bernadotte, formerly a marshall in Napoleon's army.
3. *A History of Norway*, p. 369; E. E. Reynolds, *Nansen*, Harmonsdworth, Middlesex: Penguin Books, 1932, p. 168.
4. H. E. Pauli, *Alfred Nobel, Dynamite King—Architect of Peace*. New York: L.B. Fischer, 1942, p. 275.
5. J. Sørenson, *The Saga of Fridtjof Nansen*. New York: The American Scandinavian Foundation and W.W. Morrow, 1942, p. 231.
6. Before he had reached his twenty-seventh birthday Fridtjof Nansen led a small party in successfully crossing Greenland over ice-capped and foreboding mountains. Previous attempts by more experienced explorers from several nations had led to failure. Five years later, with a crew of twelve, he traveled northward aboard the *Fram*, a ship designed under his direction to withstand the crushing pressure of Arctic ice. The *Fram* became embedded in the ice-pack north of Siberia, and in perfect accord with Nansen's calculations, was carried northward as it moved above the Asian and European continents. After reaching 84°N, a point further north than ever reached by man Fridtjof Nansen left the ship accompanied by Hjalmar Johansen. Although the intent of the trip was purely scientific, Fridtjof Nansen felt some purpose might be

served by traveling northward towards the pole. The travelers found the ice rough, the going difficult and progress slow. Nansen was too wise an explorer to put two lives in jeopardy to reach a goal he considered less important than that he had already achieved. After reaching 86° 13.6'N, two hundred miles further north than ever achieved before, Nansen and Johansen headed homeward. The *Fram* had been carried onward by the current as planned, so the two were left on their own. They crossed the Arctic ice by ski and sailed across the open waters by kayak aiming for Spitzbergen twelve hundred miles away. Half-way to their goal they were forced to winter on the island of Franz Josef Land, surviving on the diet of polar bear and walrus they had frozen in preparation. Late in the spring they met up with the British explorer, Frederick Jackson, who sent them back to northern Norway aboard his ship the *Windward*. In little more than a week Nansen received word that the *Fram* had arrived safely in Norway as well.

7. P. Noel-Baker, "Nansen and Norway" in *Fridtjof Nansen—Explorer—Scientist —Humanitarian*, ed. P. Vogt, Oslo: Dreyers Forlag, 1961, p. 138.
8. J. Sørenson, *The Saga of Fridtjof Nansen*, p. 231.
9. O. Sundet, *Johan Scharffenberg*. Oslo: Tanum-Norli, 1977, p. 68.
10. *The Saga of Fridtjof Nansen*, p. 257.

Chapter 3

1. K. Birkhaug, *One Man's Medicine*. Easley, SC: Southern Historical Press, 1979.
2. Ibid., p. 61.
3. Ibid., p. 92.
4. Ibid., p. 88.
5. Ibid., p. 110.
6. Ibid., p. 111.
7. Ibid., p. 114.
8. Ibid., p. 125.
9. Ibid., p. 125.
10. Ibid., p. 125.

Chapter 4

1. J. Sørensen, *The Saga of Fridtjof Nansen*. New York: American Scandinavian Foundation and W.W. Morrow, 1942, p. 276.
2. L. Nansen Høyer. *Nansen: A Family Portrait*. London: Longmans, Green and Co., 1957.
3. J. Sørenson, *The Saga of Fridtjof Nansen*, p. 293.
4. Ibid., p. 293.

5. Ibid., p. 297.
6. Ibid., p. 297.
7. P. M. Hayes, *Quisling: The Career and Political Ideas of Vidkun Quisling 1887–1945*. Bloomington and London: Indiana University Press, 1972, p. 17.
8. Ibid., p. 22.
9. Ibid., p. 28.
10. Ibid., p. 19.
11. J. Sørensen, *The Saga of Fridtjof Nansen*, p. 303.
12. Ibid., p. 304.
13. Ibid., p. 305.

Chapter 5

1. F. Nansen, *Armenia and the Near East*. London: G. Allen and Unwin, 1928, p. 21.
2. Ibid., p. 267.
3. Ibid., p. 287.
4. Ibid., p. 288.
5. Ibid., p. 307.
6. L. Davis, *The Slaughterhouse Province: An American Diplomat's Report on the Armenian Genocide, 1915–1917*. New Rochelle, NY: Caratzas, 1989.
7. F. Nansen, *Armenia and the Near East*, p. 306.
8. Ibid., p. 318.
9. J. Sørenson, *The Saga of Fridtjof Nansen*. New York: American Scandinavian Foundation and W.W. Morrow, 1942, p. 315.
10. F. Nansen, *Armenia and the Near East*, Foreword.
11. Ibid., p. 186.
12. J. Sørenson, *The Saga of Fridtjof Nansen*, p. 318.
13. F. Nansen, *Through the Caucasus to the Volga*. New York: W.W. Norton, 1931.
14. J. Sørenson, *The Saga of Fridtjof Nansen*, p. 23.
15. Liv Nansen Høyer, *Nansen: A Family Portrait*. London: Longmans, Green and Co. pp. 256–57.
16. O. Nansen, *Langs Veien*, Oslo: Gyldendal Norsk Forlag, 1970, p. 77.

Chapter 6

1. P. M. Hayes, *Quisling: The Career and Political Ideas of Vidkun Quisling 1887–1945*. Bloomington and London: Indiana University Press, 1972, p. 28.
2. Ibid., p. 37.
3. H. F. Dahl, *Vidkun Quisling, En fører blir til*. Oslo: H. Aschehoug & Co, 1991, p. 38.
4. Ibid., p. 138.

5. Ibid., p. 47.

6. O. Nansen, *Langs Veien*, Oslo: Gyldendal Norsk Forlag, 1970, p. 141. H. F. Dahl, *Vidkun Quisling*, (p. 146) has written "Vi vet ikke om han besøkte Nansen paa Polhøgda denne vaaren. Noen naemere kontakt ble det i alle fall ikke. Nansen war en tur il USA i februar, fikk et illebefinde etter hjemkomsten og gikk til sengs med hjertesvikt. . . . Den 13. Mai døde han, 68 aar gammel." [We do not know if he visited Polhøgda that spring. In any case there was no close contact. Nansen was on a trip to the USA in February, became ill on returning home, and took to bed with heart failure. . . . The 13th of May he died, 68 years old.]

7. Ibid., p. 141.

8. P. M. Hayes, *Quisling*, p. 60.

9. O. Nansen, *Langs Veien*, pp. 145–47.

Chapter 7

1. O. Sundet, *Johan Scharffenberg*. Oslo: Tandum-Norli, 1977. All material in this chapter related to Johan Scharffenberg is from this biography.

2. Ibid., p. 27.

3. Ibid., p. 27.

4. Ibid., p. 121.

5. Ibid., p. 40.

6. Ibid., p. 38.

7. Ibid., p. 191.

8. Ibid., p. 192.

Chapter 8

All material related to Odd Nansen in this chapter, including quotations, is derived from "Nansenhjelp" in *Langs Veien*, pp. 77–136 and 158–64.

1. O. Nansen, *Langs Veien*, Oslo: Gyldendal Norsk Forlag, 1970.

2. Tove Filseth Tau, interviews with author, Spring 1977, May 11, 1986.

3. O. Nansen, *Langs Veien*, p. 81.

4. Ibid., p. 82; Ole Johansen in *Oss selv naermest. Norge og Jødene, 1914–1943* (Nearest to ourselves. Norway and the Jews, 1914–1943) Oslo: Gyldendal Norsk Forlag, p. 117), wrote that Konstad, a pro-Nazi, had stated, "Not a single Jew would be let into Norway regardless of the pretext."

5. L. Eitinger, All material in this chapter concerning Dr. Eitinger is derived from multiple interviews on March 14, 1977, and in May 1986 and repeated personal conversations and correspondence between 1977 and 1990.

6. G. F. Kennan, *From Prague after Munich*. Princeton N.J.: Princeton University Press, 1968.

7. O. Nansen, *Langs Veien*, p. 86.

8. Ibid., pp. 85–86.
9. Ibid., p. 90.
10. Ibid., p. 101.
11. Ibid., p. 105.
12. Ibid., p. 107.
13. Ibid., p. 110.
14. Ibid., p. 110.
15. Ibid., p. 117.
16. Tove Filseth Tau, interviews.
17. O. Nansen, *Langs Veien*, p. 126.
18. Ibid., p. 130.
19. L. Eitinger, interviews and correspondence.
20. Tove Filseth Tau, interview, May 11, 1986.
21. L. Eitinger, interview, May 1986.
22. O. Nansen, *Langs Veien*, p. 133.
23. Ibid., p. 161.
24. Ibid., p. 161.
25. Ibid., p. 163.
26. Ibid., p. 164.
27. Ibid., pp. 165–66.
28. B. Gründfeld, interviews with author, March 29, 1977 and May 14, 1986.

Chapter 9

1. L. Kreyberg, All material in this chapter is from *Efter ordre-eller uten*, Oslo: Gyldendal Norsk Forlag, 1976, supplemented by a March 9, 1977 interview and conversations and correspondence until 1984, unless otherwise indicated.
2. L. Kreyberg, *Efter ordre-eller uten*, p. 14.
3. Ibid., pp. 31–32.
4. O. Sundet, *Johan Scharffenberg*, Oslo: Tandum-Norli, 1977, pp. 195–96.
5. L. Kreyberg, *Efter ordre-eller uten*, p. 23.
6. Ibid., p. 36.
7. Ibid.
8. Ibid., p. 33.
9. Ibid., pp. 44–46.

Chapter 10

1. P. M. Hayes, *Quisling: The Career and Political Ideas of Vidkun Quisling 1887–1945.* Bloomington and London: Indiana University Press, 1972, pp. 160–64; J. Andenaes, O. Riste, and M. Skodvin. *Norway and the Second World War.* Oslo: Johan Grundt Tanum Forlag, 1974, p. 34.

2. L. Kreyberg, *Efter ordre—eller uten*. Oslo: Gyldendal Norsk Forlag, 1976, pp. 48–49.
3. Ibid., p. 46.
4. J. Sundet, *Johan Scharffenberg*. Oslo: Tandum-Norli, 1977, p. 192.
5. R. Petrow, *The Bitter Years*. New York: William Morrow and Co., 1974, pp. 18–30.
6. J. Andenaes, O. Riste, and M. Skodvin, *Norway and the Second World War*, p. 46.
7. R. Petrow, *The Bitter Years*, p. 43.
8. J. Sundet, *Johan Scharffenberg*, p. 198.
9. R. Petrow, *The Bitter Years*, p. 72.
10. O. J. Malm, interviews May 13, 1977 and June 21, 1987. Personal conversations and communications from 1977–1994.
11. Ibid.
12. O. J. Malm, *"Occupatsjonstiden i perspektiv. Staar vi foran en nytolkning?"* Seminar at the People's University, South, Sandefjord, November 14, 1988.
13. L. Kreyberg, *Efter ordre—eller uten*, Oslo: Gyldendal Norsk Forlag, 1976 and *Kast ikke kortene*, Oslo: Gyldendal Norsk Forlag, 1978; interview, Spring 1977 and personal correspondence, 1977–1984; All material in section III is from the above sources.
14. L. Kreyberg, *Efter ordre—eller uten*, p. 50.
15. Ibid., p. 51.
16. Ibid., p. 66.
17. Ibid., p. 78.
18. Ibid., p. 79.
19. Ibid., p. 82.
20. Ibid., p. 91.
21. Ibid., p. 88.
22. O. Nansen, *Langs Veien*. Oslo: Gyldendal Norsk Forlag, 1970, pp. 138–39.

Chapter 11

1. O. Sundet, *Johan Scharffenberg*. Oslo: Tanum-Norli, 1977, p. 198.
2. Ibid., p. 198.
3. Ibid., p. 200.
4. O. Nansen, *Langs Veien*, Oslo: Gyldendal Norsk Forlag, 1970, pp. 167–72.
5. Ibid., p. 171.
6. Ibid., p. 172.
7. Ibid., pp. 174–79.
8. Ibid., pp. 177–79.
9. O. Sundet, *Johan Scharffenberg*, pp. 205–6.
10. Ibid., p. 206.

11. Ibid., p. 209.
12. O. Nansen, *Langs Veien*, pp. 179–80.
13. O. Sundet, *Johan Scharffenberg*, p. 210.

Chapter 12

1. J. Andenaes, O. Riste, and M. Skodvin, *Norway and the Second World War*. Oslo: Johan Grundt Tanum Forlag, 1974, p. 76; R. Petrow, *The Bitter Years*. New York: William Morrow and Company, 1974, p. 110.
2. T. Klaveness, *Oslo kommunale sykehus i krigens tegn*, Oslo: Cammermeyers Boghandel, 1947, pp. 39–73.
3. Ibid., p. 67.
4. Ibid., p. 69.
5. O. J. Malm, interview with author, 1986.
6. Ibid.
7. A. Strøm, "Laegeforeningen under okkupasjonen." *Tidsskrift f. Norske Laege-forening* n. 11 (1961): 674.
8. O. J. Malm, interview with author, June 21, 1987.
9. T. Gjelsvik, *Hjemmefronten*, Oslo: J. W. Capellens Forlag, 1977, pp. 25–28.
10. O. J. Malm, interview with author, 1986.
11. Ibid.
12. K. Kristiansen, interview with author, May 1987.

Chapter 13

1. T. Gjelsvik, *Hjemmefronten*. Oslo: J. W. Cappellens Forlag, 1977, p. 56.
2. Ibid., p. 49.
3. Ibid., pp. 61–62.
4. O. J. Malm, interviews of May 13, 1977, May 1986, and June 21, 1987, along with personal conversations and correspondence from 1977 to 1994 all contributed to the information related to Ole Jacob Malm.
5. T. Gjelsvik, *Hjemmefronten*, p. 42.
6. Ibid., p. 69.

Chapter 14

1. L. Eitinger, All material related to Dr. Eitinger, unless otherwise indicated, is derived from interviews on March 14, 1977 and in May 1986, as well as numerous personal communications between 1977 and 1990.

2. M. Skjaeraasen, *Lege for Livet*, Oslo: J. W. Cappelens Forlag, 1988, p. 60.
3. Ibid., p. 58.
4. P. Voksø, *Krigens Dagbok*, Oslo: Forlag Det Beste, 1984, p. 107.
5. Ibid., p. 219.
6. Ibid., p. 72.
7. S. Abrahamsen, *Norway's Response to the Holocaust*. New York: Holocaust Library, 1991, p. 100.
8. The order was sent out the following morning, Sunday, October 25. See S. Abrahamsen, *Norway's Response to the Holocaust*, p. 104.
9. S. H. Lund, interview with author, May 1986.
10. M. Skjaeraasen, *Lege for Livet*, p. 76.
11. P. Voksø, *Krigens Dagbok*, p. 282.
12. Tove Filseth Tau, interview with author, May 11, 1986.
13. H. Natvig, interview with author, May 11, 1986.
14. O. J. Malm, interview with author, May 13, 1977.
15. S. H. Lund, interview.
16. H. Waal, (son of Dr. "Nic" Waal), interview with author, May 1986.
17. B. Gründfeld, interview with author, March 29, 1977, and May 14, 1986.
18. L. Eitinger, interview with author, June 20, 1987.
19. Tove Filseth Tau, interviews. Spring 1977. May 11, 1986.
20. H. Natvig, interviews with author, March 7, 1977, and May 11, 1986.
21. O. J. Malm, interview with author, June 21, 1987.

Chapter 15

1. K. Birkhaug, *One Man's Medicine*, Easley, S.C.: Southern Historical Press, 1979.
2. Ibid., p. 244.
3. Ibid., p. 245.
4. D. Howarth, *The Shetland Bus*, London: Thomas Nelson and Sons Ltd., 1951.

Chapter 16

All material in this chapter is from interviews with K. Kristiansen of March 22, 1977, and of May 1987 as well as continuing correspondence, conversations, and review of the manuscript in progress from 1977 until 1992, unless otherwise indicated.
1. N. Ørvik, *Norsk Militaer i Sverige 1943–1945*. Oslo: E. G. Mortensens Forlag, 1951.
2. K. Kreyberg, personal communication with author.
3. N. Ørvik, *Norsk Militaer i Sverige*.
4. O. J. Malm, interview with author, June 21, 1987.

Chapter 17

J. Jansen, interview Spring, 1977. Except where designated, material in the chapter is from this interview supplemented by personal conversation with Ole Jacob Malm and other participants in the Home Front.

1. T. Gjelsvik, *Hjemmefronten*, Oslo: J. W. Cappelens Forlag, 1977, pp. 183–84.
2. Ibid., p. 183.
3. Ibid., p. 144.
4. Ibid., p. 118.
5. R. Eker, interview with author, May 12, 1977.
6. O. Torgersen, interview with author, spring 1977.
7. T. Gjelsvik, *Hjemmefronten*, p. 184.

Chapter 18

1. P. Voksø, *Krigens Dagbok*. Oslo: Forlage Det Beste, 1984, p. 72.
2. Ibid., p. 79.
3. M. M. Cohen, "Georg H. Monrad-Krohn: From Norway to the World," in *Neurosciences Across the Centuries*, ed. F. C. Rose. London: Smith Gordon, 1989, pp. 157–64.
4. Ibid., p. 162.
5. P. Voksø, *Krigens Dagbok*, p. 310.
6. T. Gjelsvik, *Hjemmefronten*. Oslo: J. W. Capellens Forlag, 1977, p. 130.
7. Ibid., p. 130.
8. W. Harkmark, All remaining material in this chapter is from interviews on April 27, 1977, and in May 1986 unless otherwise specified.
9. S. Refsum, interview by author, May 7, 1977.

Chapter 19

1. P. Giertson, interview with author, May 1986. All material in this chapter is derived from this interview.

Chapter 20

1. V. Gaustad, interview with author, May 12, 1977.
2. K. Kristiansen and O. Larsen, *Ullevål sykehus i hundre år*. Oslo: Oslo Kommune, Ullevål Sykehus, 1987.
3. O. Torgerson, interview with author, March, 1977.
4. R. Eker, interview with author, May 12, 1977.

Chapter 21

1. O. Nansen, *Langs Veien*. Oslo: Gyldendal Norsk Forlag, 1970, pp. 141–57.
2. Ibid.
3. O. Nansen, *Fra dag til dag*. Oslo: Gyldendal Norsk Forlag, 1947; O. Nansen, *From Day to Day*. New York: G.P. Putnam Sons, 1949. All further information is from this translation unless otherwise noted.
4. O. Nansen, *From Day to Day*, pp. 53–54.
5. Ibid., p. 265.
6. Ibid., p. 49.
7. O. Nansen, *Langs Veien*, pp. 249–50, 261–62.
8. O. Nansen, *From Day to Day*, p. 49.
9. Ibid., pp. 53–54.
10. Ibid., p. 77.
11. Ibid., p. 81.
12. Ibid., p. 86.
13. Ibid., p. 87.
14. Ibid., p. 54.
15. Ibid., p. 19.
16. Ibid., p. 28.
17. Ibid., pp. 97–98.
18. Ibid., pp. 253–54.
19. Ibid., p. 255.
20. Ibid., p. 256.
21. Ibid., pp. 290–91.

Chapter 22

1. B. Foss, interview with author, May 6, 1977.
2. H. Natvig, interview with author, March 17, 1977.
3. R. Ulstein, *Svensktrafikken i flyktningar til Sverige 1940–1943*. Oslo: Det Norske Samlaget, 1974.
4. T. Klaveness, *Oslo kommunale sykehus in krigens tegn*. Oslo: Cammermeyers Boghandel, 1947, pp. 148–49; R. Ulstein, *Svensktrafikken i flyktningar til Sverige*.
5. M. Manus, *9 Lives before Thirty*. New York: Doubleday, 1947, pp. 65–96.
6. Ibid., 69.
7. Ibid., 70–71.

Chapter 23

1. S. Abrahamsen, *Norway's Response to the Holocaust*. New York: The Holocaust Library, 1991, p. 131.

2. L. Eitinger, All material in this chapter related to Dr. Eitinger is from interviews on March 4, 1977 and in May 1986; personal communications between 1977 and 1990; and M. Skjaeraasen, *Leget for livet*, Oslo: J. W. Cappelens Forlag, 1988.
3. M. Skjaeraasen, *Leget for livet*, p. 112.
4. Ibid., p. 123.
5. Ibid., p. 130.
6. E. Weisel, *Night*, in *Night, Dawn, Day*. Northvale, NJ; London: Jason Aronson, Inc., 1985, pp. 84–86.
7. M. Skjaeraasen, *Leget for livet*, p. 147.
8. Ibid., p. 160.
9. Ibid., p. 180.
10. Ibid., p. 186.
11. Ibid., p. 191.
12. Ibid., p. 194.

Chapter 24

1. O. Nansen, *From Day to Day*, New York: G.P. Putnam Sons, 1949. All material in this chapter is from the above book.
2. Ibid., p. 313.
3. Ibid., p. 121.
4. Ibid., p. 353.
5. Ibid., p. 322.
6. Ibid., p. 337.
7. Ibid., p. 316.
8. Ibid., p. 335.
9. Ibid., p. 387.
10. Ibid., pp. 413–15.
11. Ibid., p. 437.
12. Ibid., p. 461.
13. Ibid., p. 462.
14. Ibid., p. 467.
15. Ibid., pp. 467–68.
16. Ibid., p. 469.
17. Ibid., p. 478.
18. Ibid., pp. 482, 484, 485.

Chapter 25

1. L. Kreyberg, *Kast ikke kortene*. Oslo: Gyldendal Norsk Forlag, 1978, p. 102.
2. Ibid., p. 103.

3. L. Stowe, *Chicago Daily News*, April 10, 1940, pp. 1, 3.
4. L. Kreyberg, *Kast ikke kortene*, pp. 154–55 .
5. Ibid., p. 155; interviews in 1977.
6. B. Foss, interview with author, 1977; *Krigsinvaliden* 7 and 8 (1964): 279–91.
7. B. Foss, interview.
8. H. Söderman, *Skandinaviskt Mellanspel*, Stockholm: Forum, 1946.
9. B. Foss, interview.
10. *Krigsinvaliden* 7 and 8 (1964): 281.
11. *Krigsinvaliden*, p. 287.
12. Ibid.

Chapter 26

All material related to Professor Kreyberg in this chapter is from his book *Kast ikke kortene*. Oslo: Gyldendal Norsk Forlag, 1978, supplemented by interviews and personal communications unless otherwise indicated.
1. L. Kreyberg, *Kast ikke kortene*, p. 157.
2. Ibid., p. 157.
3. Ibid., p. 158.
4. Ibid., p. 159.
5. Ibid., pp. 168–70.
6. Ibid., p. 187.
7. Ibid., p. 188.
8. Ibid., p. 187.
9. Ibid.
10. Ibid., p. 189.
11. Ibid., p. 193.
12. Ibid., pp. 197–200.
13. L. Kreyberg. *Frigjøring av de allierte krigsfanger in nordland 1945*. Oslo: Johan Grundt Tanum, 1946, p. 7.
14. L. Kreyberg, *Kast ikke kortene*, p. 208.

Chapter 27

1. H. Wergeland, interview with author, May 7, 1977.
2. H. Söderman, *Skandinavisk Mellanspel*. Stockholm: Forum, 1946, p. 99.

Chapter 28

1. S. Stackland, telephone interview with author, 1991.
2. L. Eitinger. This reference, and all other material related to Dr. Eitinger, unless otherwise specified, is from interviews on March 14, 1977, and May 1986 and from personal communications, 1977–1990.

3. M. Skjaeraasen, *Lege for livet*, Oslo: J. W. Cappelens Forlag, 1988, p. 202.
4. Ibid.
5. Ibid., p. 205. The translation from *Nynorsk* is by Professor Johan Aarli.
6. L. Eitinger, interview with author, May 1986.
7. Ibid.

Chapter 29

1. A. Andenaes, O. Riste, and M. Skodvin, *Norway and the Second World War*. Oslo: Johan Grundt Tanum Forlag, 1974, p. 119; R. Petrow, *The Bitter Years*. New York: William Morrow, 1974, pp. 337–38; T. Gjelsvik, *Hjemmefronten*, Oslo: J. W. Cappelens Forlag, 1977, pp. 234–36.
2. P. Voksø, *Norges Krigen*, Oslo: Det Beste Forlag, 1984, pp. 530, 531.
3. Ibid., pp. 532, 533.
4. O. Sundet, *Johan Scharffenberg*. Oslo: Tanum-Norli, 1977, p. 214.
5. Ibid., p. 225.
6. R. Hayes, *Quisling: The Career and Political Ideas of Vidkun Quisling 1887–1945*. Bloomington and London: Indiana University Press, 1972.
7. J. Andenaes, et al., *Norway and the Second World War*, p. 126.
8. M. Skjaeraasen, *Lege for livet*. Oslo: J. W. Cappelens Forlag, 1988, p. 209.
9. Ibid., p. 210.
10. Ibid., pp. 209–10.
11. G. H. Monrad-Krohn, personal communication with author, 1951; S. Refsum, interview with author, 1986.
12. S. Refsum, interview with author, 1986.
13. J. Andenaes, et al., *Norway and the Second World War*, p. 127.
14. R. Hayes, *Quisling: The Career and Political Ideas of Vidkun Quisling 1887–1945*, p. 303.
15. O. Sundet, *Johan Scharffenberg*, pp. 211–12.
16. Ibid., p. 227.
17. Ibid., p. 226.
18. G. H. Monrad-Krohn, personal communication with author, 1951.

Epilogue

1. O. Nansen, *From Day to Day*. New York: G.P. Putnam's Sons, 1949, pp. 335, 414–15.
2. S. Abrahamsen, "The Holocaust in Norway." In *Contemporary Views of the Holocaust*, ed. R. Braham. Boston/The Hague: Kluwer-Nijhoff Publishing, p. 112.
3. S. Abrahamsen, *Norway's Response to the Holocaust*. New York: Holocaust Library, 1991, pp. 151–52. Four hundred were admitted in 1947, and 300 of the ill and handicapped were given entry to Norway in 1952.

4. W. S. Bøe, *The Norseman* (Oslo), (No. 2, 1963): 4–8.
5. J. Benkow, *Fra synagogen til løvebakken*. Oslo: Gyldendal Norsk Forlag, 1985; J. Benkow, interview with author, June 19, 1987.
6. R. Andersen, personal conversations with author, 1948–1961.
7. K. Birkhaug, *One Man's Medicine*. Easley, S.C.: Southern Historical Press, 1979. p. 247.
8. Ibid., p. 250.
9. Ibid., p. 266.
10. L. Eitinger, interviews with author March 14, 1977 and May 1986, and personal communications, 1977–1995.
11. R. Eker, interview with author, May 12, 1977, and letter of August 3, 1995.
12. T. F. Tau, interview with author, May 11, 1986.
13. H. Natvig, letter to the author, November 11, 1995.
14. B. Foss, interview with author, May 6, 1977. M. H. Foss, letter to author, January 2, 1996.
15. V. Gaustad, letter to author, August 10, 1995.
16. P. Giertson, interview with author, May 1986.
17. B. Gründfeld, interview with author, May 1986.
18. *Aftenposten*, January 29, 1977 and August 6, 1977.
19. W. Harkmark, interview with author, May 1986.
20. T. W. Blackstad, *Minnetaler over Jan Jansen*. Oslo: Den Norske Videnskaps-Akademi Årbook, 1985 pp. 203–11.
21. L. Kreyberg, interview with author, 1977 and personal communications; O. H. Iversen, *Minnetaler over Leiv Kreyberg*. Oslo: Den Norske Videnskaps-Akademi Årbook, 1985, pp. 171–82.
22. K. Kristiansen, interviews with author, March 22, 1977, May 1987, and personal communications, 1977–1994.
23. O. J. Malm, interview with author, June 21, 1987, and personal communications, 1977–1995.
24. L. Eitinger, telephone conversation with author, May 1995.
25. M. M. Cohen, "Georg H. Monrad-Krohn: From Norway to the World," *Neuroscience Across the Centuries*, ed. F.C. Rose. London: Smith-Gordon, 1989, pp. 157–64.
26. M. Nansen Greve, interview with author, May 1987.
27. H. Natvig, interview with author, March 1977 and letter to author, November 7, 1995.
28. M. M. Cohen, and D. Vidaver, "Sigvald Refsum: The Man Behind the Syndrome," *Journal of the History of the Neurosciences*, (October 1992) 1:277–84.
29. O. Sundet, *Johan Scharffenberg*. Oslo: Tanum-Norli, 1977, p. 216.
30. Ibid., p. 233.
31. K. Kristiansen, "In Memoriam: Professor Carl Semb." *Journal of the Oslo City Hospitals* (1971) 21:117–19.
32. S. Stackland, telephone interview with author, 1991.
33. H. Waal, interview with author, May 9 1977, and personal communication.
34. H. Wergeland, interview with author, May 7, 1977.

Bibliography

Abrahamsen, Samuel. "The Holocaust in Norway." In *Contemporary Views of the Holocaust*, edited by Randolph Braham, pp. 109–42. Boston-The Hague: Kluwer-Nijhoff, 1983.

———. "Wergeland and Article 2 of the Norwegian Constitution." *Scandinavian Studies*, 38: (1966): 102–23.

Andenaes, Johannes, Olav Riste, and Magne Skodvin. *Norway and the Second World War*. Oslo: Johan Grundt Tanum, 1974.

Benkow, Jo. *Fra synagogen til løvebakken*. Oslo: Gyldendal Norsk Forlag, 1985.

Birkhaug, Konrad. *One Man's Medicine*. Easley, S.C.: Southern Historical Press, 1979.

———. *Telavåg*. Oslo: Gyldendal Norsk Forlag, 1946.

Cohen, Maynard M. "Georg H. Monrad-Krohn: From Norway to the World," in *Neuroscience Across the Centuries*, ed. F. Clifford Rose, pp. 157–64. London: Smith-Gordon, 1989.

Cohen, Maynard M., and Doris Vidaver, "The Man Behind the Syndrome," *Journal of the History of the Neurosciences* 1 (1992): 277–84.

Dahl, Hans Fredrik. *Vidkun Quisling: En fører blir til*. Oslo: H. Aschehoug and Co., 1991.

Davis Leslie. *The Slaughterhouse Province: An American Diplomat's Report on the Armenian Genocide, 1915–1917*. New Rochelle: Caratzas, 1989.

Eitinger, Leo. *Concentration Camp Survivors in Norway and Israel*. The Hague: Martinus Nijhoff, 1972.

———. "Experiences in War and During Catastrophes and their Effect upon the Human Mind." *J Oslo City Hosp* 34:75–84, 1984.

———. Jewish Concentration Camp Survivors in Norway.

Eitinger, Leo, and Axel Strøm. *Mortality and Morbidity after Excess Stress*. Oslo: Universitetsforlaget, 1973.

Gjelsvik, Tore. *Hjemmefronten*. Oslo: J.W. Cappellens Forlag, 1977.

Gogstad, Anders Christian. *Helse og hakekors*. Bergen: Alma Mater Forlag, 1991.

Hayes, Paul M. *Quisling: The Career and Political Ideas of Vidkun Quisling 1887–1945*. Bloomington and London: Indiana University Press, 1972.

Høyer, Liv Nansen. *Nansen, A Family Portrait.* London: Longmanns, Green & Co., 1957.

Hygen, Johan B. "Fridtjof Nansen—Views on Civilization and Ethics." In *Fridtjof Nansen—Explorer—Scientist—Humanitarian*, edited by Per Vogt, pp. 191–98. Oslo: Dreyers Forlag, 1961.

Kennan, George F. *From Prague after Munich.* Princeton, NJ: Princeton University Press, 1968.

Klaveness, Thorvald. *Oslo kommunale sykehus i krigens tegn.* Oslo: Cammermeyers Boghandel, 1947.

Kreyberg, Leiv. *Efter ordre-eller uten.* Oslo: Gyldendal Norsk Forlag, 1976.

———. *Frigjøring av de allierte krigsfanger i nordland 1945.* Oslo: Johan Grundt Tanum, 1946.

———. *Kast ikke kortene.* Oslo: Gyldendal Norsk Forlag, 1978.

Kristiansen, Kristian and Ø. Larsen. *Ullevål sykehus i hundre aar.* Oslo: Oslo kommune, Ullevål sykehus, 1987.

Malm, Ole Jacob. *45 Aar etter.* Speech at Grand Hotel, Oslo, May 8, 1985.

Manus, Max. *9 Lives Before Thirty.* New York: Doubleday, 1947.

Nansen, Fridjtof. *Armenia and the Near East.* London: G. Allen & Unwin, 1928.

———. *Farthest North.* 2 vols. New York: Harper, 1897.

———. *The First Crossing of Greenland.* 2 vols. London: Longmanns, 1890.

———. *Through the Caucasus to the Volga.* New York: W.W. Norton, 1931.

Nansen, Odd. *Fra dag til dag.* Oslo: Gyldendal Norsk Forlag, 1947.

———. *From Day to Day.* New York: G.P. Putnam's Sons, 1949.

———. *Langs Veien.* Oslo: Gyldendal Norsk Forlag, 1970.

Noel-Baker, Philip. "Nansen and Norway." In *Fridtjof Nansen—Explorer—Scientist—Humanitarian*, edited by Per Vogt, pp. 132–41. Oslo: Dreyers Forlag, 1961.

Ørvik, Nils. *Norsk Militaer i Sverige 1943–1945.* Oslo: E.G. Mortensens Forlag, 1951.

Petrow, Richard. *The Bitter Years.* New York: William Morrow & Company, 1974.

Reynolds, E.E. *Nansen.* Harmondsworth: Penguin Books, 1932.

Riste, Olav, and Berit Nøkleby. *Norway 1940–1945: The Resistance Movement.* Oslo: Johan Grundt Tanum Forlag, 1973.

Sachnowitz, Herman. *Det angaar ogsaa deg.* Oslo: J.W. Cappellens Forlag, 1976.

Scharffenberg, Johan. *Johan Scharffenbergs Minne*. Oslo: Johan Grundt Tanum Forlag, 1967.

Scott, J.N. *Fridtjof Nansen*. Heron Books, 1971.

Shackleton, Edward. *Nansen the Explorer*. London: H. F. & G. Witherby, 1959.

Skjaeraasen, Magne. *Lege for livet*. Oslo: J.W. Cappelens Forlag, 1988.

Söderman, Harry. *Skandinavisk Mellanspel*. Stockholm: Forum, 1946.

Sørensen, Jon. *The Saga of Fridtjof Nansen*. New York: The American Scandinavian Foundation and W.W. Morrow, 1942.

Strøm, Axel. "Laegeforeningen under okkupasjonen." *Tidsskrift f. Norsk Laegeforening* n. 11 (1961): 674.

Sundet, Olav. *Johan Scharffenberg*. Oslo: Forlag Tanum-Norli, 1977.

Ulstein, Ragnar. *Svensketraffiken I Flyktingar til Sverige 1940–1943*. Oslo: Det Norske Samlaget, 1974.

Vogt, Per. "Fridtjof Nansen—Life and Work." In *Fridtjof Nansen— Explorer—Scientist—Humanitarian*, edited by Per Vogt, pp. 9–96. Oslo: Dreyers Forlag, 1961.

Voksø, Per, ed. *Krigens Dagbok: Norge 1940–1945*. Oslo: Forlaget Det Beste, 1984.

Interviews

Robert Andersen. Personal conversations with the author, 1948–1961.

Jo Benkow. Interview with the author, June 19, 1987.

Leo Eitinger. Interviews with the author, March 14, 1977 and May 1986. Personal correspondence from 1977 to 1990.

R. Eker. Interview with the author, May 12, 1977.

Bjørn Foss. Interview with the author, May 6, 1977.

Viktor Gaustad. Interview with the author, May 12, 1977.

Per Giertson. Interview with the author, May 1986.

Marit Nansen Greve. Interview with the author, May 1987.

Berthold Gründfeld. Interviews with the author March 29, 1977 and May 14, 1986.

Wilhelm Harkmark. Interviews with the author April 27, 1977 and May 1986.

Jan Jansen. Interview with the author Spring 1977.

Leiv Kreyberg. Interview with the author March 9, 1977 and personal correspondence until 1984.

Kristian Kristiansen. Interviews with the author March 22, 1977 and May 1987, and personal correspondence from 1977 until 1994.

Aagot Christie Løken. Personal conversations with author.

Sigrid Helliesen Lund. Interview with the author, May 1986.

Ole Jacob Malm. Interviews with the author, May 13, 1977, May 1986, and June 1987, and personal correspondence from 1977 to 1994.

George H. Monrad-Krohn. Personal conversations with the author, 1951–52, 1958.

Haakon Natvig. Interviews with the author March 7, 1977 and May 11, 1986.

Sigvald Refsum. Interview with the author May 7, 1977.

Severt Stackland. Telephone interviews with the author, 1991.

Tove Filseth Tau. Interview with the author, Spring 1977 and May 11, 1986.

Olav Torgensen. Interview with the author, March 1977.

Helge Waal. Interviews with the author, May 1977 and May 1986.

Henrik Wergeland. Interview with the author, May 7, 1977.

Index

311

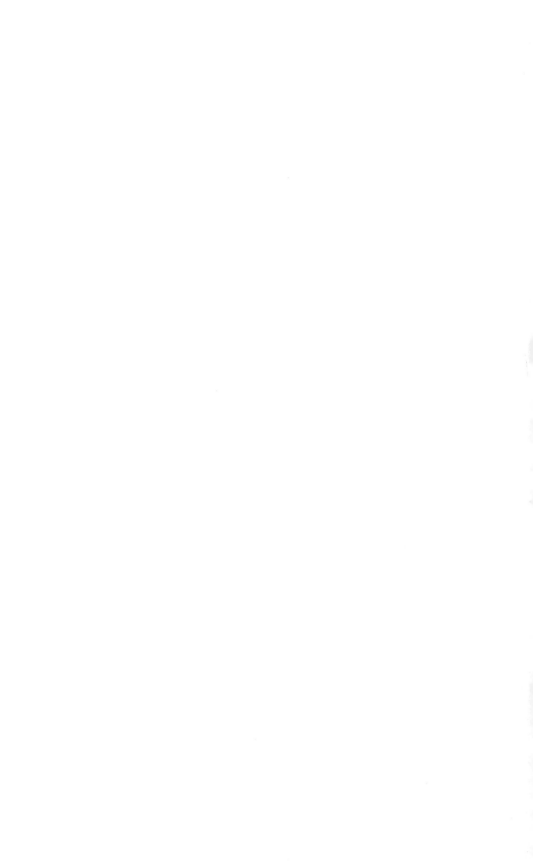